ANNALS OF THE NEW YORK ACADEMY OF SCIENCES

Volume 963

EDITORIAL STAFF

Executive Editor
BARBARA M. GOLDMAN

Managing Editor
JUSTINE CULLINAN

Associate Editor
ANGELA FINK

The New York Academy of Sciences
2 East 63rd Street
New York, New York 10021

THE NEW YORK ACADEMY OF SCIENCES
(Founded in 1817)

BOARD OF GOVERNORS, September 2001 – September 2002

TORSTEN N. WIESEL, *Chairman of the Board*
JOHN F. NIBLACK, *Vice Chairman of the Board*
BILL GREEN, *Past Chairman*

Honorary Life Governors
WILLIAM T. GOLDEN   JOSHUA LEDERBERG
JOHN T. MORGAN, *Treasurer*

Governors

ELEANOR BAUM	D. ALLAN BROMLEY	KAREN E. BURKE
	LAWRENCE B. BUTTENWIESER PRAVEEN CHAUDHARI	
JOHN H. GIBBONS	MICHAEL GOLDEN	RONALD L. GRAHAM
JACQUELINE LEO	SANDRA PANEM	RICHARD A. RIFKIND
JOHN J. ROCHE		SARA LEE SCHUPF
JAMES H. SIMONS		LEE VANCE

HELENE L. KAPLAN, *Counsel* [ex officio]

HORMONE-RELATED TUMORS

Novel Approaches to Prevention and Treatment

ANNALS OF THE NEW YORK ACADEMY OF SCIENCES
Volume 963

HORMONE-RELATED TUMORS

Novel Approaches to Prevention and Treatment

Edited by Luigi Castagnetta, Biagio Agostara, Luisa Massimo, Giuseppe Montalto, and H. Leon Bradlow

The New York Academy of Sciences
New York, New York
2002

Copyright © 2002 by the New York Academy of Sciences. All rights reserved. Under the provisions of the United States Copyright Act of 1976, individual readers of the Annals *are permitted to make fair use of the material in them for teaching or research. Permission is granted to quote from the* Annals *provided that the customary acknowledgment is made of the source. Material in the* Annals *may be republished only by permission of the Academy. Address inquiries to the Permissions Department (permissions@nyas.org) at the New York Academy of Sciences.*

Copying fees: *For each copy of an article made beyond the free copying permitted under Section 107 or 108 of the 1976 Copyright Act, a fee should be paid through the Copyright Clearance Center, Inc., 222 Rosewood Drive, Danvers, MA 01923 (www.copyright.com).*

♾ *The paper used in this publication meets the minimum requirements of the American National Standard for Information Sciences—Permanence of Paper for Printed Library Materials, ANSI Z39.48-1984.*

Library of Congress Cataloging-in-Publication Data

Course of "Biology and Biochemistry of Normal and Cancer Cell Growth"
(6th : 2001 : Erice, Italy)
  Hormone-related tumors : novel approaches to prevention and treatment
/ edited by Luigi Castagnetta ... [et al.].
       p. ; cm. — (Annals of the New York Academy of Sciences ; v.
963)
  "6th Course on Biology and Biochemistry of Normal and Cancer Cell Growth
: classical and non-classical issues from prevention to treatment of
hormone-related tumors held on May 1-6, 2001 by the Ettore Majorana
Foundation and Centre for Scientific Culture, International School of
Medical Sciences in Erice, Sicily, Italy"--E-CIP galleys.
  Includes bibliographical references and index.
  ISBN 1-57331-420-X (cloth : alk. paper) — ISBN 1-57331-421-8 (paper :
alk. paper)
  1. Cancer—Endocrine aspects—Congresses.
  [DNLM: 1. Neoplasms, Hormone-Dependent--Congresses. QZ 200 C861h
2002] I. Castagnetta, L. II. New York Academy of Sciences. III. Title.
  IV. Series.
Q11 .N5   vol. 963
  [RC268.2]   2002006997

GYAT/PCP
Printed in the United States of America
ISBN 1-57331-420-X (cloth)
ISBN 1-57331-421-8 (paper)
ISSN 0077-8923

ANNALS OF THE NEW YORK ACADEMY OF SCIENCES

Volume 963
June 2002

HORMONE-RELATED TUMORS

Novel Approaches to Prevention and Treatment

Editors and Conference Organizers
LUIGI CASTAGNETTA, BIAGIO AGOSTARA, LUISA MASSIMO,
GIUSEPPE MONTALTO, AND H. LEON BRADLOW

This volume is the result of a symposium entitled **6th Course on Biology and Biochemistry of Normal and Cancer Cell Growth: Classical and Non-Classical Issues from Prevention to Treatment of Hormone-Related Tumors** held on May 1-6, 2001 by the Ettore Majorana Foundation and Centre for Scientific Culture, International School of Medical Sciences in Erice, Sicily, Italy.

CONTENTS

Preface. *By* LUIGI CASTAGNETTA, BIAGIO AGOSTARA, LUISA MASSIMO, GIUSEPPE MONTALTO, AND H. LEON BRADLOW	xi
The Amazon Project: Helping the Patient to Become an Instrument of Her Own Recovery. *By* ANNA BARBERA AND LINA PROSA	1

Part 1. Cancer Genetics

Gene Therapy of Hepatocellular Carcinoma and Gastrointestinal Tumors. *By* BRUNO SANGRO, CHENG QIAN, VOLKER SCHMITZ, AND JESUS PRIETO	6

Part 2. Liver and Colorectal Cancer

Epidemiology, Risk Factors, and Natural History of Hepatocellular Carcinoma. *By* GIUSEPPE MONTALTO, MELCHIORRE CERVELLO, LYDIA GIANNITRAPANI, FABIO DANTONA, ANGELA TERRANOVA, AND LUIGI A. M. CASTAGNETTA	13
Genetic Alterations and Oncogenic Pathways in Hepatocellular Carcinoma. *By* LAURENCE LÉVY, CLAIRE ANGÉLIQUE RENARD, YU WEI, AND MARIE ANNICK BUENDIA	21

Hepatocellular Carcinoma: Role of Estrogen Receptors in the Liver. *By* ERICA VILLA, ANTONELLA GROTTOLA, ALESSANDRA COLANTONI, NICOLA DE MARIA, PAOLA BUTTAFOCO, ILVA FERRETTI, AND FEDERICO MANENTI... 37

Circulating IL-6 and sIL-6R in Patients with Hepatocellular Carcinoma. *By* L. GIANNITRAPANI, M. CERVELLO, M. SORESI, M. NOTARBARTOLO, M. LA ROSA, L. VIRRUSO, N. D'ALESSANDRO, AND G. MONTALTO...... 46

Expression of HIP/PAP mRNA in Human Hepatoma Cell Lines. *By* M. CERVELLO, L. GIANNITRAPANI, M. LA ROSA, M. NOTARBARTOLO, N. D'ALESSANDRO, L. VIRRUSO, J.L. IOVANNA, AND G. MONTALTO..... 53

Part 3. Neuroblastoma: A Multigenetic Disease

Neuroblastoma: A Challenge for Pediatric Oncology of the Third Millennium. *By* LUISA MASSIMO... 59

Amplified *MYCN* in Human Neuroblastoma: Paradigm for the Translation of Molecular Genetics to Clinical Oncology. *By* MANFRED SCHWAB....... 63

Linkage Analysis in Families with Recurrent Neuroblastoma. *By* PATRIZIA PERRI, LUCA LONGO, CARMEL MCCONVILLE, ROBERTO CUSANO, SALLY A. REES, MARCO SERI, MASSIMO CONTE, GIOVANNI ROMEO, MARCELLA DEVOTO, AND GIAN PAOLO TONINI.... 74

Breast Cancer Registry in Palermo and Its Province: Incidence in 1999. *By* A. TRAINA, R. CUSIMANO, M. LIQUORI, V. FERRIGNO, A. GUTTADAURO, B. RAVAZZOLO, A.M. GIAMMANCO, AND L. CASTAGNETTA............. 85

New Approaches to Breast Cancer. Oxaliplatin Combined with 5-Fluorouracil and Folinic Acid in Pretreated Advanced Breast Cancer Patients: Preliminary Reports. *By* V. LEONARDI, G. SAVIO, A. LAUDANI, L. BLASI, AND B. AGOSTARA.. 91

Ligand Binding and Cytochemical Analysis of Estrogen and Progesterone Receptors in Relation to Follow-Up in Patients with Breast Cancer. *By* L. CASTAGNETTA, A. TRAINA, B. AGOSTARA, M. MIELE, I. CAMPISI, M. CALABRÒ, L. MARASÀ, AND G. CARRUBA...................... 98

Part 4. Molecular Basis for Innovative Treatment: Receptors and Signals

Modulation of Epidermal Growth Factor Receptor in Endocrine-Resistant, Estrogen-Receptor–Positive Breast Cancer. *By* R.I. NICHOLSON, I.R. HUTCHESON, M.E. HARPER, J.M. KNOWLDEN, D. BARROW, R.A. MCCLELLAND, H.E. JONES, A.E. WAKELING, AND J.M.W. GEE... 104

Molecular Mechanisms of RET Activation in Human Cancer. *By* MASSIMO SANTORO, ROSA MARINA MELILLO, FRANCESCA CARLOMAGNO, ALFREDO FUSCO, AND GIANCARLO VECCHIO........................ 116

Part 5. Breaking Fresh Ground for Breast Cancer

Proteomic Patterns of Cultured Breast Cancer Cells and Epithelial Mammary Cells. *By* IDA PUCCI-MINAFRA, SIMONA FONTANA, PATRIZIA CANCEMI, GIUSEPPINA ALAIMO, AND SALVATORE MINAFRA.................... 122

Antiestrogenic Regulation of Transforming Growth Factor Beta Receptors I and II in Human Breast Cancer Cells. *By* M. BUCK, J. VON DER FECHT, AND C. KNABBE 140

Objective Response to Treatment as a Potential Surrogate Marker of Survival in Breast Cancer. *By* PAOLO BRUZZI 144

Part 6. Breaking Fresh Ground for Prostate Cancer

Nutrition and Prostate Cancer: A Review. *By* LEONARD A. COHEN 148

Intercellular Communication and Human Prostate Carcinogenesis. *By* GIUSEPPE CARRUBA, ROSALBA STEFANO, LETIZIA COCCIADIFERRO, FRANCESCA SALADINO, ANTONIETTA DI CRISTINA, ERIK TOKAR, SALMAAN T.A. QUADER, MUKTA M. WEBBER, AND LUIGI CASTAGNETTA . 156

Precancerous Lesions and Conditions of the Prostate: From Morphological and Biological Characterization to Chemoprevention. *By* RODOLFO MONTIRONI, ROBERTA MAZZUCCHELLI, AND MARINA SCARPELLI 169

Src Is an Initial Target of Sex Steroid Hormone Action. *By* A. MIGLIACCIO, G. CASTORIA, M. DI DOMENICO, A. DE FALCO, A. BILANCIO, AND F. AURICCHIO 185

From Castration-Induced Apoptosis of Prostatic Epithelium to the Use of Apoptotic Genes in the Treatment of Prostate Cancer. *By* YE ZHANG, BICHENG NAN, JIANG YU, TITHI SNABBOON, FRANCESCA ANDRIANI, AND MARCO MARCELLI 191

Biological Selection Criteria for Radical Prostatectomy. *By* GIOVANNI MUZZONIGRO AND ANDREA B. GALOSI 204

Connexin Expression in Nonneoplastic Human Prostate Epithelial Cells. *By* FRANCESCA SALADINO, GIUSEPPE CARRUBA, SALMAAN T.A. QUADER, MARIA AMOROSO, ANTONIETTA DI CRISTINA, MUKTA M. WEBBER, AND LUIGI A.M. CASTAGNETTA 213

Methods to Obtain More Clinical and Pathologic Information from Needle Core Biopsy of the Prostate Gland. *By* ANDREA B. GALOSI AND GIOVANNI MUZZONIGRO 218

Part 7. Molecular Basis for Innovative Treatment: Steroid Enzymes

Human Type 1 Estrogen Sulfotransferase: Catecholestrogen Metabolism and Potential Involvement in Cancer Promotion. *By* FRÉDÉRIC FAUCHER, LUCILLE LACOSTE, AND VAN LUU-THE 221

Prevention and Treatment of Breast Cancer by Suppressing Aromatase Activity and Expression. *By* SHIUAN CHEN, DUJIN ZHOU, TOMOHARU OKUBO, YEH-CHIH KAO, ELIZABETH T. ENG, BAIBA GRUBE, ANNETTE KWON, CHUN YANG, AND BIN YU 229

Anti-Aromatase Chemicals in Red Wine. *By* E.T. ENG, D. WILLIAMS, U. MANDAVA, N. KIRMA, R.R. TEKMAL, AND S. CHEN 239

Part 8. Cancer Epidemiology and Prevention

Diet and Breast Cancer. *By* H. LEON BRADLOW AND DANIEL W. SEPKOVIC.... 247

Effects of Weight Control and Physical Activity in Cancer Prevention: Role of Endogenous Hormone Metabolism. *By* RUDOLF KAAKS AND ANNEKATRIN LUKANOVA 268

The Mediet Project. *By* L. CASTAGNETTA, O.M. GRANATA, R. CUSIMANO, B. RAVAZZOLO, M. LIQUORI, L. POLITO, M. MIELE, A. DI CRISTINA, P. HAMEL, AND A. TRAINA 282

Murine Models of Paroxysmal Nocturnal Hemoglobinuria. *By* VITTORIO ROSTI 290

Molecular Genetics of Acute Myeloid Leukemia. *By* PAOLO BERNASCONI, MARINA BONI, PAOLA MARIA CAVIGLIANO, SILVIA CALATRONI, ILARIA GIARDINI, BARBARA ROCCA, AND MARILENA CARESANA 297

From Genes to Therapy: The Case of Philadelphia Chromosome-Positive Leukemias. *By* DANIELA CILLONI, ANGELO GUERRASIO, EMILIA GIUGLIANO, PATRIZIA SCARAVAGLIO, GISELLA VOLPE, GIOVANNA REGE-CAMBRIN, AND GIUSEPPE SAGLIO 306

Multidimensional Flow Cytometry Immunophenotyping of Hematologic Malignancy. *By* GUIDO PAGNUCCO, LAURA VANELLI, AND FRANCESCO GERVASI 313

Androgen Receptor Status in Nontumoral and Malignant Human Colorectal Tissues. *By* L. CASTAGNETTA, A. TRAINA, I. CAMPISI, M. CALABRÒ, A. MARATTA, A. SAETTA, B. AGOSTARA, AND N. MEZZATESTA 322

Correlation between *Helicobacter pylori* Infection and IL-18 mRNA Expression in Human Gastric Biopsy Specimens. *By* M.T. FERA, M. CARBONE, C. BUDA, M. ARAGONA, S. PANETTA, M. GIANNONE, F. LA TORRE, A. GIUDICE, AND E. LOSI 326

p53 and Anti-p53 Antibodies as Possible Markers of a Switch Towards a Neoplastic Phenotype in Patients Infected by *Helicobacter pylori*. *By* E. LOSI, A.M. MOLINARI, P. GAZZERRO, L. ORTEGA DE LUNA, M.T. FERA, M. CARBONE, M.R. CATANIA, D.L. HASTY, AND F. ROSSANO . 329

Cytokine Induction in Murine Bladder Tissue by Type 1 Fimbriated *Escherichia coli*. *By* M. CARBONE, D.L. HASTY, K.C. YI, J. RUE, M.T. FERA, F. LA TORRE, M. GIANNONE, AND E. LOSI 332

Closing Remarks. *By* THE EDITORS 336

Index of Contributors 337

Financial assistance was received from:
- **ALFA WASSERMANN**
- **AIRC**
- **ASTRA ZENECA**
- **BRISTOL-MYERS SQUIBB**
- **ECOSISTEMI**
- **ELI LILLY ITALIA**
- **GIENNE PHARMA**
- **GLAXO WELLCOME**
- **ITALFARMACO**
- **LEICA**
- **MENARINI**
- **ROCHE**
- **SCHERING PLOUGH**
- **UNIONFARMA**

> The New York Academy of Sciences believes it has a responsibility to provide an open forum for discussion of scientific questions. The positions taken by the participants in the reported conferences are their own and not necessarily those of the Academy. The Academy has no intent to influence legislation by providing such forums.

Preface

In the last decade, oncology has been distinguished by two major hallmarks: (1) the continuously increasing incidence of certain human malignancies, including hormone-related tumors, and (2) the consistent decrease in their mortality rates. The difficulty in approaching such separate issues, although featured by common traits, has greatly been eased by the expeditious increase of knowledge and the tumultuous progress of innovative, even revolutionary, technologies. Today, we live in an era in which genomics, proteomics, genetic engineering, and gene therapy have already absorbed most diagnostic procedures and are soon expected to heavily affect therapeutic strategies in oncology.

From this scenario emerges the immediate, yet unattended, need to closely connect structure and function, signaling mechanisms and biological responses, aiming to discern redundancy and heterogeneity, main and alternative pathways; in other words, to identify targets for modern diagnostic maneuvers and therapeutic measures. To obtain more information and to foster the cross-talk between *bench* and *bed*, cell biologists and geneticists, and young and mature associates, are and remain the main goals of our current and future meetings.

LUIGI CASTAGNETTA
BIAGIO AGOSTARA
LUISA MASSIMO
GIUSEPPE MONTALTO
H. LEON BRADLOW

The Amazon Project

Helping the Patient to Become an Instrument of Her Own Recovery

ANNA BARBERA AND LINA PROSA

Associazione Arlenika, Progetto Amazzone, Palermo, Italy

ABSTRACT: The Amazon Project combines science, myth, and theater to explore problems linked to cancer and its surgical management in women from a social, political, and cultural point of view. This Project is concerned with change in the hope that one day it will be possible to discuss, along with the Science of Medicine, the Science of Patients as well.

KEYWORDS: Amazon Project; breast cancer; Science of Patients

INTRODUCTION

We have both undergone breast cancer operations, and this shared experience has led us to discover the existence of a cultural emergency in the experience of cancer, especially in breast cancer, which must be recognized as coexisting with a scientific and a medical emergency.

This awareness was the cause of our unremitting commitment together in the Arlenika Association, a cultural association that regards cancer as a central theme in human processes and the languages of communication. From this association sprang the Amazon Project. This Project is concerned with change and has the ambitious aim that one day it should be possible to discuss, alongside the Science of Medicine, the Science of Patients as well. It is an ongoing project that needs constant constructive contact with all those who care about the destiny of the patient and, consequently, the destiny of all human beings.

THE AMAZON PROJECT

Before going into the structure of the Project, or *How to teach a patient the art of fighting*, which for us is the essence of the Amazon Project, we think we should first say something about the identity and the role of the patient in our programs, because this role determines the kind of action undertaken by the Project and the very nature of the rights we regard as indispensable for someone who falls ill with cancer.

In our view these rights have a twofold nature: one aspect is internal to the patient herself and concerns her own involvement in the illness, her ability to collaborate actively with the doctor in his program of treatment; the other is external to the patient and concerns the quality of the health service, the doctor-patient relationship and the sociocultural context.

Our own personal experience leads us to believe that the first aspect of this right is less observed than the second. Not enough study has been carried out, not enough work has been done to train a patient to recognize and manage her own resources in the struggle to recover. This is a shortcoming that often falls prey to improvisation, a gap filled up by a spate of philosophies of self-healing and similar experiments, alternative types of treatment, and so on.

This improvisation does not happen to the same extent at the external level, for here it is easier to achieve more effective results through the efforts of associations and organizations that form an important link between the public health system and the needs of the patient. It is obvious that the two spheres of rights must always stand on the same plane if the patient's struggle is to be effective.

We believe that it must be recognized that in the struggle against cancer a patient has a role equal to that of the doctor, so that we must all move in the same direction, but if we are to accomplish anything important, we must attain this equality of roles.

We must be aware that this conquest can only come about if we overcome a whole barrage of constraints; if we are to achieve any results, we need boldness, intelligence, and drive. In short, we must emulate Ulysses and learn what the sea teaches us, namely, that eternal movement that creates heroes, that neverending struggle that in its turn produces skilled fighters, that is what the cancer patient can become.

The Amazon Project adopts this mode of combat, and to this end it places the century-old fight against cancer in the widest possible context, ranging from hospitals and families to schools, everyday life, the media, cultural institutions, the world of work, etc., so that at the edges of the centers of suffering there should not remain active other unseen centers of infection that may seem unconnected with the problems of cancer but that nevertheless keep alive the process of multiplication.

All this is related to Culture, the site *par excellence* of the problem according to the Amazon Project, the stage where the drama of cancer unfolds in all its complexity, for it affects the body, the mind, the imagination, the law, the philosophy of life, life style, whether that of the couple or the single person, economics, social relationships, and so on. Culture is the place where our interpretation of life is worked out; therefore, it is also the place that gives rise to fear, ambiguity, prejudice, and all those types of conditioning that we know are sometimes much more dangerous than the pathology itself, affecting the patient's quality of life and hampering the diffusion of preventive measures.

The Amazon Project took stock of all these aspects, and in 1996, the year of the First International Conference, opened a cultural debate on cancer and, in particular, on breast cancer, in order to draw attention to a mode of struggle that belongs to the whole of civilized society.

We accordingly involved vast areas of the world of medicine, culture, art, the theater, education, health, work and politics, and immediately obtained a result that was to be important in establishing the credibility of what we are doing: the Project was presented to the Social Affairs Committee of the Italian Chamber of Deputies, which designated it as a pilot project for Italian cities.

The patient is the crux of the cultural complexity of which I have been speaking. Her experience of the illness affects all aspects of her life, so that medical treatment may remain only partially effective if it does not act in conjunction with all the other disciplines that can work together in constructing and completing the way to recovery. One answer to the problem, which is now universally recognized, is multidisciplinarity.

For us multidisciplinarity goes beyond the field of diagnosis, treatment, and psychological support; it refers to the possibility of getting medicine to interact with other forms of knowledge concerned with searching out the mystery of man, at least for as long as cancer remains, unfortunately, itself a mystery.

There is universal recognition of the patient's right to his or her dignity as a person. We would add that the patient, because he or she is a person, is a cultural subject and a promoter of culture. Pain and infirmity may modify languages, but they cannot abolish them. Therefore, the fundamental right we claim on behalf of the patient is that she should be given the status of a *cultural subject* and the opportunity to become a *skilled fighter* both for herself and for other patients, as well as the interlocutor of the doctor himself in the transmission of knowledge about the course of her own illness.

Another important feature of the work of the Amazon Project is the very concept of recovery. Recovery is not the reestablishment of an individual's normal way of life. This would be an enormously hypocritical attitude towards both our biological and our historical time. Recovery is rather an ongoing process that works out and recognizses within itself an inexorably new experience, something that promotes new human ventures and, consequently, new forms of human knowledge.

Consider for a moment just how persistent cancer patients are in affirming that cancer changes their lives inexorably. Through illness the patient enters into contact with the other half of life, the dark half, which is mystery, wounds, and suffering, as described by Susan Sontag in her book, "Illness as a Metaphor." The patient is "the person who knows,"[1] because, as Cioran puts it, "as long as you are well, you do not exist, or, to be more exact, you do not know that you exist."

The sick person acquires great strength in relation to both herself and her position in society. She might exercise a function similar to that of the shaman, if people would only stop dividing society into two parts, the "healthy" and the "sick." In that case, the patient might be not only the person who is treated, but also the person who renews, extends, and bears personal witness to our knowledge of the world. Viewed in this new light, the patient would be able to identify and build up her own personal resources as an important component in her program of recovery on an equal footing with the doctor and chemical or nuclear treatment.

The patient herself then is called upon to manage her own transformation and turn it into language and communication. But how can this be done? The Amazon Project indicates one way of doing this: by making use of the relationship between *Myth, Science and the Theater* to forge instruments in a "human workshop" where the workers are both "healthy" and "sick" people. Myth enables us to return to the origin of things; science pursues recovery and knowledge; and the theater seeks to restore to the mutilated body its communicative value.

The project works at two levels. The first is concerned with research and information through the **Biennial International Meetings**, which include conferences on oncology, psychooncology, theater culture, and the Assembly of Women. In October 2000 we organized the third of these meetings, which was endorsed by the Memorial Sloan-Kettering Cancer Center and the International Union Against Cancer (UICC) and UNESCO, Italian National Committee.

At a practical level the Project offers the services of the Amazon Centre, the Multidisciplinary Laboratory against Cancer, which was founded towards the end of 1999, in collaboration with the M. Ascoli Regional Oncological Centre. This is an example of how a public hospital can leave the precincts of the hospital itself and reach out towards the patient.

The spirit of our work in the Centre can be summed up in our motto, taken from Clarissa Pinkola Estés: "If you have a scar, here is a door," a superb image for someone wishing to enter the world of myth and bestow value on his or her own existence.

The Amazons, too, had a scar. These were mythical women warriors who amputated one of their breasts in order to rebel against slavery and fight more effectively. This is a metaphor of women's present-day struggle against breast cancer, but also a metaphor of women's struggle to achieve a new life project. For us the model of the Amazon warriors goes beyond the cultural stereotype that has been created in the course of time. For us it stands for women who had the courage actually to modify their own bodies in order to change their own destinies. The teaching we can draw from this is that physical mutilation, which the removal of a cancer almost always entails, should not be experienced as an impairment of the person, but as a door leading towards a source of 'female' energy, which can resurface provided that value is attributed to the experience itself.

The mythical reference to a woman's experience of cancer and its connection with mutilation underpins another great right of the patient: the right to have a body. When claimed by women, this right seems to us even more importan, because the condition of women is even more difficult in their experience of cancer. In the case of women, cancer assails and impairs not only the organ but also the symbol, what this organ represents. This "right to a body" seeks to bestow communicative value on the body's irregularity, despite the models of perfect beauty we are offered by the present-day civilization of images. Consequently, it seeks to respect a woman's freedom of choice about how to work out her own bodily identity even before she may have recourse to the reconstruction of a breast.

But there also exists a "right to the body," which concerns the dignity of the body itself, the way it is seen in the course of an illness: during a stay in the hospital, while clinical and instrumental tests are being carried out, in relationships with medical and auxiliary staff, etc. This drama must be faced by patients, whether male or female, when they are obliged to insert their bodies into that system of signs inherent in the period spent in hospital: the wearing of pyjamas (does the patient's condition coincide with her need for sleep?), the bed itself, physical proximity to other patients, smell, the taste of food, the architecture, all this is a backdrop that causes "healthy" people to experience embarrassment, fear, compassion, and the desire to escape.

THE AMAZON CENTRE

The gymnasium or training ground for the attainment and exercise of these rights is, as we said, the Amazon Centre, which for this purpose has three sectors of activity: the orientation of women both in prevention and during the course of the illness, the "Marie Curie" scientific sector, and the theater workshop.

The *Orientation* sector offers "healthy" women prevention programs including information, breast examinations, mammographies, dietary advice, etc.; women who have already undergone operations are offered general information, contact with the hospital, meetings with doctors and psychologists, and information about types of treatment and the course of the illness itself.

The *Marie Curie* sector is devoted to talks, seminars dealing with oncology, archetypal schemata, education, and sensitization campaigns against cancer, for which we have produced a video.

Knowledge and information underpin a patient's growth and the achievement of equality; they are also the key to creating a culture of prevention, towards which our activities are directed with particular attention.

The sector of the *Theatre Workshop*, directed by Lina Prosa, is devoted to drama, the use of the voice, and awareness of the body. It is open to "healthy" and sick women and has produced the plays, "The Pharmacy of Penthesilea" and "The Antigones." Integrating sick and healthy people in an artistic project is an important step towards removing the divisions that exist in our society and turning illness into an experience of shared growth, a frontier experience capable not only of fostering but also of renewing cultural and social processes.

Today Eleonora, one of the performers, can declare: "You do not die of cancer, you become an actress."

Lina Prosa does not use the theatre as a form of therapy but as a way of developing the art of using the body as an instrument to develop a person's ability to communicate, to improve body language, and therefore to become a significant cultural subject. Thus, a patient reclaims her relationship with life. She learns to tap her inner sources of energy and draw them out for the personal projects that interest her. This is what we mean when we say that a skilled fighter springs into life.

We started from breast cancer because it was our own personal experience, but we also desired to use this experience as a general observation post on cancer that might restore to us our lost horizons.

Gene Therapy of Hepatocellular Carcinoma and Gastrointestinal Tumors

BRUNO SANGRO,[a] CHENG QIAN,[a] VOLKER SCHMITZ,[b] AND
JESUS PRIETO[a]

[a]*Gene Therapy Unit, Department of Internal Medicine, Clinica Universitaria, Universidad de Navarra, Pamplona, Spain*

[b]*Department of Internal Medicine, University Hospital, Bonn, Germany*

> ABSTRACT: Primary liver cancer and liver metastases from gastrointestinal tumors lack effective therapy. Gene therapy is a promising therapeutic approach and is based on the introduction of genetic material into cells to generate a curative biological effect. Adenoviral vectors can very efficiently transduce a wide variety of malignant epithelial cells both *in vitro* and *in vivo*. A variety of gene therapy-based anticancer strategies have been effective in animal tumor models, including replacement of tumor suppressor genes, selective activation of prodrugs, genetic immunotherapy, and antiangiogenic actions. Enzymes used for genetic activation include viral thymidine kinase (tk), which may activate nucleoside analogs such as ganciclovir. We and others have demonstrated the efficacy of the tk/ganciclovir system in the treatment of hepatocellular carcinoma and metastatic colorectal cancer in experimental models. Also, this strategy can be safely applied to patients with liver tumors. Interleukin-12 (IL-12) is among the most potent cytokines in stimulating antitumor immunity. In models of primary and metastatic liver cancer we showed that intratumoral administration of recombinant adenovirus encoding IL-12 activates natural killer cells, induces specific antitumor immunity, and displays a powerful antiangiogenic effect, resulting in tumor regression. There is a synergistic effect with the gene transfer of the chemokine IP-10. Also, intratumoral injection of either dendritic cells transfected *ex vivo* with recombinant adenovirus encoding IL-12 (Ad.IL-12) or an adenovirus coding for the CD40 ligand have shown an intense antitumor effect against experimental colorectal cancer. In summary, a variety of gene therapy strategies have been effective against animal models of gastrointestinal tumors. Clinical trials should determine whether human patients can be treated safely and effectively by such strategies.
>
> KEYWORDS: gene therapy; hepatocellular carcinoma; gastrointestinal neoplasms; thymidine kinase; interleukin-12; CD40 ligand; genetic immunotherapy

GENERAL ASPECTS

Gene therapy represents a new and promising therapeutic modality. The underlying principle is based on the introduction of genetic material into cells to generate a

---

Address for correspondence: Dr. Jesus Prieto, Department of Internal Medicine, Clinica Universitaria, Ap. 4209, 31080 Pamplona, Spain. Voice: +34 948 295400; fax: +34 948 295600.
jprieto@unav.es

Ann. N.Y. Acad. Sci. 963: 6–12 (2002). © 2002 New York Academy of Sciences.

curative biological effect.[1,2] Such genetic material can be a natural or chimeric gene, or, more rarely, subgenomic particles and efficient cell transduction can be achieved by diverse natural (viruses) or artificial molecular constructs. For a gene to be expressed within a cell, its coding sequence should be linked to appropriate regulatory sequences. Gene promoters (and other regulatory elements) may allow transgene expression in every transduced cell (universal promoters) or, alternatively, only in selected cells containing transcription factors able to interact specifically with the promoter (as in tumor-specific promoters). However, promoters may determine continuous expression of the transgene in the transduced cell, or, alternatively, drugs given to the patient as inducers for transgene expression can regulate this promoter function. The most challenging issues in successful application of gene therapy to human neoplasms are the choice of a relevant therapeutic gene, an appropriate promoter and regulatory sequences, and an effective vector for delivering the transgene into target cells. Promoter and vector features determine transduction efficacy and specificity, duration of transgene expression, and the eventual appearance of side effects.

GENE TRANSFER TO TUMOR CELLS

Several approaches have been developed for transferring genes to human tissues. Plasmidic DNA can be efficiently transferred either directly, attached to cell-specific ligands, or embedded in lipidic formulations. On the other hand, viruses can be used for the same purpose, and extensive work was performed in the last decade on the use of adenoviruses, retroviruses, parvoviruses, herpesviruses, and other viruses for transferring recombinant DNA to cells.

Adenoviral vectors can very efficiently transduce a wide variety of malignant epithelial cells both *in vitro* and *in vivo*. Also, in most experimental animals, adenoviruses show a strong tropism for the liver when given systematically. The short-lived gene expression due to immunologic rejection of the infected cells represents a hurdle in the treatment of chronic diseases but not cancer. Also, the appearance of neutralizing antibodies impedes the repeated administration of adenoviral vectors when given intravascularly but not intratumorally.[3] Hence, intralesional injection of adenoviral vectors seems to be a good choice for transferring genes to liver tumors.

Retroviruses are also capable of efficiently infecting dividing cells, and, in fact, gene expression is more prolonged after retroviral-mediated transduction. However, the growth fraction of primary and most secondary liver tumors is small, which makes retroviral vectors unsuitable for human gene therapy of liver tumors. Liposomes have also been used as gene therapy vectors in various experimental models of cancer as well as in patients. Nevertheless, low transduction efficiency still limits the clinical application of liposomal formulations.

GENE THERAPY FOR NEOPLASTIC LIVER DISEASES

Malignant diseases of the liver are ranked fifth among all primary neoplastic diseases.[4] Hepatocellular carcinoma is the most common primary liver malignancy, with a rising incidence worldwide.[4,5] In addition, the liver is the most common organ in which tumor metastases occur.[5,6] Both unresectable hepatocellular carcinoma and liver metastases of digestive tumors lack effective therapy.[4,7] For these conditions, there is an urgent need for efficient alternative therapeutic approaches, and gene therapy has emerged as a new and promising method to treat human tumors. This article focuses on recent gene therapeutic strategies in the treatment of liver cancer.

Transfer of therapeutic genes to the tumor mass or peritumoral tissue provides a promising new approach to cancer therapy.[8–10] A variety of gene therapy-based anticancer strategies have been effective in animal tumor models, including replacement of tumor suppressor genes (e.g., wild-type p53), antisense strategies to inhibit oncogene expression, drug sensitization by transduction of tumor cells with suicide genes, genetic immunotherapy to stimulate the host's antitumoral immune response (e.g., immunostimulatory cytokines, chemokines, costimulatory molecules, combination of cytokines and chemokines, and genetic vaccination), and transfer of genes that interfere with the biological program of tumor growth (e.g., antiangiogenic substances). In the following paragraphs we concentrate mainly on suicide genes and genetic immunotherapy.

PRODRUG ACTIVATION THERAPY

This therapy consists of the transfer of a gene encoding a foreign enzyme that converts a nontoxic prodrug into an agent cytotoxic to the tumor cells. Antitumor selectivity can be achieved by either transferring the suicide gene exclusively to the tumor cells, using tumor-specific promoters to govern transgene expression (for instance, alpha-fetoprotein), or activating agents that can kill tumor cells selectively. Enzymes used for genetic activation include viral thymidine kinase, which may activate ganciclovir; cytosine deaminase, which can activate the antifungal 5-flucitosine into 5-fluorouracil; silimarase, which can activate silimarin; and many others. The herpes simplex virus thymidine kinase (HSV-tk) is the best-characterized suicide gene. Expression of functional HSV-tk in transduced tumor cells induces the conversion of the nontoxic prodrug ganciclovir into a toxic phosphorylated compound that terminates DNA chain elongation and inhibits DNA polymerase.[11] A characteristic trait of the suicide gene is the so-called bystander effect caused by diffusion of the activated metabolite from the transduced cells to the surrounding tissue, thus increasing the number of tumor cells destroyed by the procedure. Because of this effect, significant tumor regression can be achieved even when only a limited percentage of neoplastic cells has been transduced.[12,13] *In vivo*, the bystander effect also derives from necrosis of tumoral tissue inducing local inflammation, attraction of dendritic cells, and stimulation of antitumoral immunity. Thus, a synergistic antitumor effect was observed between suicide gene-based therapy and gene transfer of immunostimulatory molecules.[14]

Several studies have demonstrated the efficacy of the tk/ganciclovir system in the treatment of hepatocellular carcinoma[12,15,16] and metastatic colorectal cancer.[17,18] Also, a phase I clinical trial has shown that this tk/ganciclovir strategy can be safely applied to patients with liver metastases from colorectal cancer by intratumoral injection of an adenoviral vector.[19] Whether tk-based gene therapy of primary or secondary liver tumors is effective is yet to be shown.

GENETIC IMMUNOTHERAPY

The host's immunity fails to eliminate malignant tumor tissue because of either the lack of recognizable tumor antigens or the inability of tumor antigens to stimulate an effective immune response.[20,21] Defective antitumor immunity can be attributed partly to the lack of expression of MHC molecules by the tumor cells and to the secretion of immunosuppressive factors by the tumor (such as transforming growth factor-beta or vascular endothelial growth factor).[20] Gene transfer of cytokines that are important in the regulation of the immune system can overcome the immune tolerance to tumor antigens and facilitate tumor rejection. Many different cytokines (IL-2, IL-4, IL-6, IL-7, IL-12, gamma-interferon [INF-γ], tumor necrosis factor-alpha, and GM-CSF) have been used to modulate the host's immune response by either *ex vivo* or *in vivo* gene transfer.[22–25] IL-12, which is among the most potent cytokines at stimulating antitumor immunity, acts by inducing a TH1 type of response, activating natural killer cells and cytotoxic T lymphocytes, enhancing the expression of adhesion molecules on endothelial cells, thus facilitating the traffic of lymphocytes to the tumor, and inducing a potent antiangiogenic effect.

In an orthotopic model of primary liver cancer in Buffalo rats we showed that intratumoral administration of recombinant adenovirus encoding IL-12 (Ad.IL-12) caused complete tumor eradication in most animals and increased long-term survival.[25] Interestingly, when two tumors were separately implanted in the same liver, treatment of only one resulted in regression of both. This effect has been attributed to the fact that a proportion of adenoviruses injected into a neoplastic nodule escapes into the general circulation and, because of their strong liver tropism, infects the entire liver. IL-12 produced by the tumor and the hepatocytes surrounding the neoplastic nodules strongly activates natural killer cells, induces specific antitumor immunity and enhanced expression of adhesion molecules in tumor vessels, and displays a powerful antiangiogenic effect with resulting tumor regression.[25] Ad.IL-12 given by the intrahepatic arterial route has also been effective in the treatment of a very aggressive model of multifocal hepatocellular carcinoma in rats (induced by diethylnitrosamine), significantly reducing the tumor burden and prolonging survival.[25] Ad.IL-12 also induced potent antitumor effects in animal models of colorectal cancer metastatic to the liver by either intratumoral injection or systemic administration, resulting in peritumoral gene transfer.[26]

Although IL-12–based gene therapy showed an intense antitumor effect, it may also cause systemic toxic effects mainly derived from the ability of this cytokine to induce IFN-γ production. To enhance the antineoplastic activity of IL-12 while reducing the risk of toxicity, we tested the therapeutic effect of injecting intratumorally a suboptimal dose of Ad.IL-12 when given in combination with an adenovirus expressing the chemokine IP-10. The rationale was to attract immunoeffector cells to the neoplasm through IP-10 production and to activate the attracted lymphocytes with IL-12. We found that this combined therapy allows the dose of Ad.IL-12 to be reduced without losing antitumor efficacy but with less risk of toxicity.[27]

Dendritic cells are the most efficient antigen-presenting cells. Because activation of dendritic cells is critical for the induction of antitumor immunity, another possible way to take advantage of the therapeutic effect of IL-12 is to infect dendritic cells with AdIL-12 *ex vivo* and to inject these engineered dendritic cells into the tumor.[28]

In animal models of colon cancer this strategy was extremely potent at eliminating tumor lesions and eliciting antitumor immune responses.

Stimulation of dendritic cells is widely dependent on activation by costimulatory molecules such as B7 and the CD40 ligand.[29,30] We observed that adenovirus-mediated gene transfer of the CD40 ligand completely abolished the tumorigenicity of *ex vivo* infected rat hepatocellular carcinoma cells and that intratumoral injection of this adenovirus into established intrahepatic tumor nodules in rats resulted in tumor regression and prolonged survival.[31] Treatment of rat liver cancer with an adenovirus coding for the CD40 ligand induced protective antitumor immunity and was devoid of significant toxicity.[30,31]

OUTLOOK

Gene therapy has emerged as a powerful and very plastic tool for governing biological functions in diseased tissues. Animal models of human disease and pilot clinical studies clearly show a future for genes to be used as curative drugs. Much remains to be done in various fields concerning gene therapy. New vectors with improved transduction efficiency, transgene capacity, toxicity profile, and duration of expression should be developed. Systems to control gene expression must be improved. The ideal therapeutic gene or combination of genes for treating each specific medical condition has to be identified. Different routes and procedures for vector administration should be tested. A regulatory policy to ensure both safety and functionality needs to be established. Innovative methods of large-scale industrial production are to be implemented to allow cheap dispensation of these new drugs. The field is new but wide open, and it will certainly represent a great step in the progress of medical therapy.

ACKNOWLEDGMENTS

This work was supported by grants from MJ Huarte, J. Vidal, M. Mendez, Arburua Aspiunza, Fundacion Echebano, Fundacion Areces, and CICYT (Grants SAF98-0146, SAF99-0039, and SAF99-0084). One of the authors (V.S.) was partly supported by VERUM Foundation, Germany.

REFERENCES

1. MILLER, A.D. 1992. Human gene therapy comes of age. Nature **357:** 455–460.
2. MULLIGAN, R.C. 1993. The basic science of gene therapy. Science **260:** 926–932.
3. LAMBRIGHT, E.S., S.D. FORCE, M.E. LANUTI, *et al.* 2000. Efficacy of repeated adenoviral suicide gene therapy in a localized murine tumor model. Ann. Thorac. Surg. **70:** 1865–1870.
4. LAU, W.Y. 2000. Primary liver tumors. Sem. Surg. Oncol. **19:** 135–144.
5. CHOTI, M.A. & G.B. BULKLEY. 1999. Management of metastatic disease. *In* Schiff's Disease of the Liver. E.R. Schiff, M.F. Sorrell & W.C. Maddrey, eds. :134. Lippincott- Raven. Philadelphia.
6. MCCARTER, M.D. & Y. FONG. 2000. Metastatic liver tumors. Sem. Surg. Oncol. **19:** 177–188.

7. LAI, E.C., S.T. FAN, C.M. LO, et al. 1995. Hepatic resection for hepatocellular carcinoma. An audit of 343 patients. Ann. Surg. **221:** 291–298.
8. QIAN, C., M. DROZDZIK, W.H. CASELMANN & J. PRIETO. 2000. The potential of gene therapy in the treatment of hepatocellular carcinoma. J. Hepatol. **32:** 344–351.
9. RUIZ, J., C. QIAN, M. DROZDZIK & J. PRIETO. 1999. Gene therapy of viral hepatitis and hepatocellular carcinoma. J. Viral Hepat. **6:** 17–34.
10. HEIDEMANN, D.A.M., W.R. GERRITSEN & M.E. CRAANEN. 2000. Gene therapy for gastrointestinal tract cancer: a review. Scand. J. Gastroenterol. **232**(suppl): 93–100.
11. MOOLTEN, F.L. 1994, Drug sensitivity ("suicide") genes for selective cancer chemotherapy. Cancer Gene Ther. **1:** 279–287.
12. QIAN, C., R. BILBAO, O. BRUÑA & J. PRIETO. 1995. Induction of sensitivity to ganciclovir in human hepatocellular carcinoma cells by adenovirus-mediated gene transfer of herpes simplex virus thymidine kinase. Hepatology **22:** 118–123.
13. BI, W.L., L.M. PARYSEK, R. WARNICK & P.J. STAMBROOK. 1993. In vivo evidence that metabolic cooperation is responsible for the bystander effect observed with HSV tk retroviral gene therapy. Hum. Gene Ther. **4:** 725–731.
14. DROZDZIK, M., C. QIAN, X. XIE, et al. 2000. Combined gene therapy with suicide gene and interleukin-12 is more efficient than therapy with one gene alone in a murine model of hepatocellular carcinoma. J. Hepatol. **32:** 279–286.
15. KURIYAMA, S., T. NAKATANI, K. MASUI, et al. 1996. Evaluation of prodrugs' ability to induce effective ablation of cells transduced with viral thymidine kinase gene. Anticancer Res. **16:** 2623–2628.
16. QIAN, C., IODATE, M, BILBAO, R, et al. 1997. Gene transfer and therapy with adenoviral vector in rats with diethylnitrosamine-induced hepatocellular carcinoma. Hum. Gene Ther. **8:** 349–358.
17. HAYASHI, S., N. EMI, I. YOKOYAMA, et al. 1997. Effect of gene therapy with the herpes simplex virus-thymidine kinase gene on hepatic metastasis in murine colon cancer. Surg. Today **27:** 40–43.
18. HAYASHI, S., N. EMI, I. YOKOYAMA, et al. 1997. Inhibition of establishment of hepatic metastasis in mice by combination gene therapy using both herpes simplex virus-thymidine kinase and granulocyte macrophage-colony stimulating factor genes in murine colon cancer. Cancer Gene Ther. **4:** 339–344.
19. SUNG, M.W., H.C. YEH, S.N. THUNG, et al. 2001. Intratumoral adenovirus-mediated suicide gene transfer for hepatic metastases from colorectal adenocarcinoma: results of a phase I clinical trial. Mol. Ther. **4:** 182–191.
20. ROTH, C., C. ROCHLITZ & P. KOURILSKY. 1994. Immune response against tumors. Adv. Immunol. **57:** 281–351.
21. GABRILOVICH, D.I., H.L. CHEN, K.R. GIRGIS, et al. 1996. Production of vascular endothelial growth factor by human tumors inhibits the functional maturation of dendritic cells. Nature Med. **2:** 1096–1103.
22. MUSIANI, P., A. MODESTI, M. GIOVARELLA, et al. 1997. Cytokine, tumor-cell death and immunogenicity: a question of choice. Immunol. Today **18:** 32–36.
23. SCHMIDT-WOLF, G. & G.H. SCHMIDT-WOLF. 1995. Cytokines and gene therapy. Immunol. Today **16:** 173–175.
24. COLOMBO, M. & G. FORNI. 1994. Cytokine gene transfer in tumor inhibition and tumor therapy: where are we now? Immunol. Today **15:** 48–51.
25. BARAJAS, M., G. MAZZOLINI, G. GENOVÉ, et al. 2001. Gene therapy of orthotopic hepatocellular carcinoma in rats using adenovirus coding for interleukin-12 (IL-12). Hepatology **33:** 52–61.
26. BRUNDA, M.J., L. LUISTRO, R.R. WARRIER, et al. 1993. Antitumor and antimetastatic activity of interleukin 12 against murine tumors. J. Exp. Med. **178:** 1223–1230.
27. NARVAIZA, I., G. MAZZOLINI, M. BARAJAS, et al. 2000. Intratumoral coinjection of two adenoviruses, one encoding the chemokine IFN-gamma-inducible protein-10 and another encoding IL-12, results in marked antitumoral synergy. J. Immunol. **164:** 3112–3122.
28. MAZZOLINI, G., C. QIAN, I. NARVAIZA, et al. 2000. Adenoviral gene transfer of interleukin 12 into tumors synergizes with adoptive T cell therapy both at the induction and effector level. Hum. Gene Ther. **11:** 113–125.

29. SUN, Y., C. QIAN, D. PENG & J. PRIETO. 2000. Gene transfer to liver cancer cells of B7-1 plus interleukin 12 changes immunoeffector mechanisms and suppresses helper T cell type 1 cytokine production induced by interleukin 12 alone. Hum. Gene Ther. **11:** 127–138.
30. SCHMITZ, V., M. BARAJAS, L. WANG, *et al.* 2001. Adenovirus mediated CD40 ligand gene therapy in a rat model of orthotopic hepatocellular carcinoma. Manuscript submitted.
31. SCHMITZ, V., M. BARAJAS, Y. SUN, *et al.* 2000. Gene therapy of colon carcinomas (CC) and hepatocellular carcinomas (HCC) by adenovirus-mediated *in vivo* gene transfer of CD40 ligand [abstr]. Mol. Ther. **1:** S268.

Epidemiology, Risk Factors, and Natural History of Hepatocellular Carcinoma

GIUSEPPE MONTALTO, MELCHIORRE CERVELLO,[a] LYDIA GIANNITRAPANI, FABIO DANTONA, ANGELA TERRANOVA, AND LUIGI A. M. CASTAGNETTA[b]

Institute of Internal Medicine, Institute of Development Biology, [a]CNR and [b]Institute of Oncology, University of Palermo, Palermo, Italy

ABSTRACT: The incidence of hepatocellular carcinoma is increasing in many countries. The estimated number of new cases annually is over 500,000, and the yearly incidence comprises between 2.5 and 7% of patients with liver cirrhosis. The incidence varies between different geographic areas, being higher in developing areas; males are predominantly affected, with a 2:3 male/female ratio. The heterogeneous geographic distribution reflects the epidemiologic impact of the main etiologic factors and environmental risk, which are the hepatitis B (HBV) and hepatitis C (HCV) viruses. The percentage of cases of hepatocellular carcinoma attributable to HBV worldwide is 52.3% and is higher in Asia where the seroprevalence of HBsAg in the population is high. However, the vaccination campaign against this virus in some eastern countries has tended to lower the incidence of new cases of hepatocellular carcinoma. The percentage of cases of hepatocellular carcinoma attributable to HCV is 25%, and it is more prevalent in Japan, Spain, and Italy where the association between hepatocellular carcinoma and antibodies to HCV ranges between 50 and 70%. In most cases hepatocellular carcinoma develops in cirrhotic livers, where the persistent proliferation of liver cells represents the key factor of progression to hepatocellular carcinoma independent of the etiology. Another minor risk factor is aflatoxin B1 consumption, which is responsible for most cases of hepatocellular carcinoma in Africa, where the consumption of contaminated foods is common. Other known risk factors are some hereditary diseases, such as hemochromatosis, porphyria cutanea tarda, hereditary tyrosinemia, and α_1 anti-trypsin deficiency. The natural history of hepatocellular carcinoma is heterogeneous and is influenced by nodule dimension, the mono- or plurifocality of lesions at diagnosis, the growth rate of the tumor, and the stage of the underlying cirrhosis. Available data to date suggest that tumor growth in a cirrhotic liver is variable and that the time in which a lesion in undetectable until it becomes 2 cm is between 4 and 12 months. Therefore, the suggested interval for surveillance screening with ultrasound in patients with liver cirrhosis has been set at 6 months. Patients who should benefit from screening programs are those who would be treated with curative therapy if diagnosed with hepatocellular carcinoma. Thus, the ideal target population should be limited to Child-Pugh's class A cirrhotic patients without significant comorbidity.

KEYWORDS: hepatocellular carcinoma; liver cirrhosis; hepatitis B; hepatitis C

Address for correspondence: Giuseppe Montalto, M.D., Istituto di Medicina Interna e Geriatria, via del Vespro 141, 90127 Palermo, Italy. Voice: 39 091 6552991; fax: 39 091 6552936.
gmontal@unipa.it

EPIDEMIOLOGY

Hepatocellular carcinoma (HCC) in recent years has become one of the most frequently occurring tumors worldwide, occupying fifth place (average of men and women) in the classification of all malignancies.[1] The estimated incidence of new cases is about 500,000 per year, and since the prevalence is estimated to be similar, the survival of patients on the whole is 1 year.[1] With few exceptions its occurrence is increasing all over the world, but important differences have been noted between countries. Areas with a very high incidence (>20 cases/100,000 inhabitants) include sub-Saharan Africa, the western coast of Africa, which includes Gambia, Guinea, and Mali, and South Africa; in Asia a very high incidence is found in the southeastern countries (Korea, Hong Kong, Thailand, and Mongolia) and in large areas of China and Japan. European countries at high risk (11–20 cases/100,000) include Italy and Spain, and those at intermediate risk (5–10 cases/100,000) include France, United Kingdom, and Germany. A low incidence (<5 cases/100,000) is found in the United States, Canada, and Scandinavia. The Latin American countries are included in the areas of high incidence. There are large areas of the world, however, where the prevalence and incidence are still unknown.[2,3] Asia has the highest number of cases (about 76% globally) followed by Africa, Europe, United States, and Australia. Incidence adjusted by age and sex has yielded estimated values of 18 cases/100,000 males and 6 cases/100,000 females in developing countries, these estimates being 2.5-fold those reported in developed countries.[1] In the United States the incidence of HCC increased from 1.4/100,000 per year from 1976–1980 to 2.4/100,000 per year from 1991–1995.[4] Similar increases have also been registered in Italy, the United Kingdom, Canada, Japan, and Australia. In the same study the increase was reported mainly among blacks and was accompanied by a parallel increase in hospitalization and mortality for HCC.[4]

Changes in incidence have also involved age. In fact, from 1981–1985 the peak incidence of HCC occurred in patients aged 80–84 years, whereas from 1991–1995 the peak was noted in subjects aged 74–79 years. A shift in incidence towards younger persons was noted in the last two decades. A characteristic of HCC is to grow on cirrhotic liver; in fact, in western countries it develops on cirrhotic livers in more than 90% of cases, whereas in Asia and Africa the percentage of cases of HCC is higher in noncirrhotic than in cirrhotic liver.[5]

RISK FACTORS

The main risk factors of HCC are the hepatitis B (HBV) and the hepatitis C (HCV) viruses, which together account for three quarters of all cases worldwide. Other risk factors include aflatoxin B1 intake, alcohol consumption, and some hereditary diseases, among which are hereditary hemochromatosis, hereditary tyrosinemia, and α_1 anti-trypsin deficiency.

The attributable risk fraction for each risk factor varies according to the country examined. Whereas HCV has the greatest attributable risk in developed countries (60% in the USA, Europe, and Japan), it is responsible for a limited number of cases in most areas of Asia and Africa, where, on the contrary, HBV is mainly responsible.[6] Aflatoxin B1 probably does not play a role in developed countries, whereas it is definitely responsible, with a risk, however, not quantifiable, for numerous cases in Africa and Asia.[7]

ROLE OF THE HEPATITIS C VIRUS

Many epidemiologic studies have shown that many patients with HCC (as high as 70%) have anti-HCV antibody in the serum.[8–10] HCV therefore represents the most important risk factor for HCC in western countries. In almost all cases, neoplastic degeneration occurs in patients with liver cirrhosis, whereas only a few cases of HCV-associated HCC have been reported in the noncirrhotic liver,[11,12] indicating that this virus possibly has a mutagenic effect. The time lapse for the development of HCC in patients infected with HCV is much longer and includes all intermediate steps from mild chronic hepatitis, to severe chronic hepatitis, to liver cirrhosis, and finally to HCC.

The natural history of HCV infection has been examined in several studies. We refer, in particular, to a Japanese[13] and an American study,[14] which reported similar results. The Japanese study reported that it takes 13 years from a presumed infection, which was produced by a blood transfusion infected with HCV, to the development of chronic hepatitis. It was reported to be about 10 years in the American study. It took almost 20 years for the same patients to develop liver cirrhosis; the mean time for developing HCC was reported to be 28 years in the American study and 29 in the Japanese one. The annual risk of developing HCC in HCV-infected patients depends on the presence and severity of the underlying liver disease. Whereas the risk of HCC is rare in carriers of HCV infection,[15] it reaches 1.2–1.7% in patients with underlying chronic hepatitis[16,17] and can reach 1.4–2.5% in subjects with liver cirrhosis.[18,19] The risk of developing HCC becomes more significant in subjects with liver cirrhosis in whom hepatocytes show irregular growth,[20] with a high index of proliferation[21,22] or with signs of liver dysplasia.[23] The role of the HCV genotype, however, is still undefined. Whereas some reports indicate the greater responsibility of genotype 1b,[24] others refute this hypothesis.[25,26]

ROLE OF THE HEPATITIS B VIRUS

Epidemiologic studies associate HBV, as well as HCV, with the development of HCC. One study of a Taiwanese population reported that the relative risk of developing HCC was 102, because among carriers of HBV, 473 cases/100,000 per year developed HCC compared to only 4.6 cases/100,000 per year among noncarriers.[27] Another study performed on HBV carriers in Alaska reported similar data.[28] The role of the HBV in the development of HCC was also confirmed by the fact that after the vaccination campaign in Taiwan in the 1980s, there was an important reduction in HCC cases, and this reduction is ongoing.[29]

The annual incidence of developing HCC, like that for the HCV, is conditioned by the presence and severity of the underlying liver disease. As with HCV infection, it has been reported that, at least in western countries, carriers of HBsAg rarely develop HCC,[30] but the incidence with increasing severity of liver disease reaches 0.5–0.8% per year in patients with underlying chronic hepatitis[17,31] and 1.5–6.6% in patients with liver cirrhosis.[32,33]

Unfortunately, some persons become infected with both viruses. These patients have a higher risk of developing HCC than do those with a single infection. A study that attempted to quantify the risk of single versus double infection showed that the cumulative risk of a patient with double infection is greater than that in those with a single infection, whether infected by HBV or HCV.[34] Furthermore, the same patients followed up over time had a cumulative risk of developing HCC of 10, 21, and 23%, respectively, after 5 years and of 16, 28, and 45%, respectively, after 10 years.

ROLE OF AFLATOXIN B1

Aflatoxin B1 (AFB1) has long been associated with the development of HCC, because areas with a large consumption of this toxin coincide with areas with a high incidence of HCC. It is produced by a fungus of the genus *Aspergillus* in large areas of Asia and sub-Saharan Africa where, for climatic reasons (heat and humidity) and because of storage techniques, the fungus represents a common contaminant of foods (grain, corn, peanuts, legumes, etc.), producing large quantities of toxin. However, it was recently observed that areas that have a high incidence of HCC and high aflatoxin intake correspond to areas in which HBV infection is endemic and that patients at higher risk of developing HCC are those who are exposed to both HBV and AFB1 risk factors.[35] A case control study using biomarkers of exposure to AFB1, such as urinary metabolites of AFB1 or the blood concentration of AFB1 adducts, did not confirm the responsibility of AFB1 in the development of HCC;[36] for this reason it has been proposed that in addition to a high intake of AFB1, patients who previously were exposed to HBV should be considered at higher risk of developing HCC.[37] One possible means by which AFB1 can lead to HCC is to provoke a specific mutation of codon 249 of the p53 tumor suppressor gene.[38] However, this mutation has almost always been found in patients who had previous contact with the HBV.

ROLE OF ALCOHOL

Alcohol has not been proved experimentally to be mutagenic and therefore directly responsible for neoplastic degeneration. Nevertheless, it is a frequent etiologic agent of liver cirrhosis, through which it can favor the development of HCC. Whatever the etiology of cirrhosis, once it has been diagnosed, it is the main cause of neoplastic degeneration of the liver. However, high alcohol intake (70–80 g/day) over a long period (at least 5 years) is necessary for liver cirrhosis to develop. Low or moderate intake of alcohol is not associated with the development of liver cirrhosis and consequently of HCC.

NATURAL HISTORY OF HEPATOCELLULAR CARCINOMA

It is difficult to outline the natural history of HCC, because it depends on a series of variables that, when combined, can evolve into the disease, not only in different subjects, but also sometimes within the same subject. The natural history depends on the number and size of neoplastic nodules at diagnosis, the growth speed pattern of the nodule(s), and the severity of the underlying liver disease.

Currently, with improvement in diagnostic tools (ultrasound, helicoidal CT), HCC is more often found as a single nodule or nodules of small size, allowing patients to be treated radically (resection, transplantation, and thermoablation). Consequently, they are excluded from the group of untreated patients, which is the group in which the natural history of the disease can be delineated. However, when patients have numerous nodules or signs of extrahepatic disease at diagnosis, they have access only to symptomatic treatment and therefore they are not even ideal candidates for delineating the natural history of the disease.

Currently, more patients are being found to have a treatable nodule at diagnosis than in the past. However, after more extensive investigation, some of them show satellite nodules and/or intra- or extrahepatic diffusion of the disease, which nullifies attempts at radical treatment.

Also, the growth pattern of a neoplastic nodule can vary from one patient to another. Even in the same patient periods of faster growth can alternate with periods of slower growth. The doubling time of a nodule of small dimensions has been estimated within a period of 1–19 months,[39–41] thus indicating the great variability, and there are some small nodules that after a long period of stability can grow rapidly. On the contrary, some nodules with initial fast growth can subsequently stop growing. Nodules with fast initial growth are those that nullify attempts to screen for HCC in patients with liver cirrhosis, because within a time lapse of 6 months ultrasound can reveal a neoplastic liver that has developed beyond the limits of radical treatment. However, Italian guidelines indicate an interval of 6 months for the screening of HCC in cirrhotic patients,[42] which is the estimated median of doubling time for a neoplastic nodule of small dimensions.[39–41]

Another variable conditioning the natural history of HCC is the severity of the underlying liver disease. The discovery of a neoplastic nodule in Child's class C patients does not modify the natural history of liver cirrhosis, and for this reason these patients are excluded from screening programs. Untreated patients with HCC in Child's class A or B, who are historical or belong to the control arm of ramdomized controlled trials, have a different prognosis, which is better in those patients with better underlying hepatic function.[43,44]

Another variable that seems to affect the survival of patients with unresectable liver neoplasia is the state of the estrogen receptor on the surface of the hepatocytes. Patients with the wild-type estrogen receptor live longer than do patients with a variant form of estrogen receptor on the hepatocyte surface.[45]

CONCLUSIONS

Hepatocellular carcinoma is currently one of the most frequently occurring tumors worldwide and it has a highly negative prognosis. The main risk factors are HCV and HBV. Each one is prevalent in different areas of the world, HCV in western countries, Japan, and Australia, and HBV in large areas of Africa and Asia. They are responsible for neoplastic degeneration of the liver, mainly through cirrhosis. Alcohol is also considered a risk factor for HCC, but only indirectly after progression of liver cirrhosis and only in heavy drinkers. AFB1 has recently been redimensioned as an etiologic factor in HCC, because although its consumption is high in those countries, such as Africa and Asia, where the incidence of HCC is high, it seems to be only a cofactor of neoplastic degeneration.

What should health professionals do in the next few years to reduce the incidence of HCC? They should: (1) extend the universal campaigns of vaccination against HBV, which is the most frequent etiologic factor of HCC, above all in developing countries where the virus is endemic; (2) reduce AFB1 intake through the appropriate storage and treatment of foods; (3) reduce the incidence of HCV infection through diffusion of educational programs on the knowledge of contaminated materials and, above all, targeting groups at high risk, such as drug users, people practicing body piercing, and homosexuals, awaiting the implementation of a vaccine to prevent HCV infection; and (4) limit the availability of alcoholic beverages.

Some of these preventive measures, such as the vaccination campaign against HBV in Taiwan, are already in place. With awareness, our generation can assist in decreasing the incidence of this neoplasia, probably within the next 20 years, which will make HCC drop to a more acceptable position in the table of malignancies.

ACKNOWLEDGMENTS

This work was supported in part by MURST (Ministero dell'Università e della Ricerca Scientifica e Tecnologica) 40%, year 2000, to G.M.

REFERENCES

1. PARKIN, D.M., P. PISANI & J. FERLAY. 1999. Estimates of the worldwide incidence of twenty-five major cancers in 1990. Int. J. Cancer **80:** 827–841.
2. FERLAY, J., D.M. PARKIN & P. PISANI. 1998. GLOBOCAN Graphical Package 1: Cancer Incidence and Mortality Worldwide. IARC Press. Lyon.
3. BOSCH, F.X., J. RIBES & J. BORRÀS. 1999. Epidemiology of primary liver cancer. Semin. Liver Dis. **19:** 271–285.
4. EL-SERAG, H.B. & A.C. MASON. 1999. Rising incidence of hepatocellular carcinoma in the United States. N. Engl. J. Med. **340:** 745–750.
5. OKUDA, K. 2000. Hepatocellular carcinoma. J. Hepatol. **32:** 225–237.
6. PISANI, P., D.M. PARKIN, M. MUNOZ, et al. 1997. Cancer and infection: estimates of the attributable fraction in 1990. Cancer Epidemiol. Biomark Prev. **6:** 387–400.
7. FAO, WHO, Expert Committee, JECFA, and Bosch FX. 1996. Toxicological evaluation of certain food additives. WHO Food Additives. Series 37. WHO/IPCS. Geneva.
8. NISHIOKA, K., J. WATANABE, S. FURUTA, et al. 1991. A high prevalence of antibody to the hepatitis C virus in patients with hepatocellular carcinoma in Japan. Cancer **67:** 429–433.
9. BRUIX, J., X. CALVET, J. COSTA, et al. 1989. Prevalence of antibody to hepatitis C virus in Spanish patients with hepatocellular carcinoma and hepatic cirrhosis. Lancet **2:** 1004–1006.
10. COLOMBO, M., Q.L. CHOO, E. DEL NINNO, et al. 1989. Prevalence of antibody to hepatitis C virus in Italian patients with hepatocellular carcinoma. Lancet **2:** 1006–1008.
11. DE MITRI, M.S., K. POUSSIN, P. BACCARINI, et al. 1995 HCV–associated liver cancer without cirrhosis. Lancet **345:** 413–415.
12. EL-REFAIE, A., K. SAVANE, S. BHATTACHARYA, et al. 1996. HCV-associated hepatocellular carcinoma without cirrhosis. J. Hepatol. **4:** 277–285.

13. KIYOSAWA, K., T. SODEYAMA, E. TANAKA, et al. 1990. Interrelationship of blood transfusion, non-A, non-B hepatitis and hepatocellular carcinoma: analysis by detection of antibody to hepatitis C virus. Hepatology **12:** 671–675.
14. TONG, M.J., N.S. EL-FARRA, A.R. REIKES, et al. 1995. Clinical outcomes after transfusion-associated hepatitis C. N. Engl. J. Med. **332:** 1463–1466.
15. TRADATI, F., M. COLOMBO, P.M. MANNUCCI, et al. 1998. A prospective multicenter study of hepatocellular carcinoma in Italian hemophiliacs with chronic hepatitis C. Blood **91:** 1173–1177.
16. TSUKUMA, H., T. HIYAMA, S. TANAKA, et al. 1993. Risk factors for hepatocellular carcinoma among patients with chronic liver disease. N. Engl. J. Med. **328:** 1797–1801.
17. TAKANO, S., O. YOKOSUKA, F. IMAZEKI, et al. 1995. Incidence of hepatocellular carcinoma in chronic hepatitis B and C: a prospective study of 251 patients. Hepatology **21:** 650–665.
18. FATTOVICH, G., G. GIUSTINA, F. DEGOS, et al. 1997. Effectiveness of interferon alfa on incidence of hepatocellular carcinoma and decompensation in cirrhosis type C. J. Hepatol. **27:** 201–205.
19. BRUNO, S., E. SILINI, A. CROSIGNANI, et al. 1997. Hepatitis C virus genotypes and risk of hepatocellular carcinoma in cirrhosis: a prospective study. Hepatology **25:** 754–758.
20. SHIBATA, M., S. TAKEDA, T. KUDO, et al. 1991. Minus strand RNA of hepatitis C virus in liver tissues. J. Hepatol. **13:** 379–380.
21. BORZIO, M., S. BRUNO, M. RONCALLI, et al. 1995. Liver cell dysplasia is a major risk factor for hepatocellular carcinoma in cirrhosis: a prospective study. Gastroenterology **108:** 812–817.
22. DONATO, M.F., E. AROSIO, E. DEL NINNO, et al. 2001. High rates of hepatocellular carcinoma in cirrhotic patients with high liver cell proliferative activity. Hepatology **34:** 523–528.
23. CARRIÈ, N., C. CHASTANG, F. CHAPEL, et al. 1996. Predictive score for the development of hepatocellular carcinoma and additional value of liver large cell dysplasia in western patients with cirrhosis. Hepatology **23:** 1112–1118.
24. SILINI, E., R. BOTTELLI, M. ASTI, et al. 1996. Hepatitis C virus genotypes and risk of hepatocellular carcinoma in cirrhosis: a case–control study. Gastroenterology **111:** 199–205.
25. TANAKA, K., T. HIROHATA, H. IKEMATSU, et al. 1996. Hepatitis C virus infection and risk of hepatocellular carcinoma among Japanese: possible role of type 1b (II) infection. J. Natl. Cancer Inst. **88:** 742–746.
26. BENVEGNU, L., P. PONTISSO, D. CAVALLETTO, et al. 1997. Lack of correlation between hepatitis C virus genotypes and clinical course of hepatitis C virus-related cirrhosis. Hepatology **25:** 211–215.
27. BEASLEY, R.P., L.Y. HWANG, C.C. LIN, et al. 1981. Hepatocellular carcinoma and hepatitis B virus: a prospective study of 22,707 men in Taiwan. Lancet **2:** 1129–1133.
28. MCMAHON, B.J., S.R. ALBERTS, R.B. WAINWRIGHT, et al. 1990. Hepatitis B related sequelae. Prospective study in 1400 hepatitis B surface antigen–positive Alaska native carriers. Arch. Intern. Med. **150:** 1051–1054.
29. CHANG, M.H., C.J. CHEN, M.S. LAI, et al. 1997. Universal hepatitis B vaccination in Taiwan and the incidence of hepatocellular carcinoma in children. N. Engl. J. Med. **336:** 1855–1859.
30. DE FRANCHIS, R., G. MEUCCI, M. VECCHI, et al. 1993. The natural history of asymptomatic hepatitis B surface antigen carriers. Ann. Intern. Med. **118:** 191–194.
31. LIAW, Y.F., D.I. TAI, C.M. CHU, et al. 1986. Early detection of hepatocellular carcinoma in patients with chronic type B hepatitis. A prospective study. Gastroenterology **90:** 263–267.
32. FATTOVICH, G. 1998. Progression of hepatitis B and C to hepatocellular carcinoma in western countries. Hepato-gastroenterology **45:** 1206–1213.
33. TSAI, J.F., J.E. JENG, M.S. HO, et al. 1997. Effect of hepatitis C and B virus infection on risk of hepatocellular carcinoma: a prospective study. Br. J. Cancer **76:** 968–974.
34. CHIARAMONTE, M., T. STROFFOLINI, A. VIAN, et al. 1999. Rate of incidence of hepatocellular carcinoma in patients with compensated viral cirrhosis. Cancer **85:** 2132–2137.

35. GROOPMAN, J.D., P. SCHOOL & J.S. WANG. 1996. Epidemiology of human aflatoxin exposures and their relationship to liver cancer. Progr. Clin. Biol. Res. **395:** 211–222.
36. CAMPBELL, T.C., J.S. CHEN, C.B. LIU, *et al.* 1990. Nonassociation of aflatoxin with primary liver cancer in a cross-sectional ecological survey in the People's Republic of China. Cancer Res. **50:** 6882–6893.
37. BRUIX, J., M. SHERMAN, J.M. LLOVET, *et al.* 2001. Clinical management of hepatocellular carcinoma. Conclusion of the Barcelona–2000 EASL conference. J. Hepatol. **35:** 421–430.
38. BRESSAC, B., M. KEW, J. WANDS & M. OZTURK. 1991. Selective G to T mutations of p53 gene in hepatocellular carcinoma from southern Africa. Nature **350:** 429–431.
39. EBARA, M., M. OHITO & T. SHINAGAWA. 1986. Natural history of minute hepatocellular carcinoma smaller that three centimeters complicating cirrhosis. Gastroenterology **90:** 289–298.
40. COLOMBO, M. & A. SANGIOVANNI. 1992. Natural history of hepatocellular carcinoma. Ital. J. Gastroenterol. **24:** 95–99.
41. OKAZAKY, N., M. YOSHINO & T. YOSHIDA. 1989. Evaluation of the prognosis for small hepatocellular carcinoma based on tumor volume doubling time. A preliminary report. Cancer **63:** 2207–2210.
42. COLOMBO, M. 1992. Early diagnosis of hepatocellular carcinoma in Italy. A summary of a consensus development conference held in Milan, 16 November 1990 by the Italian Association for the Study of the Liver. J. Hepatol. **14:** 401–403.
43. LIVRAGHI, T., L. BOLONDI, L. BUSCARINI, *et al.* 1995. No treatment, resection and ethanol injection in hepatocellular carcinoma: a retrospective analysis of survival in 391 patients with cirrhosis. J. Hepatol. **22:** 522–526.
44. LLOVET, J.M., J. BUSTAMANTE, A. CASTELLS, *et al.* 1999. Natural history of untreated nonsurgical hepatocellular carcinoma: rationale for the design and evaluation of therapeutic trials. Hepatology **29:** 62–67.
45. VILLA, E., A. MOLES, I. FERRETTI, *et al.* 2000. Natural history of inoperable hepatocellular carcinoma: estrogen receptors' status in the tumor is the strongest prognostic factor for survival. Hepatology **32:** 233–238.

Genetic Alterations and Oncogenic Pathways in Hepatocellular Carcinoma

LAURENCE LÉVY, CLAIRE ANGÉLIQUE RENARD, YU WEI, AND
MARIE ANNICK BUENDIA

*Unité de Recombinaison et Expression Génétique, INSERM U163,
Département des Rétrovirus, Institut Pasteur, 75015 Paris, France*

ABSTRACT: Hepatocellular carcinoma (HCC) is a major type of primary liver cancer and one of the rare human neoplasms etiologically linked to viral factors. Chronic infections with the hepatitis B virus (HBV) and the hepatitis C virus (HCV) have been implicated in about 80% of cases worldwide, and other known environmental risk factors, including alcohol abuse and dietary intake of aflatoxin B1, might synergize with viral infections. Recent insight into the molecular mechanisms leading to HCC development has been provided by the identification of major genetic abnormalities revealed by genomewide allelotype studies and molecular cytogenetic analysis. Moreover, several oncogenic pathways have been implicated in malignant transformation of liver cells. Inactivation of the p53 tumor suppressor gene by mutations and allelic deletions in about 30% of HCC cases has been associated predominantly with exposure to aflatoxin B1 and HBV infection. By contrast, a mutation in the β-catenin gene in around 22% of HCCs is more rare in HBV-associated tumors. Activation of cyclin D1 and disruption of the Rb pathway are also commonly involved in liver tumorigenesis. New major challenges include the identification of candidate genes located in frequently altered chromosomal regions and that of oncogenic pathways driven by different risk factors. This search might shed some light on the tumorigenic role of HBV and HCV. It might also permit accurate evaluation of major targets for prognostic and therapeutic intervention.

KEYWORDS: hepatocellular carcinoma; loss of heterozygosity; LOH; comparative genomic hybridization; CGH; beta-catenin; hepatitis virus

INTRODUCTION

Hepatocellular carcinoma (HCC) is among the eight most common cancers worldwide, and its incidence is still rising in different countries.[1,2] Extensive epidemiologic studies have identified multiple risk factors, including chronic infection with hepatitis B virus (HBV) and hepatitis C virus (HCV), alcoholic cirrhosis, environmental carcinogens such as aflatoxin B1 (AFB1), and some inherited metabolic diseases, including hemochromatosis, tyrosinemia, and α_1-antitrypsin deficiency.

Address for correspondence: Marie Annick Buendia, Inserm U163, Department of Retroviruses, Institut Pasteur, 28 rue du Dr. Roux, 75724 Paris Cedex 15, France. Voice: 33/145 688 866; fax: 33/145 688 943.
 mbuendia@pasteur.fr

Furthermore, a synergistic interplay between HBV and AFB1 and between HCV and alcohol abuse has been shown. The question of whether other viral or chemical agents are responsible for the recently observed increase in HCC rates in some countries is still debated.

Recent investigations have revealed insights into the complex role of HBV in malignant transformation of liver cells. The major chromosomal abnormalities in HCC have been unraveled, and recent data on new oncogenic pathways and tumor suppressor networks have accumulated. However, many challenges remain, because most of the tumor genes that map to frequently affected regions have yet to be identified.

DIRECT AND INDIRECT ROLES OF HEPATITIS B VIRUS IN LIVER ONCOGENESIS

Chronic HBV infection remains a major risk factor for HCC worldwide, not only in endemic areas but also in Europe where cryptic HBV infections are frequently detected in patients with HCC.[3,4] The complex role of this virus in liver carcinogenesis through direct and indirect mechanisms is still being debated.[5] Integration of HBV DNA sequences into the host cell genome can activate cellular genes by a cis-acting mechanism in a minority of HCC cases (FIG. 1). Chromosomal instability may also result from HBV DNA integration, as exemplified by frequent chromosomal translocations and deletion or amplification of large chromosomal regions at the site of HBV integration. More indirectly, liver cell injury mediated by cellular immune responses may be sufficient to cause liver cancer by promoting cell death and proliferation, and genetic mutations may accumulate in the context of necroinflammatory disease. This hypothesis has been strongly supported by the finding that HBV transgenic mice develop chronic hepatitis and ultimately HCC after stimulation of the immune response by adoptive transfer of activated T lymphocytes.[6]

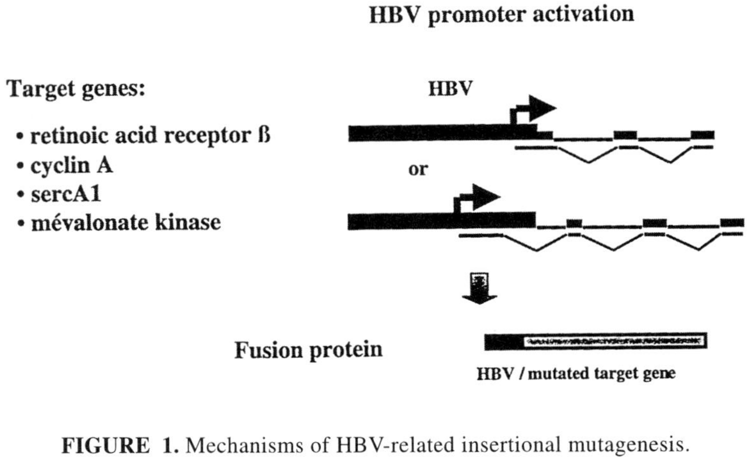

FIGURE 1. Mechanisms of HBV-related insertional mutagenesis.

Whether long-term expression of viral genes plays a part in the malignant transformation process is also a debated issue. The HBV genome encodes a 16.5-kDa protein, termed HBx, that harbors weak transcriptional transactivation activity. HBx might be a prime candidate for mediating HBV pathologic effects. The X gene is conserved among tumorigenic mammalian hepadnaviruses, and it is required for viral replication in the woodchuck host.[7,8] The 16.5-kDa HBx protein is a multifunctional transactivator that upregulates a variety of viral and cellular genes (reviewed in Ref. 9). This protein has no direct DNA-binding activity, and it modulates the expression of target genes through protein-protein interactions (reviewed in Ref. 10). HBx may function as a coactivator by interacting in the nucleus with transcription factors (CREB/ATF) and with elements of the basal transcription machinery (TFIIB, TBP, and RPB5).[11–13] In a cytoplasmic location, HBx activates the Src pathway, thereby stimulating the intracellular viral replication process[14] and the Ras/Raf signaling pathway, leading to the activation of several oncogenes such as c-myc, c-jun, and c-fos.[15–18] In addition, HBx activates two different transcription factors,, NF-KB and NF-AT, implicated in the regulation of cytokine expression (interleukin [IL]-6, IL-8, and tumor necrosis factor-alpha [TNF-α]).[19–22]

HBx has been implicated in liver tumorigenesis by several lines of evidence. Expression of HBx is generally maintained through all stages of the tumorigenic process, and viral RNAs containing X but not surface or core sequences have been detected, even in HCCs from HBsAg-negative patients.[23,24] Integrated HBV sequences in tumor DNA frequently contain X gene sequences.[25–27] In a transgenic mouse lineage generated in the CD1 background, liver expression of the X transgene was reported to induce frequent liver tumors.[28] In other lineages, however, HBx has no obvious pathologic effect, but it sensitizes liver cells to the carcinogenic effects of diethylnitrosamine.[29,30] Moreover, expression of HBx in Myc transgenic mice accelerates liver tumorigenesis in bitransgenic animals.[31] These data suggest that the X protein has no acutely transforming activity by itself, but its overexpression might cooperate with activated cellular oncogene(s) in multistep hepatic transformation. Finally, studies in established cell lines have demonstrated that HBx expression can transform SV40 TAg-immortalized rodent hepatocytes and fibroblasts,[32,33] and stimulate cell cycle progression, DNA synthesis, and apoptosis.[19,34–36] Physical interactions of HBx with a variety of cellular proteins might also be relevant to the HBx oncogenic potential (FIG. 2). Notably, HBx has been reported to bind the DNA repair protein UVDDB, the p53 tumor suppressor protein, and proteasome subunits.[37–43] Although HBx might interfere with DNA repair in established cell lines,[44] its expression in transgenic mouse liver is not associated with an increased rate of spontaneous genomic mutations.[45] More recently, a contribution of HBx in hepatic fibrosis was suggested by the finding that HBx amplifies TGF-β signaling through direct interaction with Smad4.[46]

There is increasing evidence that the HBx protein interacts with regulatory pathways controlling apoptosis. The hypothesis that HBx might play a role as a "sensitizer" to other proapoptotic stimuli has notably been supported by its ability to increase cell sensitivity to apoptotic death induced by TNF-α, a proinflammatory cytokine activated in chronic liver diseases.[19,47] The association of HBx with mitochondria results in decreased mitochondrial membrane potential, cytochrome c release, and eventual apoptosis.[8] However, in different studies, HBx was reported to

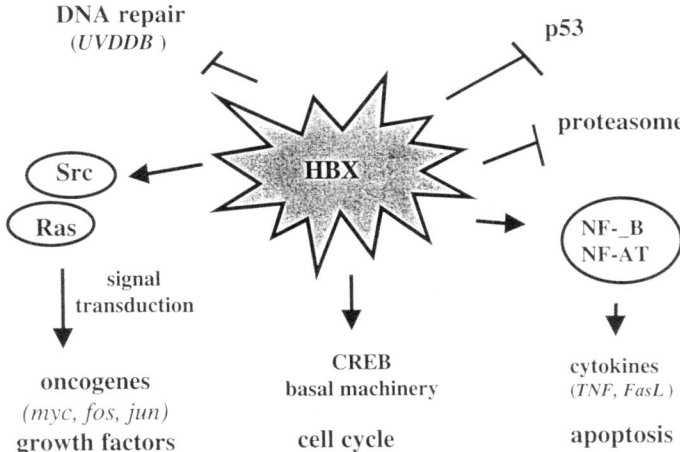

FIGURE 2. Multiple interactions of the HBX regulatory protein.

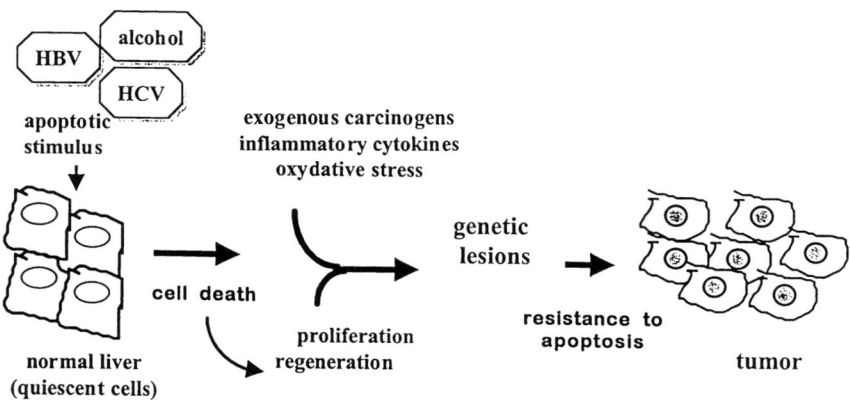

FIGURE 3. Deregulation of apoptosis control in hepatocarcinogenesis.

either induce or repress cell death.[35,36,49–52] These apparent discrepancies might be explained by the large variety of experimental conditions used in different studies, and they suggest that the fate of HBx-expressing cells might be determined by different parameters, including the level of HBx expression and the cellular context. All together, these data suggest that HBx expression participates in the pathogenesis of chronic hepatitis B. At tumoral stages, loss of apoptotic activity of HBx mutants might be an important step in the escape of tumor cells from apoptosis.[25,53,54] These studies strongly support the notion that deregulated control of apoptosis plays a crucial role at different steps of liver tumorigenesis (FIG. 3).

CHROMOSOMAL ABNORMALITIES IN HEPATOCELLULAR CARCINOMA

Cancer proceeds through the accumulation of mutations in genes that govern cell proliferation and death. The long latency period of tumor development has led some to postulate that at least five different genetic events may be required to reach the fully malignant phenotype.[55] Recently, it was proposed that six essential alterations in cell physiology may dictate malignant transformation, including independence towards growth, anti-growth and apoptotic signals, unlimited division, and angiogenetic and metastatic capacities.[56] Mutations in critical genes may result from different types of genetic alterations, ranging from subtle sequence changes at a few nucleotides to gross chromosomal abnormalities including deletions, amplifications, and translocations of large DNA fragments. It is generally accepted that recurrent allelic deletions at specific chromosomal regions denote the presence of a tumor suppressor gene. Although small genetic lesions can be detected only by selective molecular analysis, large chromosomal abnormalities can be visualized through different approaches, which are listed below.

Conventional cytogenetic methods were first used for genetic analysis of hepatoma cell lines and primary liver tumors, and they revealed that most HCCs are aneuploid and harbor multiple different chromosomal abnormalities, with recurrent deletions of the short arm of chromosome 1.[57,58] However, the number of tumors analyzed has remained limited, and strategies based on molecular analyses of genomic DNA have been more widely developed.

The development of a polymerase chain reaction-based approach allowing genomewide scans for loss of heterozygosity (LOH) has greatly improved our understanding of HCC genetics. Short tandem repeats, called microsatellites, are 2–6 bp repeated sequences (a common repeat motif is CA) spread throughout the genome. They represent an abundant class of human polymorphisms, which can be typed using the polymerase chain reaction. It is estimated that the human genome carries at least 100,000 microsatellites, and presently, about 10–15,000 markers positioned over all human chromosomes have been made available in databanks. These sequences represent an ideal tool for LOH studies, because their chromosomal location is precisely known, and they are highly polymorphic, with most individuals carrying paternal and maternal alleles of different sizes in more than 70% of cases. In addition, this method requires a small amount of DNA, allowing the analysis of few selected tumor cells. It must be emphasized, however, that the presence of contaminating normal cells in the tumor sample can lead to a pattern of allelic imbalance rather than true allelic loss. Recent allelotype studies using polymorphic microsatellite markers have demonstrated LOH at multiple chromosomal loci. It suggests that a variety of tumor suppressor genes might be inactivated during the tumoral process, which is consistent with the multifactorial etiology of HCC (reviewed in Refs. 59 and 60). In comprehensive allelotype studies of HCCs associated with different risk factors, it was shown that chromosomal loci localized on chromosomes 1p, 4q, 6q, 7p, 8p, 9p, 10q, 13q, 16pq, and 17p are frequently involved in human hepatocarcinogenesis.[61,62] Among known cancer genes, LOH has been reported for the p53 locus at 17p13, Rb at 13q14, axin at 16p13, and mannose-6-phosphate/IGF II receptor at 6q27.[63–65] Tumor suppressor genes localized in other frequently deleted chromosomal regions in HCC remain currently unknown. LOH at chromosome 1p might represent an early event in HCC,[66] whereas LOH at 16q is frequently associated with HBV markers, advanced tumor stage, and poor prognosis.[67,68] The absence of obvious genetic predisposition to HCC development recognized so far has greatly hindered the identification of tumor suppressor genes involved in liver tumorigenesis. To obtain further insight into the candidate genes localized on different chromosomes, fine mapping analysis of LOH loci on these chromosomal arms has been performed.[69] These studies have revealed in all cases several frequently affected regions, suggesting that more than one tumor suppressor gene might be located along the chromosomal arms.

Comparative genomic hybridization is a global, sensitive method based on the labeling of tumor and matched normal DNA with two different fluorochromes and simultaneous hybridization of normal metaphase spread chromosomes. This method, allowing a survey of the entire genome, has a major advantage over microsatellite analysis in that it can reveal DNA copy gains and small amplified regions, which may be suspected of containing dominant oncogenes. However, it can detect only deleted or amplified regions more than 10–20 megabases in size. Different comparative genomic hybridization analyses have confirmed DNA copy losses at chromosomal arms affected by LOH, and they have shown frequent DNA copy gains or amplification on chromosomes 1q, 8q, 6p, and 17q.[67,70–73] Chromosome gains at these locations are also frequently observed in other human malignancies. Besides the c-myc oncogene localized at 8q22-24, it is likely that oncogenes present on chromosomal arms 1q, 6p, and 17q are implicated in the development of liver cancer. A summary of average chromosomal gains and losses from different LOH and comparative genomic hybridization studies is shown in FIGURE 4.

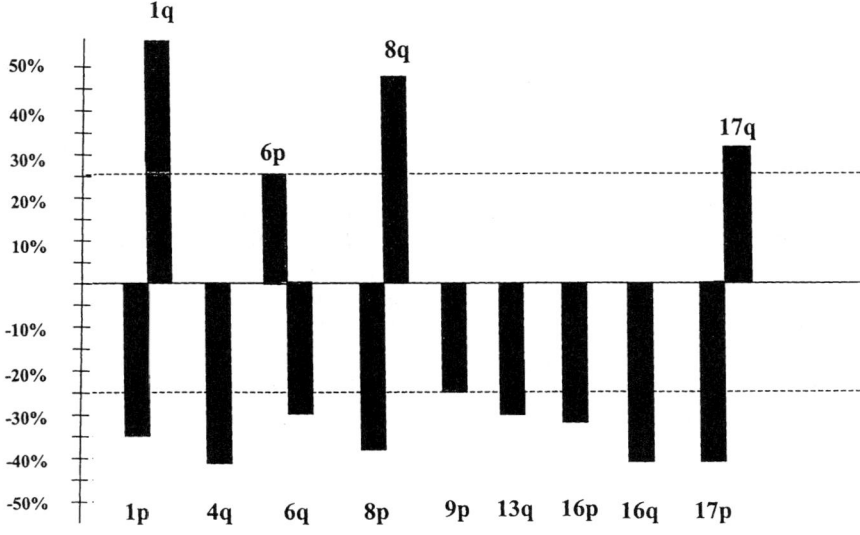

FIGURE 4. Chromosome gains and losses in hepatocellular carcinoma.

GENETIC INSTABILITY IN HEPATOCELLULAR CARCINOMA

Genetic instability plays a central role in cancer development. Different types of instabilities have been described in human cancer. Microsatellite instability is associated with a mutator phenotype at the nucleotide level; it is caused by defects in the DNA mismatch repair genes MSH2 and MLH1 located on chromosomes 2 and 3.[74] In HCC, however, these chromosomal regions are not frequently affected by allelic losses, and microsatellite instability has not been detected by microsatellite marker analysis. Furthermore, very few mutations have been detected in the mononucleotide repeats in Bax, IGF-IIR, or MLH genes in HCC.[75,76]

Chromosomal instability manifests as a high variation in chromosome numbers among cells from individual tumor clones. It has been associated with defects in chromosome segregation resulting from loss of p53, BUB-1, or APC functions.[77] Whether HBV infection and integration of HBV DNA play a role in chromosomal instability is an interesting issue. It has been shown that peripheral blood cells of HBV chronic carriers present a higher incidence of chromosome breaks than matched uninfected populations and that HBV-transfected hepatoma cells HepG2 have de novo genetic alterations at several chromosomal sites.[78,79] Large rearrangements of genomic DNA frequently accompany HBV DNA integration in host chromosomes.[80] These data support the hypothesis that HBV infection and/or HBV DNA integration might contribute in cellular transformation by interfering with cellular processes responsible for the stability of the genome.

TUMOR SUPPRESSOR GENES

Allelotype studies have revealed multiple allelic deletions on different chromosomal arms in HCC, most of which cannot precisely be attributed to a known tumor suppressor gene. In some cases, however, mutational or biological analysis has demonstrated the involvement of a few tumor suppressor genes, including the p53, Rb, IGF-II receptor, and axin genes.

The p53 gene is probably the most common molecular target involved in human carcinogenesis.[81] Also called "guardian of the genome" and "cellular gatekeeper," p53 is activated in response to DNA damage, inducing either cell cycle arrest to permit DNA repair or apoptosis. Loss of p53 function occurs mainly through allelic deletions at chromosome 17p13, where the gene is located, and missense mutations in the four highly conserved regions located within the specific DNA-binding domain. These mutations select mainly against the DNA-binding activity of p53, and they are critical for correct folding of the protein. Additionally, they are associated with a prolonged half-life of the protein, which accumulates in the cell nuclei, suggesting that it has acquired an oncogenic gain of function.[81] In human HCC, LOH at chromosome 17p13 has been observed in 25–60% of tumors, and the worldwide prevalence of p53 mutations is around 28% with, however, important geographic variations. HBV infection or the presence of HBV DNA in the tumor has been associated with an increased rate of p53 mutations, and it has been reported that the p53 mutational profile differs between HBV- and HCV-positive tumors.[82] It is now well established that codon 249 p53 mutation in HCC is mostly seen in some regions of Africa (Mozambique, Senegal) and the southeast coast of Asia (Qidong, Vietnam), where chronic HBV infection is highly endemic and the aflatoxin content of the diet is high.[83,84] Aflatoxin B1 is a fungal metabolite found in grain crops, known to be transformed into a 8,9 epoxyde that binds DNA and forms adducts. It has been shown that AFB1 adducts result frequently in G:C to T:A transversions in human hepatocytes, mainly at codon 249.[85] P53 codon 249 mutations occur occasionally in regions showing low to moderate AFB1 exposure (Beijin, Taiwan, Hong-Kong, and Thailand), and they are rare in European countries and in the United States where no evidence for food contamination has been provided. Thus, the specific "hot spot" 249 mutation appears to be a hallmark of dietary exposure to AFB1.

Allelic deletions at chromosome 13q in human cancer have been associated with the inactivation of two tumor suppressor genes, Rb and BRCA2 located at 13q14 and 13q12-13. The Rb gene plays a major role in cell cycle control, and its disruption renders cells insensitive to antiproliferative signals that induce growth arrest at the G1 phase. Rb can be inactivated by different ways, including mutations in the gene itself, loss of TGF-β responsiveness, and inactivation of $p16^{INK4A}$, $p15^{INK4B}$, or CDK4.[56] In HCC, LOH at the Rb locus has been found in 25–48% of cases,[64,66] and it has been shown that pRb expression is strongly downregulated in 30–50% of tumors.[86] However, the gene itself is rarely mutated, and silencing of p16 by promoter methylation represents a major mechanism for inactivation of Rb. A low frequency of mutations in the Smad2, Smad4, and TGF-β RII genes might implicate a disruption of the TGF-β pathway in a minority of HCCs.[87,88] The finding of a new oncogene, termed gankyrin, defines a novel pathway leading to pRb inactivation.[89] Gankyrin is an ankyrin-repeat protein homologous to the p28 subunit of the 26S proteasome. It is overexpressed in all HCCs; it binds pRb and promotes its degradation by the ubiquitin-proteasome pathway.

The finding of frequent allelic deletions at chromosome 6q26-27[90] has led to investigation into the involvement of the mannose-6-phosphate/IGF-II receptor (M6P/IGF2R). This gene is implicated as a tumor suppressor by its ability to activate TGF-β signaling and to promote the degradation of IGF-II, a potent growth factor for liver cells. In tumors harboring a 6q LOH, mutations of the M6P/IGF2R gene on the remaining allele have been detected in 25% of cases, leading to major amino acid substitutions or premature truncation of the protein.[63] However, a recent search for mutations of the M6P/IGF2R gene in 43 HCCs was unsuccessful.[91] The reasons for these discrepancies need to be clarified.

Recurrent LOH at both the short and the long arms of chromosome 16 in HCC is well documented. On 16p, a major candidate is the axin gene. Axin is part of a cytoplasmic multiprotein complex that contains β-catenin, APC, and GSK3β, and it acts as a scaffolding protein in phosphorylation-dependent ubiquitination and degradation of β-catenin.[92] Loss of function of axin promotes β-catenin accumulation in the nucleus in the absence of mutation in the β-catenin gene itself.[65]

ACTIVATION OF THE β-CATENIN ONCOGENE IN HEPATOCELLULAR CARCINOMA

β-catenin is an important multifunctional protein involved in Wingless/Wnt signaling during embryonic development and in cell-cell adhesion.[93,94] In normal adult epithelial cells, in the absence of Wnt signaling, β-catenin is localized at the cell

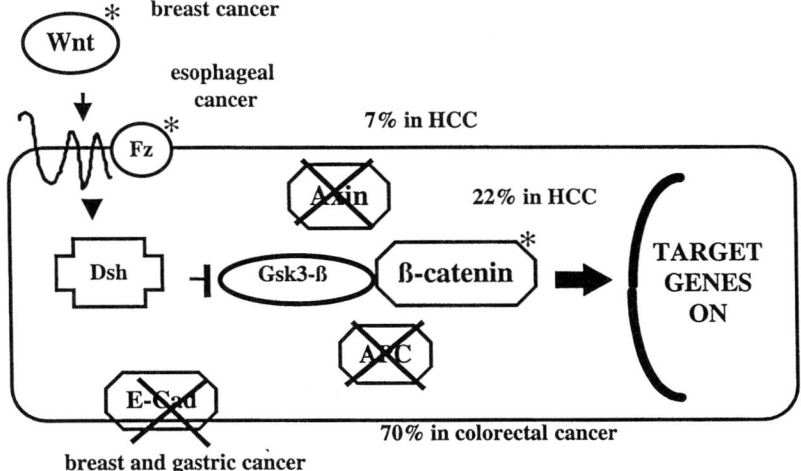

FIGURE 5. Activation of the Wnt/β-catenin pathway in human cancer.

membrane in a complex with E-cadherin and α-catenin at the sites of adherens junctions. The excess β-catenin is phosphorylated at N-terminal serine-threonine residues by functional interactions with glycogen synthase kinase (GSK)-3β, axin, and the adenomatous polyposis coli protein (APC), and subsequently targeted to degradation by the ubiquitin-proteasome system.[95] Activation of the Wnt signal inhibits GSK-3β activity and induces β-catenin stabilization. Translocation of β-catenin to the nucleus and its association with high mobility group domain factors Tcf/LEF causes transcriptional activation of target genes,[96] including the c-myc and cyclin D1 genes.[97,98]

Deregulated expression of β-catenin has been implicated as an important step in carcinogenesis, through activating mutations in the β-catenin gene, APC or axin defects, or other alterations in the Wnt pathway, as summarized in FIGURE 5. Mutant β-catenins that are resistant to downregulation by GSK-3β phosphorylation and ubiquitination were first characterized in human colorectal cancers and then in a variety of carcinomas (reviewed in Ref. 99). Recently, oncogenic mutations in the β-catenin gene were evident in human and mouse liver tumors.[100,101] β-catenin mutations have been found in 19–41% (average 22%) of human HCCs of different etiologic origin.[100–105] The strong correlation between nuclear β-catenin staining and somatic mutations of the β-catenin gene in tumor cells indicates that activation of the Wnt/β-catenin pathway in HCC occurs predominantly through mutations in the β-catenin gene itself.[103] It differs from colorectal cancers in which APC mutations are responsible for β-catenin stabilization in 70–80% of the cases. HCCs harboring intense nuclear expression of β-catenin are characterized by high proliferative rate, and their prognosis might be more severe.[103] By contrast in nontumorous livers, dysplastic lesions, and cirrhotic nodules, β-catenin immunostaining is restricted to the cell membrane. It has been shown that β-catenin mutations are more prevalent in HCCs that are not related to HBV infection. HCCs carrying a β-catenin mutation harbor otherwise a limited number of chromosomal aberrations detected by microsatellite marker analysis.[105,106] This suggests that the oncogenic activity of β-catenin overrides the need for multiple genetic events in the multistep process of hepatocarcinogenesis and that different oncogenic pathways may lead to the appearance of the malignant phenotype. In mouse models of hepatocarcinogenesis, the incidence of β-catenin mutations is highly variable between tumors induced by different carcinogenic agents[107] or developed on different p53 backgrounds.[108] Further studies of human HCCs are required to better characterize the molecular mechanisms leading to the appearance of β-catenin mutations and their oncogenic impact.

CONCLUSIONS

Consistent with the multifactorial etiology of HCC and the long latency period of tumor formation, multiple oncogenes, growth factors, and tumor suppressors have been implicated in human hepatocarcinogenesis[59] (FIG. 6). The question of whether HBV and other etiologic factors and cofactors may trigger different tumorigenic pathways can now be addressed, owing to the development of novel technologies for genomewide scans of genetic alterations. Indeed, increased frequency of p53 mutations has been associated with AFB1 exposure and chronic HBV infection, and mutation at the p53 codon 249 is considered the hallmark of AFB1 contamination in the diet.[83] Moreover, tumors from HBsAg-positive patients harbor increased rates of deletion at different chromosomes.[68,109] By contrast, activating mutations of the β-catenin gene are rare in HBV-associated HCCs compared with tumors associated with other risk factors.[106] So far, however, attempts to correlate a number of genetic alterations with a direct role of HBV (such as integration) have remained unsuccessful. Besides genetic alterations, epigenetic factors, such as methylation-associated gene silencing, play an important role in the deregulation of cell cycle control and

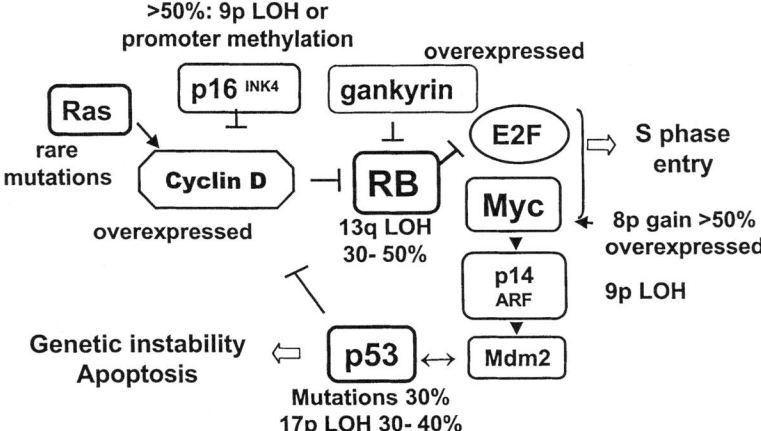

FIGURE 6. Network of oncogenic and tumor suppressor pathways in hepatocellular carcinoma.

proliferation. Large studies of gene expression in HCC and chronic hepatitis by microarray screening have recently been reported.[110–112] These studies will undoubtedly contribute to a better understanding of the complex role of HBV in liver tumorigenesis.

REFERENCES

1. BOSCH, F.X. 1997. Global epidemiology of hepatocellular carcinoma. *In* Liver Cancer. K. Okuda & E. Tabor, eds. :13-28. Churchill Livingstone. New York.
2. MURRAY, C.J.L. & A.D. LOPEZ. 1997. Mortality by cause for eight regions of the world: global burden of disease study. Lancet **349:** 1269–1276.
3. BRÉCHOT, C., F. JAFFREDO, D. LAGORCE, *et al.* 1998. Impact of HBV, HCV, and GBV-C/HGV on hepatocellular carcinomas in Europe: results of an European concerted action. J. Hepatol. **29:** 173–183.
4. CHEMIN, I., F. ZOULIM, P. MERLE, *et al.* 2001. High incidence of hepatitis B virus infections among chronic hepatitis cases of unknown etiology. J. Hepatol. **34:** 447–454.
5. BRECHOT, C., D. GOZUACIK, Y. MURAKAMI, *et al.* 2000. Molecular bases for the development of hepatitis B virus (HBV)-related hepatocellular carcinoma (HCC). Semin. Cancer Biol. **10:** 211–231.
6. NAKAMOTO, Y., L.G. GUIDOTTI, C.V. KUHLEN, *et al.* 1998. Immune pathogenesis of hepatocellular carcinoma. J. Exp. Med. **188:** 341–350.
7. CHEN, H.S., S. KANAKO, R. GIRONES, *et al.* 1993. The woodchuck hepatitis virus X gene is important for establishment of virus infection in woodchucks. J. Virol. **67:** 1218–1226.
8. ZOULIM, F., J. SAPUTELLI & C. SEEGER. 1994. Woodchuck hepatitis virus X protein is required for viral infection *in vivo.* J. Virol. **68:** 2026–2030.
9. CASELMANN, W.H. 1996. Trans-activation of cellular genes by hepatitis virus proteins: a possible mechanism of hepatocarcinogenesis. Adv. Virus Res. **47:** 253–302.
10. ANDRISANI, O.M. & S. BARNABAS. 1999. The transcriptional function of the hepatitis B virus X protein and its role in hepatocarcinogenesis. Int. J. Oncol. **15:** 373–379.
11. QADRI, I., H.F. MAGUIRE & A. SIDDIQUI. 1995. Hepatitis B virus transactivator protein X interacts with the TATA-binding protein. Proc. Natl. Acad. Sci. USA **92:** 1003–1007.
12. CHEONG, J., M. YI, Y. LIN, *et al.* 1995. Human RPB5, a subunit shared by eukaryotic nuclear RNA polymerases, binds human hepatitis B virus X protein and may play a role in X transactivation. Embo J. **14:** 143–150.
13. HAVIV, I., M. SHAMAY, O. DOITSH, *et al.* 1998. Hepatitis B virus pX targets TFIIB in transcription coactivation. Mol. Cell. Biol. **18:** 1562–1569.
14. KLEIN, N.P., M.J. BOUCHARD, L.H. WANG, *et al.* 1999. Src kinases involved in hepatitis B virus replication. Embo J. **18:** 5019–5027.
15. CROSS, J.C., P. WEN & W.J. RUTTER. 1993. Transactivation by hepatitis B virus X protein is promiscuous and dependent on mitogen-activated cellular serine/threonine kinases. Proc. Natl. Acad. Sci. USA **90:** 8078–8082.
16. NATOLI, G., M.L. AVANTAGGIATI, P. CHIRILLO, *et al.* 1994. Ras- and Raf-dependent activation of c-Jun transcriptional activity by the hepatitis B virus transactivator pX. Oncogene **9:** 2837–2843.
17. BENN, J. & J. SCHEIDER. 1994. Hepatitis B virus HBx protein activates Ras-GTP complex formation and establishes a Ras, Raf, MAP kinase signaling cascade. Proc. Natl. Acad. Sci. USA **91:** 10350–10354.
18. SU, P. & R.J. SCHNEIDER. 1996. Hepatitis B virus HBx protein activates transcription factor NF-KB by acting on multiple cytoplasmic inhibitors of rel-related proteins. J. Virol. **70:** 4558–4566.
19. SU, F. & R.J. SCHNEIDER. 1997. Hepatitis B virus HBx protein sensitizes cells to apoptotic killing by tumor necrosis alpha. Proc. Natl. Acad. Sci. USA **94:** 8744–8749.
20. LARA-PEZZI, E., A.L. ARMESILLA, P.L. MAJANO, *et al.* 1998. The hepatitis B virus X protein activates nuclear factor of activated T cells (NF-AT) by a cyclosporin A-sesitive pathway. Embo J. **17:** 7066–7077.

21. LARA-PEZZI, E., P.L. MAJANO, M. GOMEZ-GONZALO, *et al.* 1998. The hepatitis B virus X protein up-regulates tumor necrosis factor alpha gene expression in hepatocyte. Hepatology **28:** 1013–1021.
22. WEIL, R., H. SIRMA, C. GIANNINI, *et al.* 1999. Direct association and nuclear import of the hepatitis B virus X protein with the NF-kappaB inhibitor IkappaBalpha. Mol. Cell Biol. **19:** 6345–6354.
23. SU, Q., C.H. SCHRÖDER, W.J. HOFMAN, *et al.* 1998. Expression of hepatitis B virus X protein in HBV-infected human livers and hepatocellular carcinoma. Hepatology **27:** 1109–1120.
24. PATERLINI, P., K. POUSSIN, M. KEW, *et al.* 1995. Selective accumulation of the X transcript of hepatitis B virus in patients negative for hepatitis B surface antigen with hepatocellular carcinoma. Hepatology **21:** 313–321.
25. SIRMA, H., C. GIANNINI, K. POUSSIN, *et al.* 1999. Hepatitis B virus X mutants, present in hepatocellular carcinoma tissue abrogate both the antiproliferative and transactivation effects of HBx. Oncogene **18:** 4848–4859.
26. WEI, Y., J. ETIEMBLE, G. FOUREL, *et al.* 1995. Hepnavirus integration generates virus-cell cotranscripts carrying 3′ truncated X genes in human and woodchuck liver tumors. J. Med. Virol. **45:** 82–90.
27. WOLLERSHEIM, M., U. DEBELKA & P.H. HOFSCHNEIDER. 1988. A transactivating function encoded in the hepatitis B virus X gene is conserved in the integrated state. Oncogene **3:** 545–552.
28. KIM, C.M., K. KOIKE, I. SAITO, *et al.* 1991. HBx gene of hepatitis B virus induces liver cancer in transgenic mice. Nature **351:** 317–320.
29. DANDRI, M., P. SCHIRMACHER & C.E. ROGLER. 1996. Woodchuck hepatitis virus X protein is present in chronically infected woodchuck liver and in woodchuck hepatocellular carcinomas which are permissive for viral replication. J. Virol. **70:** 5246–5254.
30. SLAGLE, B.L., T.H. LEE, D. MEDINA, *et al.* 1996. Increased sensitivity to the hepatocarcinogen diethylnitrosamine in transgenic mice carrying the hepatitis B virus x gene. Molec. Carcinogenesis **15:** 261–269.
31. TERRADILLOS, O., O. BILLET, C.A. RENARD, *et al.* 1997. The hepatitis B virus X gene potentiates c-myc-induced liver oncogenesis in transgenic mice. Oncogene **14:** 395–404.
32. HÖHNE, M., S. SCHAEFER, M. SEIFER, *et al.* 1990. Malignant transformation of immortalized transgenic hepatocytes after transfection with hepatitis B virus DNA. Embo J. **9:** 1137–1145.
33. GOTTLOB, K., S. PAGANO, M. LEVRERO, *et al.* 1998. Hepatitis B virus X protein transcription activation domains are neither required nor sufficient for cell transformation. Cancer Res. **58:** 3566–3570.
34. BENN, J. & R.J. SCHNEIDER. 1995. Hepatitis B virus HBx protein deregulates cell cycle checkpoint controls. Proc. Natl. Acad. Sci. USA **92:** 11215–11219.
35. CHIRILLO, P., S. PAGANO, G. NATOLI, *et al.* 1997. The hepatitis B virus X gene induces p53-mediated programmed cell death. Proc. Natl. Acad. Sci. USA **94:** 8162–8167.
36. ELMORE, L.W., A.R. HANCOCK, S.-F. CHANG, *et al.* 1997. Hepatitis B virus X protein and p53 tumor suppressor interactions in the modulation of apoptosis. Proc. Natl. Acad. Sci. USA **94:** 14707–14712.
37. LEE, T.-H., S.J. ELLEDGE & J.S. BUTEL. 1995. Hepatitis B virus X protein interacts with a probable DNA repair protein. J. Virol. **69:** 1107–1114.
38. SITTERLIN, D., T.H. LEE, S. PRIGENT, *et al.* 1997. Interaction of the UV-damaged DNA-binding protein with hepatitis B virus X protein is conserved among mammalian hepadnaviruses and restricted to transactivation-proficient X-insertion mutants. J. Virol. **71:** 6194–6199.
39. SIRMA, H., R. WEIL, O. ROSMORDUC, *et al.* 1998. Cytosol is the prime compartment of hepatitis B virus X protein where it colocalizes with the proteasome. Oncogene **16:** 2051–2063.
40. HU, Z., Z. ZHANG, E. DOO, *et al.* 1999. Hepatitis B virus X protein is both a substrate and a potential inhibitor of the proteasome complex. J. Virol. **73:** 7231–7240.
41. FEITELSON, M.A., M. ZHU, L.X. DUAN, *et al.* 1993. Hepatitis B x antigen and p53 are associated *in vitro* and in liver tissues from patients with primary hepatocellular carcinoma. Oncogene **8:** 1109–1117.

42. UEDA, H., S.J. ULLRICH, J.D. GANGEMI, et al. 1995. Functional inactivation but not structural mutation of p53 causes liver cancer. Nature Genet. **9:** 41–47.
43. LIN, Y., T. NOMURA, T. YAMASHITA, et al. 1997. The transactivation and p53-interacting functions of hepatitis B virus X protein are mutually interfering but distinct. Cancer Res. **57:** 5137–5142.
44. BECKER, S.A., T.H. LEE, J.S. BUTEL, et al. 1998. Hepatitis B virus X protein interferes with cellular DNA repair. J. Virol. **72:** 266–272.
45. MADDEN, C.R., M.J. FINEGOLD & B.L. SLAGLE. 2000. Expression of hepatitis B virus X protein does not alter the accumulation of spontaneous mutations in transgenic mice. J. Virol. **74:** 5266–5272.
46. LEE, D.K., S.H. PARK, Y. YI, et al. 2001. The hepatitis B virus encoded oncoprotein pX amplifies TGF-beta family signaling through direct interaction with Smad4: potential mechanism of hepatitis B virus-induced liver fibrosis. Genes Dev. **15:** 455–466.
47. SU, F., C.N. THEODOSIS & R.J. SCHNEIDER. 2001. Role of NF-kappaB and myc proteins in apoptosis induced by hepatitis B virus HBx protein. J. Virol. **75:** 215–225.
48. TAKADA, S., Y. SHIRAKATA, N. KANENIWA, et al. 1999. Association of hepatitis B virus X protein with mitochondria causes mitochondrial aggregation at the nuclear periphery, leading to cell death. Oncogene **18:** 6965–6973.
49. WANG, X.W., M.K. GIBSON, W. VERMEULEN, et al. 1995. Abrogation of p53-induced apoptosis by the hepatitis B virus X gene. Cancer Res. **55:** 6012–6016.
50. LEE, S.G. & H.M. RHO. 2000. Transcriptional repression of the human p53 gene by hepatitis B viral X protein. Oncogene **19:** 468–471.
51. KLEIN, N.P. & R.J. SCHNEIDER. 1997. Activation of Src family kinases by hepatitis B virus HBx protein and coupled signaling to Ras. Mol. Cell. Biol. **17:** 6427–6436.
52. KIM, H., H. LEE & Y. YUN. 1998. X-gene product of hepatitis B virus induces apoptosis in liver cells. J. Biol. Chem. **273:** 381–385.
53. STRAND, S., W.J. HOFMANN, H. HUG, et al. 1996. Lymphocyte apoptosis induced by CD95 (APO-1/Fas) ligand-expressing tumor cells: a mechanism of immune evasion? Nature Med. **2:** 1361–1366.
54. YEH, C.T., C.H. SHEN, D.I. TAI, et al. 2000. Identification and characterization of a prevalent hepatitis B virus X protein mutant in taiwanese patients with hepatocellular carcinoma. Oncogene **19:** 5213–5220.
55. FEARON, E.R. & B. VOGELSTEIN. 1990. A genetic model for colorectal tumorigenesis. Cell **61:** 759–767.
56. HANAHAN, D. & R.A. WEINBERG. 2000. The hallmarks of cancer. Cell **100:** 57–70.
57. PARADA, L.A., M. HALLEN, K.G. TRANBERG, et al. 1998. Frequent rearrangements of chromosomes 1, 7, and 8 in primary liver cancer. Genes Chrom. Cancer **23:** 26–35.
58. SIMON, D., B.B. KNOWLES & A. WEITH. 1991. Abnormalities of chromosome 1 and loss of heterozygosity on 1p in primary hepatomas. Oncogene **6:** 765–770.
59. NAGAI, H. & M.A. BUENDIA. 1998. Oncogenes, tumor suppressors and co-factors in hepatocellular carcinoma. *In* Hepatitis B Viruses: Molecular Mechanisms in Disease and Novel Strategies for Therapy. R. Koshy & W. Caselman, eds. :182–218. Imperial College Press. London.
60. BUENDIA, M.A. 2000. Genetics of hepatocellular carcinoma. Semin. Cancer Biol. **10:** 185–200.
61. NAGAI, H., P. PINEAU, P. TIOLLAIS, et al. 1997. Comprehensive allelotyping of human hepatocellular carcinoma. Oncogene. **14:** 2927–2933.
62. BOIGE, V., P. LAURENT-PUIG, P. FOUCHET, et al. 1997. Concerted nonsyntenic allelic losses in hyperploid hepatocellular carcinoma as determined by a high-resolution allelotype. Cancer Res. **57:** 1986–1990.
63. DE SOUZA, A.T., G.R. HANKINS, M.K. WASHINGTON, et al. 1995. M6P/IGF2R gene is mutated in human hepatocellular carcinomas with loss of heterozygosity. Nature Genet. **11:** 447–449.
64. MURAKAMI, Y., K. HAYASHI, S. HIROHASHI, et al. 1991. Aberrations of the tumor suppressor p53 and retinoblastoma genes in human hepatocellular carcinomas. Cancer Res. **51:** 5520–5525.
65. SATOH, S., Y. DAIGO, Y. FURUKAWA, et al. 2000. AXIN1 mutations in hepatocellular carcinomas, and growth suppression in cancer cells by virus-mediated transfer of AXIN1. Nature Genet. **24:** 245–250.

66. KUROKI, T., Y. FUJIWARA, E. TSUCHIYA, *et al.* 1995. Accumulation of genetic changes during development and progression of hepatocellular carcinoma: loss of heterozygosity of chromosome arm 1p occurs at an early stage of hepatocarcinogenesis. Genes Chrom. Cancer. **13:** 163–167.
67. LIN, Y.W., J.C. SHEU, G.T. HUANG, *et al.* 1999. Chromosomal abnormality in hepatocellular carcinoma by comparative genomic hybridisation in Taiwan. Eur. J. Cancer **35:** 652–658.
68. SHEU, J.C., Y.W. LIN, H.C. CHOU, *et al.* 1999. Loss of heterozygosity and microsatellite instability in hepatocellular carcinoma in Taiwan. Br. J. Cancer **80:** 468–476.
69. PINEAU, P., H. NAGAI, S. PRIGENT, *et al.* 1999. Identification of three distinct regions of allelic deletions on the short arm of chromosome 8 in hepatocellular carcinoma. Oncogene **18:** 3127–3134.
70. MARCHIO, A., M. MEDDEB, P. PINEAU, *et al.* 1997. Recurrent chromosomal abnormalities in hepatocellular carcinoma detected by comparative genomic hybridization. Genes Chrom. Cancer **18:** 59–65.
71. KUSANO, N., K. SHIRAISHI, K. KUBO, *et al.* 1999. Genetic aberrations detected by comparative genomic hybridization in hepatocellular carcinomas: their relationship to clinicopathological features. Hepatology **29:** 1858–1862.
72. SAKAKURA, C., A. HAGIWARA, H. TANIGUCHI, *et al.* 1999. Chromosomal aberrations in human hepatocellular carcinomas associated with hepatitis C virus infection detected by comparative genomic hybridization. Br. J. Cancer **80:** 2034–2039.
73. WONG, N., P. LAI, S.W. LEE, *et al.* 1999. Assessment of genetic changes in hepatocellular carcinoma by comparative genomic hybridization analysis: relationship to disease stage, tumor size, and cirrhosis. Am. J. Pathol. **154:** 37–43.
74. LENGAUER, C., K.W. KINZLER & B. VOGELSTEIN. 1998. Genetic instabilities in human cancers. Nature **396:** 643–649.
75. KONDO, Y., Y. KANAI, M. SAKAMOTO, *et al.* 1999. Microsatellite instability associated with hepatocarcinogenesis. J. Hepatol. **31:** 529–536.
76. SALVUCCI, M., A. LEMOINE, R. SAFFROY, *et al.* 1999. Microsatellite instability in European hepatocellular carcinoma. Oncogene **18:** 181–187.
77. FODDE, R., J. KUIPERS, C. ROSENBERG, *et al.* 2001. Mutations in the APC tumour suppressor gene cause chromosomal instability. Nat. Cell Biol. **3:** 433–438.
78. SIMON, D., T. LONDON, H.W. HANN, *et al.* 1991. Chromosome abnormalities in peripheral blood cells of hepatitis B virus chronic carriers. Cancer Res. **51:** 6176–6179.
79. LIVEZEY, K.W. & D. SIMON. 1997. Accumulation of genetic alterations in a human hepatoma cell line transfected with hepatitis B virus. Mutat. Res. **377:** 187–198.
80. PINEAU, P., A. MARCHIO, M.G. MATTEI, *et al.* 1998. Extensive analysis of duplicated-inverted hepatitis B virus integrations in human hepatocellular carcinoma. J. Gen. Virol. **79:** 591–600.
81. LEVINE, A.J. 1997. p53, the cellular gatekeeper for growth and division. Cell **88:** 323–331.
82. TERAMOTO, T., K. SATONAKA, S. KITAZAWA, *et al.* 1994. p53 gene abnormalities are closely related to hepatoviral infections and occur at a late stage of hepatocarcinogenesis. Cancer Res. **54:** 231–235.
83. BRESSAC, B., M. KEW, J. WANDS, *et al.* 1991. Selective G to T mutations of p53 gene in hepatocellular carcinoma from southern Africa. Nature **350:** 429–431.
84. HSU, I.C., R.A. METCALF, T. SUN, *et al.* 1991. Mutational hotspot in the p53 gene in human hepatocellular carcinomas. Nature **350:** 427–428.
85. AGUILAR, F., S.P. HUSSAIN & P. CERUTTI. 1993. Aflatoxin B1 induces the transversion of G-->T in codon 249 of the p53 tumor suppressor gene in human hepatocytes. Proc. Natl. Acad. Sci. USA **90:** 8586–8590.
86. HSIA, C.C., A.M. DI BISCEGLIE, D.E. KLEINER, *et al.* 1994. RB tumor suppressor gene expression in hepatocellular carcinoma from patients infected with the hepatitis B virus. J. Med. Virol. **44:** 67–73.
87. KAWATE, S., S. TAKENOSHITA, S. OHWADA, *et al.* 1999. Mutation analysis of transforming growth factor beta type II receptor, Smad2, and Smad4 in hepatocellular carcinoma. Int. J. Oncol. **14:** 127–131.

88. YAKICIER, M.C., M.B. IRMAK, A. ROMANO, et al. 1999. Smad2 and Smad4 gene mutations in hepatocellular carcinoma. Oncogene **18:** 4879–4883.
89. HIGASHITSUJI, H., K. ITOH, T. NAGAO, et al. 2000. Reduced stability of retinoblastoma protein by gankyrin, an oncogenic ankyrin-repeat protein overexpressed in hepatomas. Nat. Med. **6:** 96–99.
90. DE SOUZA, A.T., G.R. HANKINS, M.K. WASHINGTON, et al. 1995. Frequent loss of heterozygosity on 6q at the mannose 6-phosphate/insulin-like growth factor II receptor locus in human hepatocellular tumors. Oncogene **10:** 1725–1729.
91. WADA, I., H. KANADA, K. NOMURA, et al. 1999. Failure to detect genetic alteration of the mannose-6-phosphate/insulin-like growth factor 2 receptor (M6P/IGF2R) gene in hepatocellular carcinomas in Japan. Hepatology **29:** 1718–1721.
92. NAKAMURA, T., F. HAMADA, T. ISHIDATE, et al. 1998. Axin, an inhibitor of the Wnt signalling pathway, interacts with beta-catenin, GSK-3beta and APC and reduces the beta-catenin level. Genes Cells **3:** 395–403.
93. ABERLE, H., H. SCHWARTZ & R. KEMLER. 1996. Cadherin-catenin complex: protein interactions and their implications for cadherin function. J. Cell. Biochem. **61:** 514–523.
94. CADIGAN, K.M. & R. NUSSE. 1997. Wnt signaling: a common theme in animal development. Genes Dev. **11:** 3286–3305.
95. POLAKIS, P. 1997. The adenomatous polyposis coli (APC) tumor suppressor. Biochim. Biophys. Acta **1332:** F127–147.
96. CLEVERS, H. & M. VAN DE WETERING. 1997. TCF/LEF factor earn their wings. Trends Genet. **13:** 485–489.
97. HE, T.C., A.B. SPARKS, C. RAGO, et al. 1998. Identification of c-MYC as a target of the APC pathway. Science **281:** 1509–1512.
98. TETSU, O. & F. MCCORMICK. 1999. Beta-catenin regulates expression of cyclin D1 in colon carcinoma cells. Nature **398:** 422–426.
99. POLAKIS, P. 1999. The oncogenic activation of beta-catenin. Curr. Opin. Genet. Dev. **9:** 15–21.
100. DE LA COSTE, A., B. ROMAGNOLO, P. BILLUART, et al. 1998. Somatic mutations of the beta-catenin gene are frequent in mouse and human hepatocellular carcinomas. Proc. Natl. Acad. Sci. USA **95:** 8847–8851.
101. MIYOSHI, Y., K. IWAO, G. NAWA, et al. 1998. Frequent mutations in the beta-catenin gene in desmoid tumors from patients without familial adenomatous polyposis. Oncol. Res. **10:** 591–594.
102. TERRIS, B., P. PINEAU, L. BREGEAUD, et al. 1999. Close correlation between beta-catenin gene alterations and nuclear accumulation of the protein in human hepatocellular carcinomas. Oncogene **18:** 6583–6588.
103. TRAN VAN NHIEU, J., C.A. RENARD, Y. WEI, et al. 1999. Nuclear accumulation of mutated beta-catenin in hepatocellular carcinoma is associated with increased cell proliferation. Am. J. Pathol. **155:** 703–710.
104. HUANG, H., H. FUJII, A. SANKILA, et al. 1999. Beta-catenin mutations are frequent in human hepatocellular carcinomas associated with hepatitis C virus infection. Am. J. Pathol. **155:** 1795–1801.
105. LEGOIX, P., O. BLUTEAU, J. BAYER, et al. 1999. Beta-catenin mutations in hepatocellular carcinoma correlate with a low rate of loss of heterozygosity. Oncogene **18:** 4044–4046.
106. HSU, H.C., Y.M. JENG, T.L. MAO, et al. 2000. Beta-catenin mutations are associated with a subset of low-stage hepatocellular carcinoma negative for hepatitis B virus and with favorable prognosis. Am. J. Pathol. **157:** 763–770.
107. DEVEREUX, T.R., C.H. ANNA, J.F. FOLEY, et al. 1999. Mutation of beta-catenin is an early event in chemically induced mouse hepatocellular carcinogenesis. Oncogene **18:** 4726–4733.
108. RENARD, C.A., G. FOUREL, M.P. BRALET, et al. 2000. Hepatocellular carcinoma in WHV/N-myc2 transgenic mice: oncogenic mutations of beta-catenin and synergistic effects of p53-null alleles. Oncogene **19:** 2678–2686.
109. MARCHIO, A., P. PINEAU, M. MEDDEB, et al. 2000. Distinct chromosomal abnormality pattern in primary liver cancer of non-B, non-C patients. Oncogene **19:** 3733–3738.

110. SHIROTA, Y., S. KANEKO, M. HONDA, *et al.* 2001. Identification of differentially expressed genes in hepatocellular carcinoma with cDNA microarrays. Hepatology **33:** 832–840.
111. HONDA, M., S. KANEKO, H. KAWAI, *et al.* 2001. Differential gene expression between chronic hepatitis B and C hepatic lesion. Gastroenterology **120:** 955–966.
112. OKABE, H., S. SATOH, T. KATO, *et al.* 2001. Genome-wide analysis of gene expression in human hepatocellular carcinomas using cDNA microarray: identification of genes involved in viral carcinogenesis and tumor progression. Cancer Res. **61:** 2129–2137.

Hepatocellular Carcinoma

Role of Estrogen Receptors in the Liver

ERICA VILLA, ANTONELLA GROTTOLA, ALESSANDRA COLANTONI, NICOLA DE MARIA, PAOLA BUTTAFOCO, ILVA FERRETTI, AND FEDERICO MANENTI

Department of Internal Medicine, Division of Gastroenterology, University of Modena and Reggio Emilia, 41100 Modena, Italy

ABSTRACT: Experimental and clinical evidence indicates that estrogens have a relevant role in the pathogenesis of cancer of hormone-sensitive organs. Estrogen receptors (ERs) are present in liver cells. Normal liver expresses almost exclusively wild-type ERs derived from the full-length transcript of the gene. During progression of liver disease to hepatocellular carcinoma, variant forms of ERs have been demonstrated that greatly influence the course of the disease and the possibility of palliative treatment. Peritumoral cirrhotic tissue of patients with hepatocellular carcinoma, especially males, expresses a variant form of ER (vER) with an exon 5 deletion. In hepatocellular carcinoma, vER largely predominates and sometimes becomes the only form expressed. That the occurrence of vER alone is limited almost exclusively to males suggests that it could be one of the molecular events that eventually lead to the preferential development of hepatocellular carcinoma in males. In addition, the presence of vER appears most frequently in patients infected with the hepatitis B virus. The growth rate of hepatocellular carcinoma in patients with vER is also significantly higher than that in patients with tumors expressing wtER.

KEYWORDS: hepatocellular carcinoma; estrogen receptors; hepatitis B

INTRODUCTION

Hepatocellular carcinoma (HCC) is a leading cause of death worldwide. Its incidence has increased in the last few years not only in the Eastern but also in the Western world.[1] Many different factors (hepatitis B virus, HBV; hepatitis C virus, HCV; aflatoxin; alcohol; and sex hormones) have been implicated in the pathogenesis of HCC, but no definite conclusion on the predominant mechanisms leading to its development has been reached. A common characteristic in the different geographic areas is the striking prevalence of HCC in males.[2,3] This observation led to investigations on the circulating levels of sex hormones and the pattern of their receptors in the liver in order to elucidate the relation between gender and prevalence of HCC. Both androgen and estrogen receptors were studied; however, the results of quanti-

---

Address for correspondence: Erica Villa, M.D., Department of Internal Medicine, Division of Gastroenterology, University of Modena and Reggio Emilia, Via del Pozzo 71, 41100 Modena, Italy. Voice: +39-59-4224 359; fax: +39-59-4224 363.
villa.erica@unimo.it

tative analysis are not conclusive.[4–9] Elements in human HCC, such as the association between HCC and cirrhosis, further complicate the study of hepatic carcinogenesis. The etiologic factors in cirrhosis and the pathologic processes involved in the cirrhotic transformation likely contribute in many different ways to the carcinogenic process. An approach as broad as possible can therefore be helpful even when investigating single pathways to HCC.

The role of estrogen receptors (ERs) in hepatic carcinogenesis is herein reviewed. In particular, the relation between ERs and the etiologic factors that likely contribute to differentiate human from experimental carcinogenesis is addressed

EPIDEMIOLOGY OF HEPATOCELLULAR CARCINOMA: LINK WITH VIRAL INFECTIONS

Among the factors implicated in human carcinogenesis, such as HBV, HCV, aflatoxin, alcohol, and sex hormones, none seems able to directly determine the development of HCC (except aflatoxin, which is implicated, however, in the pathogenesis of a small fraction of HCC in eastern countries).

Epidemiologic data from Asia and Africa have linked HBV infection to an increased risk of HCC. Both case-control[10–12] and cohort studies[13–15] have shown a substantial increase in the relative risk for HCC. The mechanism whereby HBV may cause HCC is not fully understood. Integration of HBV DNA into host genome may be an important step in the development of liver cancer. Some of the proteins encoded by HBV (namely, preS/S and HBx) may determine critical modifications of the biochemical pathways that permit extended survival, resistance to immune-mediated apoptosis, and perhaps growth advantage.[16]

Data on a direct oncogenic role for HCV are less consistent, although studies on an HCV transgenic mouse model have indicated a possible role for HCV core antigen in hepatic carcinogenesis.[17]

Overall, the most constant data in all series in the literature are the development of HCC in preexisting chronic liver disease (CLD), mostly cirrhosis, regardless of the etiology of CLD. Hepatocellular carcinoma may develop even in patients with CLD, such as primary biliary cirrhosis, which was thought not to be a risk factor for HCC. Therefore, chronic hepatocytic death and regeneration are factors that contribute to neoplastic modification of liver cells.

The second finding common to all reported series is the prevalence of HCC in men. Overall, the male/female ratio for HCC usually ranges between 3:1 and 5:1. The male/female ratio is further unbalanced whenever the prevalent etiologic factor for CLD and HCC is HBV infection. When this is the case, the male/female ratio increases to 8:1.[2,18] During the last two decades, the observation of the preferential occurrence of HCC in men has prompted investigation of the relation between sex hormones and HCC. Results of studies on circulating hormones remain controversial. The first studies failed to show a significant correlation with HCC development due in part to the presence of confounding factors such as HBV infection and cirrhosis, which per se determine sex hormone imbalance.[19–22] Recently, two studies from Korea and Japan suggested that elevated serum testosterone levels or an imbalanced testosterone/estradiol rate is associated with an increased risk of HCC.[23,24] Although the association was clear-cut, the mechanism by which elevated levels of testosterone determined an increased incidence of HCC were only suggested but not demonstrated.

EARLY STUDIES ON SEX STEROID RECEPTORS IN THE LIVER

The liver is a hormone-sensitive organ. Human liver from both male and female patients expresses ERs[4,5] as well as androgen receptors (ARs).[7–9] Experimental studies showed that sequential modifications in the pattern of circulating sex hormone levels and sex hormone receptors within the liver progressively occur during hepatocarcinogenesis. Some reports suggest that estrogens may promote carcinogenesis, whereas androgens may maintain the proliferation of liver tumors. Several antiestrogenic drugs were studied for the palliative treatment of unresectable HCC. Studies with antiandrogens produced negative results due to either a lack of activity or excessive toxicity.

Estrogen receptor concentration increases in males during the progression of CLD, especially when it is due to alcohol.[25] Variable results, depending also on the heterogeneity of the methods used to quantitate sex steroid hormone receptors, are reported when HCC develops.[6,7,24,26] Although ERs in HCC are evidently functional, their specific role in promoting or maintaining carcinogenesis is not clear. Data on ARs are not clear as well. In particular, tumor tissue seems to have slightly elevated AR levels compared with those of the surrounding tissue. Quantitative studies on ERs and ARs suggested involvement of sex steroids in HCC, but the mechanisms were not clear. It should be remembered, however, that the inconsistencies found in different studies may reflect the technical difficulty of the binding assays in human liver, particularly for elevated levels of endogenous proteases that need to be inactivated in order to have a reliable assay.[5] An additional indication that a simple increase in ER or AR levels may not be sufficient to determine relevant biological consequences comes from the recognition of the substantial inefficacy of palliative treatment of HCC with antiestrogenic drugs.[27–31]

ESTROGEN RECEPTORS AND THE DEVELOPMENT OF HEPATOCELLULAR CARCINOMA

Although the liver is not a classical target for sex hormones, evidence apart from the presence of their receptors indicates that it responds to them by increasing or decreasing protein synthesis and modulating cell growth.[26]

In breast cancer, which often depends on estrogen for growth, the progression from hormone dependence to hormone independence and the contemporary development of a more aggressive phenotype are associated with the onset of a variant form of ER.[32–34] Among these variant forms of ER is a variant derived by an exon 5-deleted transcript that lacks the hormone-binding domain of the receptor but maintains constitutive transcriptional activity, being intact in the DNA-binding domain (FIG. 1).[35] Normal liver expresses almost exclusively the wild-type ER, derived from the full-length transcript. Only occasionally the variant form is present as a minor component. Once HCC has developed, the difference between tumor tissue and the surrounding hepatic parenchyma emerges. In particular, in nontumor tissue the 438-

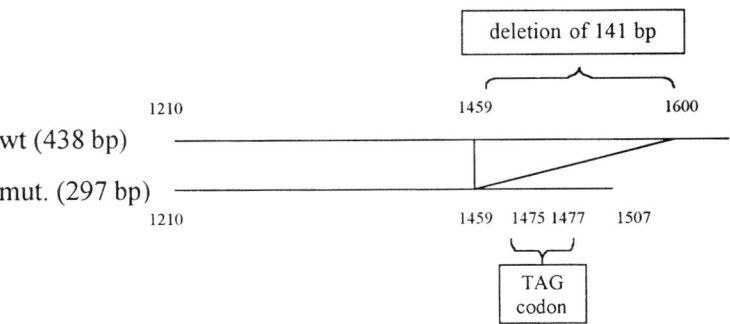

FIGURE 1. Schematic representation of wild-type and variant estrogen receptor transcript and resulting translated protein in the liver. *Underlined sequence* represents the part of the protein diverging from wt ER protein. *Asterisk* represents the newly created stop codon.

base pair band is still the predominant form of ER, whereas the variant form has about half the level of expression of the wild-type form. In tumor tissue, the variant form is largely predominant especially in males, and sometimes it becomes the only form expressed.[36] The presence of wild-type ER (wtER) positively relates with measured levels of ER by ligand binding assay in both normal liver and cirrhotic, nontumoral tissue (ER levels range between 13 ± 4 fmol/mg cytosol protein in normal male liver, 15 ± 5 fmol/mg cytosol protein in nontumor liver tissue from male patients with HCC, and 18 ± 4 fmol/mg cytosol protein in tumor tissue from female patients with HCC). No specific binding is usually obtained from HCC samples when the variant ER form (vER) predominates, as these receptors do not bind the hormone.

The greatly increased expression of the vER transcript in peritumoral cirrhotic tissue of patients with HCC, especially males, compared with normal liver tissue suggests that a gradual transformation may take place during the progression of the cirrhotic process. The marked difference between males and females, the occurrence

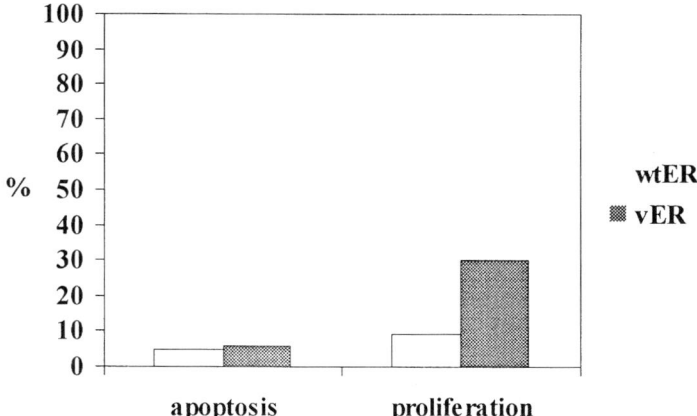

FIGURE 2. Proliferation and apoptosis in human hepatocellular carcinoma, classified according to the presence of the type of estrogen receptor (ER). Proliferation was assessed by immunohistochemical detection of Ki67, whereas apoptosis was assessed by the presence of DNA fragmentation (FragEl). Results are expressed as a percentage of positive cells per total cells counted in five adjacent fields at 25× magnification. $N = 15$ in each group. Estrogen receptor transcripts were measured by RT-PCR. vER, variant estrogen receptor; wtER, wild-type estrogen receptor.

of the variant transcript alone being limited almost exclusively to males, suggests that this could be one of the molecular events that could eventually lead to the preferential development of HCC in males.

The expression of vER occurs in all chronic liver diseases independent of their etiology, but it is significantly more frequent in chronic HBV infection. This is most evident in patients with chronic active hepatitis and HCC, whereas in cirrhosis the vER is expressed more frequently in HBV-positive than in HCV-positive patients, but not to a statistically significant level.[37] We have shown that vER clusters preferentially in HBsAg-positive patients. The ability of HBV, as a DNA virus, to integrate into host genome and therefore to interfere with gene transcription may constitute one factor influencing the formation of ER variants. In a large series of patients with HCC in whom we analyzed the DD5 variant, we recently confirmed that a high percentage of HBsAg-positive patients bear vER, whereas anti-HCV–positive patients more often have the wild type. This difference is statistically significant ($p <0.04$). The result suggests that vER may be one factor contributing to the rapid course of HCC in HBsAg-positive patients than in anti-HCV–positive ones.[39]

The growth rate of HCC in patients with vER is also significantly higher than that of tumors expressing wtER, as determined *in vivo* by magnetic resonance.[38] Further support of a higher proliferation rate in tumors with variant ERs comes from an evaluation of the proliferation in tumor tissue by immunohistochemistry. The percentage of proliferating cells is significantly higher in HCC with vER than in those characterized by wtERs. Interestingly, apoptosis is not significantly different in the two types of tumor (A. Colantoni and E. Villa, in preparation) (FIG. 2).

NATURAL HISTORY OF HEPATOCELLULAR CARCINOMA IN RELATION TO ESTROGEN RECEPTOR STATUS IN THE LIVER AND THERAPEUTIC OPTIONS

Stratification of patients with HCC by hepatic ER transcript status shows that spontaneous survival in patients expressing the wtER is exceedingly better than that of patients with HCC characterized by vER, even patients with inoperable disease at presentation. The median survival of patients with wild-type ERs is approximately 36 months compared with 13 months in patients with vER. Spontaneous survival in these two groups of patients is remarkably different ($p = 0.0000$).[39] The influence of variant ERs on survival is also evident when the population under study is stratified by viral etiology. Anti-HCV–positive subjects with wtERs have a surprisingly long survival, whereas survival is significantly shorter when the variant form of ER is present. Interestingly, the difference in survival between wtER-positive and vER-positive HCC patients does not reach statistical significance among HBsAg-positive patients. This is likely attributable to an elevated mortality rate in HBsAg-positive subjects with wtERs; HBV is a significant independent variable in the stepwise discriminant analysis to identify factors affecting the onset of HCC and survival.[2,14] HBV infection *per se*, therefore, can determine short-term survival in HCC patients, but the contemporary presence of HBV infection and vERs identifies the subgroup of patients with the worst prognosis (median survival, 8 months). It is noteworthy that vERs have been associated significantly more often with HBV infection than with HCV infection.[37] A possible explanation for this association could reside in the preferential mechanism of altered splicing, which is believed to be the preferential cause of vERs,[40] possibly facilitated by the integration of HBV sequences in the host DNA.

The importance of identifying factors involved in the development of HCC expressing variant ER resides in the finding that, apart from having a tumultuous clinical course, these cancers are not sensitive to palliative treatment with tamoxifen. The variant receptor does not bind the hormone as well as the antihormones with the same sterical structure of estradiol, such as tamoxifen,. This has suggested an alternative approach using a progestin drug in an attempt to slow down tumor growth. Megestrol has significantly improved survival in these patients at 1 year; unfortunately, the effect was short-lived.[41]

FUTURE DEVELOPMENTS

The role of estrogen receptors and their variant forms should be investigated in an *in vitro* system in an attempt to elucidate whether they can actually act as potent inducers of proliferation, as suggested by *in vivo* data. Furthermore, it is extremely relevant to understand the factors that could trigger modifications of the estrogen-dependent pathways. Diet is certainly among these factors; food contains many substances that are structurally similar to estradiol and have an estrogenic effect, such as the fito-estrogens. Their role in development of HCC has not been investigated yet, but it is likely that these substances may play a role in HCC as they do in other tumors, such as breast and prostate cancer. Preliminary data from a case-control study of patients with cirrhosis and HCC matched with nonhepatic chronic disease or tumors, have shown that patients with HCC ingest significantly less fito-estrogens (namely, genistein) than do cirrhotic patients without tumor or matched controls (E. Villa, personal communication).

ACKNOWLEDGMENTS

The experimental work was supported by Grant "40% Cofin 2000" of the Ministry of University and of Scientific and Technological Research (MURST), Progetti di ricerca con ricaduta assistenziale Azienda Policlinico di Modena, and Associazione Italiana per la Ricerca sul Cancro (AIRC).

REFERENCES

1. EL-SERAG, H.B. & A.C. MASON. 1999. Rising incidence of hepatocellular carcinoma in the United States. N. Engl. J. Med. **340:** 745–750.
2. VILLA, E., G.M. BALDINI, C. PASQUINELLI, et al. 1988. Risk factors for hepatocellular carcinoma in Italy. Male sex, hepatitis B virus, non-A, non-B infection, alcohol. Cancer **62:** 611–615.
3. INTERNATIONAL AGENCY FOR RESEARCH ON CANCER. 1997. Cancer Incidence in Five Continents. Vol. VII. IARC. Lyon.
4. PORTER, L.E., M.S ELM, D.H. VAN THIEL, et al. 1983. Characterization and quantitation of human hepatic estrogen receptors. Gastroenterology **84:** 704–712.
5. ROSSINI, G.P., G.M. BALDINI, E. VILLA et al. 1989. Characterization of estrogen receptors from human liver. Gastroenterology **96:** 1102–1109.
6. NAGASUE, N., A. ITO, H. YUKAYA, et al. 1986. Estrogen receptors in hepatocellular carcinoma. Cancer **57:** 87–91.
7. OHNISHI, S., T. MURAKAMI, T. MORIYAMA, et al. 1986. Androgen and estrogen receptors in hepatocellular carcinoma and in the surrounding non-cancerous liver tissue. Hepatology **6:** 440–443.
8. NAGASUE, N., A. ITO, H. YUKAYA, et al. 1985. Androgen receptors in hepatocellular carcinoma and surrounding parenchyma. Gastroenterology **89:** 643–647.
9. WILKINSON, M.L., M.J. IQBAL & R. WILLIAMS. 1985. Characterisation of high affinity binding sites of androgens in primary hepatocellular carcinoma Clin. Chim. Acta **152:** 105–113.
10. TSUKUMA, H., T. HIYAMA, A. OSHIMA, et al. 1990. A case-control study of hepatocellular carcinoma in Osaka, Japan. Int. J. Cancer **45:** 231–236.
11. AUSTIN, H., E. DELZELL, S. GRUFFERMAN, et al. 1986. A case-control study of hepatocellular carcinoma and the hepatitis B virus, cigarette smoking, and alcohol consumption. Cancer Res. **46:** 962–966.
12. ZHANG, J.Y., M. DAI, X. WANG, et al. 1998. A case-control study of hepatitis B and C virus infection as risk factors for hepatocellular carcinoma in Henan, China. Int. J. Epidemiol. **27:** 574–578.
13. OBATA, H., N. HATASHI, Y. MOTOIKE, et al. 1980. A prospective study on the development of hepatocellular carcinoma from liver cirrhosis with persistent hepatitis B virus infection. Int. J. Cancer **24:** 741–747.
14. ZAMAN, S.N., W.M. MELIA, R.D. JOHNSON, et al. 1985. Risk factors in development of hepatocellular carcinoma in cirrhosis: prospective study of 613 patients. Lancet **1:** 1357–1360.
15. BEASLEY, R.P., L.Y. HWANG, C.C. LIN, et al. 1982. Hepatocellular carcinoma and hepatitis B virus. Lancet **2:** 1129–1132.
16. FEITELSON, M.A. 1999. Hepatitis B virus in hepatocarcinogenesis. J. Cell. Physiol. **181:** 188–201.
17. RAY, R.B., K. MEYER & R. RAY. 2000. Hepatitis C virus core protein promotes immortalization of primary human hepatocytes. Virology **271:** 197–204.

18. LEROSE, R., R. MOLINARI, E. ROCCHI, et al. 2000. Prognostic features and survival of hepatocellular carcinoma in Italy: impact of stage of disease. Eur. J. Cancer **37:** 239–245.
19. YU, M.W. & C.J. CHEN. 1993. Elevated serum testosterone levels and risk of hepatocellular carcinoma. Cancer Res. **53:** 790–794.
20. YUAN, J.M., R.K ROSS, F.Z. STANCZYK, et al. 1995. A cohort study of serum testosterone and hepatocellular carcinoma in Shanghai, China. Int. J. Cancer **63:** 441–493.
21. GANNE-CARRIE, N., C. CHASTANG, B. UZZAN, et al. 1997. Predictive value of serum sex hormone binding globulin for the occurrence of hepatocellular carcinoma in male patients with cirrhosis. J. Hepatol. **26:** 96–102.
22. NAGASUE, N., Y. OGAWA, H. YAKAYA, et al. 1985. Serum levels of estrogen and testosterone in cirrhotic men with and without hepatocellular carcinoma. Gastroenterology **88:** 768–777.
23. YU, M.W., S.W. CHENG, M.W. LIN, et al. 2000. Androgen-receptor gene CAG repeats, plasma testosterone levels, and risk of hepatitis B-related hepatocellular carcinoma. J. Natl. Cancer Inst. **92:** 2023–2928.
24. TANAKA, K., H. SAKAI, M. HASHIZUME, et al. 2000. Serum testosterone:estradiol ratio and the development of hepatocellular carcinoma among male cirrhotic patients. Cancer Res. **60:** 5106–5110.
25. VILLA, E., G.M. BALDINI, G.P. ROSSINI, et al. 1989. Ethanol-induced increase in cytosolic estrogen receptors in human male liver: a possible explanation for biochemical feminization in chronic liver disease due to alcohol. Hepatology **8:** 1610–1614.
26. EAGON, P.K., A. FRANCAVILLA, A. DILEO, et al. 1991. Quantitation of estrogen and androgen receptors in hepatocellular carcinoma and adjacent normal human liver. Digest. Dis. Sci. **36:** 1303–1308.
27. CASTELLS, A., J. BRUIX, C. BRU, et al. 1995. Treatment of hepatocellular carcinoma with tamoxifen: a double-blind trial in 120 patients. Gastroenterology **109:** 917–922.
28. GALLO, C. & CLIP STUDY GROUP. 1998. Tamoxifen in the treatment of hepatocellular carcinoma: a randomised controlled trial. Lancet **352:** 17–19.
29. RAVOET, C., H. BLEIBERG & B. GERARD. 1993. Non-surgical treatment of hepatocarcinoma. J. Surg. Oncol. **3:** 104–111.
30. GRIMALDI, C., H. BLEIBERG, F. GAY, et al. 1998. Evaluation of antiandrogen therapy in unresectable hepatocellular carcinoma: results of a European organization for research and treatment of cancer: multicentric double-blind trial. J. Clin. Oncol. **16:** 411–417.
31. MANESIS, E.K., G. GIANNOULIS, P. ZOUMBOULIS, et al. 1995. Treatment of hepatocellular carcinoma with combined suppression and inhibition of sex hormones: a randomized, controlled trial. Hepatology **21:** 1535–1542.
32. RAAM, S., N. ROBERT, C.A PAPPAS, et al. 1988. Defective estrogen receptors in human mammary cancers: their significance in defining hormone dependence. J. Natl. Cancer Inst. **80:** 756–761.
33. GRAHAM, M.L., II, N.L. KRETT, L.A MILLER, et al. 1990. T4DCO cells, genetically unstable and containing estrogen receptors mutations, are a model for the progression of breast cancers to hormone resistance. Cancer Res. **50:** 6208–6217.
34. MCGUIRE, W.L., G.C. CHAMNESS, S.A FUQUA, et al. 1991. Estrogen receptors variants on clinical breast cancer. Mol. Endocrinol. **5:** 1571–1577.
35. FUQUA, S.A.W., S.D. FITZGERALD, D.C ALRED, et al. 1992. Inhibition of estrogen receptors action by naturally occurring variant in human breast tumors. Cancer Res. **52:** 483–486.
36. VILLA, E., L. CAMELLINI, A. DUGANI, et al. 1995. Variant estrogen receptors mRNA species detected in human primary hepatocellular carcinoma. Cancer Res. **55:** 498–500.
37. VILLA, E., A. DUGANI, A. MOLES, et al. 1998. Variant liver estrogen receptor transcripts already occur at an early stage of chronic liver disease. Hepatology **27:** 983–988.
38. VILLA, E., L. CAMELLINI, E. FANTONI, et al. 1996. Type of estrogen receptor determines response to antiestrogen therapy in hepatocellular carcinoma. Cancer Res. **56:** 3883–3885.

39. VILLA, E., I. FERRETTI, P. BUTTAFOCO, et al. 2000. Natural history of inoperable hepatocellular carcinoma: estrogen receptor status in the tumor is the strongest prognostic factor for survival. Hepatology **32:** 233–238.
40. ZHANG, Q.X., S.G. HILSENBECK, S.A.W. FUQUA, et al. 1996. Multiple splicing variants of the estrogen receptor are present in individual human breast tumors. J. Steroid Biochem. Mol. Biol. **59:** 251–260.
41. VILLA, E., I. FERRETTI, A. GROTTOLA, et al. 2001. Hormonal therapy with megestrol in inoperable hepatocellular carcinoma characterised by variant estrogen receptors: a prospective, randomised, controlled trial. Br. J. Cancer **84:** 881–885.

Circulating IL-6 and sIL-6R in Patients with Hepatocellular Carcinoma

L. GIANNITRAPANI,[a] M. CERVELLO,[b] M. SORESI,[a] M. NOTARBARTOLO,[c]
M. LA ROSA,[b] L. VIRRUSO,[b] N. D'ALESSANDRO,[c] AND G. MONTALTO[a]

[a]*Istituto di Medicina Interna e Geriatria, Università di Palermo, Palermo, Italy*
[b]*Istituto di Biologia dello Sviluppo, C.N.R., Palermo, Italy*
[c]*Dipartimento di Scienze Farmacologiche, Università di Palermo, Palermo, Italy*

> ABSTRACT: Interleukin-6 plays a central role in regulating the immune system, hematopoiesis, and acute phase reaction. It interacts with a receptor complex consisting of a specific ligand-binding protein (IL-6R, gp80) and a signal transduction protein (gp130). In this report, serum levels of IL-6 and a soluble form of the interleukin-6 receptor (sIL-6R) were evaluated in patients with hepatocellular carcinoma. The correlation between IL-6 and sIL-6R values, the stage of hepatocellular carcinoma, and main liver function tests was also studied.
>
> KEYWORDS: hepatocellular carcinoma; interleukin-6; signal transduction protein; gp130; liver function tests; receptor

INTRODUCTION

Interleukin-6 (IL-6) is a multifunctional cytokine that plays a central role in the regulation of the immune system, hematopoiesis, and acute phase reaction.[1] It mediates its diverse biological effects by interacting with a receptor complex consisting of a specific ligand-binding protein (IL-6R, gp80) and a signal transduction protein (gp130).[1] A key feature in our understanding of the regulation of IL-6 responses has been the identification of a soluble form of the interleukin-6 receptor (sIL-6R).[2] When the IL-6/sIL-6R complex associates with the membrane-bound signal-transducing chain, it can induce the signal transduction cascade, acting as an agonist and stimulating a variety of cellular responses including proliferation, differentiation, and activation of inflammatory processes. The mechanism of production of the soluble form of IL-6R is believed to involve either proteolytic cleavage of the cell surface receptor (shedding) or differential splicing of IL-6R mRNA. Elevated IL-6 and sIL-6R levels have been documented in numerous clinical conditions. In particular, elevation of circulating levels of IL-6 in various neoplastic diseases (such as multiple myeloma, ovarian and prostate cancers, and lung, renal cell, stomach, and colorectal carcinomas) has been described.[3–9] Elevated sIL-6R levels have also been observed in different pathologic conditions, thus indicating that this production is coordinated

---

Address for correspondence: Dr. G. Montalto, Istituto di Medicina Interna e Geriatria, Università di Palermo, Palermo, Italy. Voice: 091-655-2991; fax: 091-655-2936.
gmontal@unipa.it

as part of a response to disease.[10] In fact, sIL-6R may have the potential to regulate both local and systemic IL-6–mediated events.

Previous studies have concentrated only on the behavior of IL-6 circulating levels in various liver diseases.[11–14] In this report we evaluated serum levels of IL-6 and sIL-6R in patients with hepatocellular carcinoma (HCC). We also studied the correlation between IL-6 and sIL-6R values, the stage of HCC, and main liver function tests (LFTs).

MATERIAL AND METHODS

Patients

One hundred fifteen subjects were included in this study and divided into two groups. Group 1 included 87 patients (60 male and 27 female, mean age 62.2 ± 9.0 years) with HCC. Diagnosis was based on biopsy or cytologic findings in 41 cases. In the other cases, there were unequivocal clinical and serologic data with at least two concordant examinations including ultrasound or CT scan and alpha-fetoprotein (AFP) assay. Most of the patients with HCC had liver cirrhosis and were being followed up at our outpatients clinic for chronic liver disease, whereas others had been referred to our center already diagnosed with HCC. The disease was associated with serum hepatitis C virus (HCV) antibodies in all cases.

Patients were divided into three stages according to Okuda's classification.[15] In brief, stage I is an initial stage in which the neoplasia (or the sum of nodules, if present) measures less than 50% of the whole liver section on CT scan, there is no ascites, albumin levels are over 3 g/dl, and bilirubin levels are below 3 mg/dl; stage II is moderately advanced, with two or more indices of advanced disease; stage III is very advanced, with three or all indices of advanced disease.

The control group was composed of 28 healthy asymptomatic subjects (19 male, and 9 female, mean age 55.4 ± 2 years) recruited from donors at the blood bank of our hospital. Liver disease was excluded on the basis of anamnestic, biochemical, and instrumental data. There were no cases of neoplastic disease, evaluated by a follow-up of at least six months. In none of the two groups was daily alcohol consumption greater than 30 g/day.

Serum Sampling and Determination of Interleukin-6 (IL-6) and sIL-6R Concentrations

Blood samples were taken after overnight fasting. After centrifugation, part of the serum sample was used to assay the main parameters of liver function by routine methods; the remainder was frozen at –40°C for IL-6 and sIL-6R measurements. Serologic testing for anti-HCV was performed using commercial third-generation enzyme-linked immunosorbent assay (ELISA, Orthodiagnostic System, Raritan, NJ, USA), in accordance with the manufacturer's instructions. The positivity of anti-HCV–reacting samples was confirmed using a third generation anti-HCV recombinant immunoblot assay (RIBA III, Chiron Corporation, Emeryville, CA, USA). Markers of HBV were tested using the Abbott radioimmunoassay kit.

TABLE 1. Median and range of serum values of interleukin-6 (IL-6, pg/ml), sIL-6R (ng/ml), and sIL-6R/IL-6 ratio (both expressed in pg/ml) in patients with hepatocellular carcinoma and a control group

	Hepatocellular carcinoma ($n = 87$) median (min-max)	Controls ($n = 28$) median (min-max)
IL-6	14^a (3-301)	3^a (3-17)
sIL-6R	42.4 (17.6-80)	36.4 (7.2-58)
sIL-6R/IL-6	$3,000^b$ (5,980-31,333)	$10,866^b$ (2,400-19,066)

[a] $z = 5.92$; $p < 0.0001$.
[b] $z = 2.35$; $p < 0.0001$.

Serum concentrations of IL-6 and sIL-6R were determined using a commercially available ELISA kit (Quantikine, human IL-6 and sIL-6R, R&D Systems, Minneapolis, MN, USA) in accordance with the manufacturer's instructions.

Statistical Analysis

Data were expressed as mean, standard deviation, median, and range (min-max). Groups were compared using the Mann-Whitney U test. Chi-square test was used for frequency analyses. Simple linear regression and Spearman's rank correlation test were used where appropriate. The cut-off values for IL-6 and sIL-6R were established as the highest value found in the control subjects. Results were considered significant if $p < 0.05$.

RESULTS

TABLE 1 shows the median, range, and ratio of serum IL-6 and sIL-6R values in the two study groups. In the HCC group, the median of IL-6 levels was significantly higher than that in the control group ($p < 0.0001$). No significant difference in sIL-6R levels was found between the two groups. As for the sIL-6R/IL-6 ratio, the value for HCC was significantly lower than that in the controls ($p < 0.0001$).

TABLE 2 shows the median and range of serum IL-6 and sIL-6R levels and the sIL-6R/IL-6 ratio in the group of HCC patients divided according to Okuda's classification and compared with controls. Values of IL-6 in stage III patients were significantly higher than those in stage I and II patients. By contrast, the sIL-6R/IL-6 ratio in the HCC patients divided according to stage was significantly lower in all stages than in the controls.

Spearman's rank correlation test showed a significant increase in both IL-6 and sIL-6R levels from stage I to stage III ($r = 0.27$, $p < 0.02$; $r = 0.38$, $p < 0.0005$, respectively) and a negative, but not significant, correlation for the sIL-6R/IL-6 ratio ($r = -0.17$, $p = $ n.s.).

TABLE 2. Median and range of serum values of interleukin-6 (IL-6, pg/ml), sIL-6R (ng/ml), and sIL-6R/IL-6 ratio (both expressed in pg/ml) in patients with hepatocellular carcinoma divided according to stage of disease

	Stage I ($n = 22$) median (min-max) (a)	Stage II ($n = 45$) median (min-max) (b)	Stage III ($n = 18$) median (min-max) (c)	Controls ($n = 28$) median (min-max) (d)	z	p
IL-6	5.5 (3–270)	12 (3–301)	32 (3–110)	3 (3–17)	a-d:3.9 b-d:5.2 c-d:5.3 a-c:2.3 b-c:2.7	0.0001 0.0001 0.0001 0.03 0.01
sIL-6R	34 (17.6–64)	39.6 (18–80)	56 (30–80)	36.4 (7.2–58)	c-d:3.5 a-c:3.1 b-c:2.8	0.0004 0.002 0.005
sIL-6R/IL-6	4,840 (115.5–21,333)	4,033 (59.8–2,933)	1,860 (384.6–10,666)	10,866 (2,400–19,006)	a-d:2.9 b-d:4.3 c-d:4.9	0.004 0.0001 0.0001

TABLE 3. Number of patients with hepatocellular carcinoma with serum levels of interleukin-6 (IL-6), sIL-6R, and AFP above the cut-off values

	Hepatocellular carcinoma ($n = 87$)
IL-6 (cut-off = 17 pg/ml)	43 (49%)
sIL-6R (cut-off = 58 ng/ml)	21 (24%)
AFP (cut-off = 166 IU/l)	28/71 (40%)

TABLE 4. Correlation between individual values of interleukin-6 (IL-6), sIL-6R, and sIL-6R/IL-6 ratio in patients with hepatocellular carcinoma with the main parameters of liver function and AFP

	IL-6 r	sIL-6R r	sIL-6R/IL-6 r
Albumin	−0.18	−0.09	0.38[b]
GOT	−0.157	0.32[a]	0.17
GPT	−0.132	0.15	0.13
Bilirubin	−0.02	0.21	0.17
Prothrombin	0.12	0.02	0.10
Alpha-fetoprotein	0.037	0.33[c]	0.11

[a] $p < 0.01$; [b] $p < 0.005$; [c] $p < 0.004$.

Analysis of TABLE 3 shows that 49% of patients with HCC had higher IL-6 values than the cut-off value, whereas only 40% of these patients had alpha-fetoprotein values above the cut-off level.

TABLE 4 shows the correlations between individual serum values of IL-6, sIL-6R, and the sIL-6R/IL-6 ratio and the main parameters of liver function in patients with HCC. No significant correlation was noted between IL-6 and liver function parameters, whereas sIL-6R significantly correlated with glutamic oxalacetic transaminase (GOT, $p < 0.01$) and AFP ($p < 0.005$). By contrast, the sIL-6R/IL-6 ratio was significantly correlated only with serum albumin values ($p < 0.004$).

DISCUSSION

Elevated levels of both IL-6 and sIL-6R proteins have been detected in the blood stream and in other biological fluids, such as ascites and urine, of patients with different neoplastic diseases.[16,17] Higher levels of IL-6 and/or sIL-6R have generally been reported to correlate with a more advanced stage of disease and a worse outcome.[3–5,7] In liver diseases, previous studies have reported that circulating IL-6 levels are elevated in patients with chronic hepatitis,[12] alcoholic liver diseases,[13] and liver cirrhosis.[14] In patients with HCC, higher levels of IL-6 have been correlated with tumor mass and cancer invasiveness.[11,18] Currently, no data on the behavior of circulating sIL-6R levels in subjects with HCC are available. The aim of our study was to evaluate serum IL-6 and sIL-6R levels in a group of patients with HCC associated with liver cirrhosis. Moreover, we correlated IL-6 and sIL-6R values with stage of HCC and main liver function tests. Only HCC patients with HCV infection were selected to exclude the possible interference of different etiologic factors in the production of the cytokine.

Interleukin-6 levels in our group of patients with liver cirrhosis-associated HCC were higher than those in controls, perhaps indicating an increase in the production of this cytokine by tumor cells. This finding is supported by the higher values we found in Okuda's stage III, in which the neoplastic mass is more extensive than that in stages I and II.

No significant differences in values of the soluble receptor were noted between control subjects and patients with HCC, but when the HCC group was divided according to Okuda's classification, stage III patients had significantly higher levels. This may indicate an increase in sIL-6R release only in advanced HCC.

Results in TABLE 3 suggest that an IL-6 assay could be more efficacious than AFP in detecting patients with HCC. It would therefore be interesting to evaluate the behavior of IL-6 levels in a population of cirrhosis subjects, using the same cut-off value established for HCC patients, in order to evaluate the degree of sensitivity of the assay. However, if these results are confirmed in a larger patient population, they would be of considerable importance because currently it is quite rare to find elevated AFP levels in HCV-associated HCC subjects, especially in the initial phases of the disease.

No correlation was found with liver synthesis indices (albumin and prothrombin activity). Data on other types of tumors have, instead, reported an inverse correlation with albumin.[3]

Among the indices of cytolysis, only GOT correlated positively with sIL-6R levels. However, in the literature, data referring to chronic hepatitis subjects reported a positive correlation between GOT and IL-6 values.[12] This result could depend on the fact that in liver tumors associated with cirrhosis the inflammatory phenomena may disappear or the functioning liver mass may be reduced and therefore cytolysis be decreased. We might also suggest, however, that the increases in levels of IL-6 and sIL-6R are the result not only of the active phase of the disease, and thus of an increased production, but also of insufficient clearance from the circulation due to liver failure.

Interestingly, sIL-6R levels were higher only in patients with a more advanced stage of disease, so that when we analyzed their correlations with AFP levels, we found a positive correlation. Finally, correlations between sIL-6R and AFP and liver function tests suggest a relation between the soluble IL-6 receptor and the neoplastic mass or the residual functioning tissue.

ACKNOWLEDGMENT

This study was supported in part by Progetto Finalizzato Assessorato Sanità-Regione Siciliana and MURST 40% (to G.M.).

REFERENCES

1. HIRANO, T. 1998. Interleukin 6 and its receptor: ten years later. Int. Rev. Immunol. **16:** 249–284.
2. ROSE-JOHN, S. & P.C. HEINRICH. 1994. Soluble receptors for cytokines and growth factors: generation and biological function. Biochem. J. **300:** 281–290.
3. WIERZBOWSKA, A., H. URBANSKA-RYS & T. ROBAK. 1999. Circulating IL-6 cytokines and sIL-6R in patients with multiple myeloma. Br. J. Haematol. **105:** 412–419.
4. BEREK, J.S., C. CHUNG, K. KALDI, et al. 1991. Serum Interleukin 6 levels correlate with disease status in patients with epithelial ovarian cancer. Am. J. Obstet. Gynecol. **164:** 1038–1043.
5. NAKASHIMA, J., M. TACHIBANA, Y. HORIGUCHI, et al. 2000. Serum interleukin 6 as a prognostic factor in patients with prostatic cancer. Clin. Cancer Res. **6:** 2702–2706.
6. YANAGAWA, H., S. SONE, Y. TAKAHASHI, et al. 1995. Serum levels of interleukin 6 in patients with lung cancer. Br. J. Cancer **71:** 1095–1098.
7. TSUKAMOTO, T., Y. KUMANOTO, N. MIYAO, et al. 1992. Interleukin 6 in renal cell carcinoma. J. Urol. **148:** 1778–1782.
8. WU, C.W., S.R. WANG, M.F. CHAO, et al. 1996. Serum interleukin 6 levels reflect disease status of gastric cancer. Am. J. Gastroenterol. **91:** 1417–1422.
9. KINOSHITA, T., H. ITO & C. MIKI. 1999. Serum interleukin 6 level reflects the tumor proliferative activity in patients with colorectal carcinoma. Cancer **85:** 2526–2531.
10. JONES, S.A., S. HORIUCHI, N. TOPLEY, et al. 2001. The soluble interleukin 6 receptor: mechanisms of production and implications in disease. FASEB J. **15:** 43–58.
11. GOYDOS, J.S., A.M. BRUMFIELD, E. FREZZA, et al. 1998. Marked elevation of serum interleukin 6 in patients with cholangiocarcinoma. Ann. Surg. **227:** 398–404.
12. MALAGUARNERA, M., I. DI FAZIO, M.A. ROMEO, et al. 1997. Elevation of interleukin 6 levels in patients with chronic hepatitis due to hepatitis C virus. J. Gastroenterol. **32:** 211–215.
13. DIVIERE, J., J. CONTENT & C. DENYS. 1989. High interleukin 6 serum levels and increased production by leukocytes in alcoholic liver cirrhosis: correlation with IgA serum levels and lymphokine production. Clin. Exp. Immunol. **77:** 221–225.
14. GENESCA, J., A. GONZALES, R. SEGURA, et al. 1999. Interleukin 6, nitric oxide and the clinical and hemodynamic alterations of patients with liver cirrhosis. Am. J. Gastroenterol. **94:** 169–177.
15. OKUDA, K., T. OHTSUKI, H. OBATA, et al. 1985. Natural history of hepatocellular carcinoma and prognosis in relation to treatment. Cancer **56:** 918–928.
16. PLANTE, M., S.C. RUBIN, G.Y. WONG, et al. 1994. Interleukin 6 level in serum and ascites as a prognostic factor in patients with epithelial ovarian cancer. Cancer Res. **73:** 1882–1888.
17. SEGUCHI, T., K. YOKOKAWA, H. SUGAO, et al. 1992. Interleukin 6 activity in urine and serum in patients with bladder carcinoma. J. Urol. **148:** 791–794.
18. MALAGUARNERA, M., I. DI FAZIO, A. TAURINI, et al. 1996. Role of interleukin 6 in hepatocellular carcinoma. Bull. Cancer **83:** 379–384.

Expression of HIP/PAP mRNA in Human Hepatoma Cell Lines

M. CERVELLO,[a] L. GIANNITRAPANI,[b] M. LA ROSA,[a] M. NOTARBARTOLO,[c] N. D'ALESSANDRO,[c] L. VIRRUSO,[a] J.L. IOVANNA,[d] AND G. MONTALTO[b]

[a]*Istituto di Biologia dello Sviluppo, C.N.R., Palermo, Italy*

[b]*Istituto di Medicina Interna e Geriatria, Università di Palermo, Palermo, Italy*

[c]*Dipartimento di Scienze Farmacologiche, Università di Palermo, Palermo, Italy*

[d]*Unité 315, INSERM, Marseille, France*

ABSTRACT: The present study attempts to shed more light on the role of hepatocarcinoma-intestine-pancreas/pancreatic associated protein (HIP/PAP) in hepatoma cells. We initially examined, by reverse transcription-polymerase chain reaction (RT-PCR), the HIP/PAP transcripts present in human hepatoma cell lines of different origins and with different grades of differentiation and genetic profiles. We also used DNA sequencing analysis to investigate the structure of the HIP/PAP gene. Further investigation is necessary to define the role of HIP/PAP during the development of human hepatocellular carcinoma and to ascertain whether the use of different transcripts is helpful in regulating HIP/PAP expression in transformed liver cells.

KEYWORDS: hepatoma; carcinoma; HIP/PAP; pancreatitis; protein

INTRODUCTION

Hepatocarcinoma-intestine-pancreas/pancreatic associated protein (HIP/PAP), a C-type lectin, has been described as an acute phase secretory protein expressed during acute pancreatitis in humans and rats. However, induction of the HIP/PAP gene has been also described in some cases of liver, stomach, and colorectal cancer. Furthermore, increased serum levels of HIP/PAP protein have been shown in patients with hepatocellular carcinoma.[1–3]

Although the biological function of HIP/PAP in the liver remains elusive, evidence supports HIP/PAP involvement in hepatocyte differentiation and proliferation.[3] On the other hand, it has been shown that in pancreatic cells the antiapoptotic mechanisms triggered by tumor necrosis factor-alpha (TNF-α) are mediated by HIP/PAP overexpression, suggesting that HIP/PAP might be an effector of apoptosis inhibition.[4]

At the molecular level a detailed analysis of the size of HIP/PAP transcripts has shown that the HIP/PAP mRNA expressed in some stomach cancer tissues is longer

Address for correspondence: Dr. M. Cervello, Istituto di Biologia dello Sviluppo, C.N.R., Palermo, Italy.
cervello@ibs.pa.cnr.it

than the mRNA detected in some hepatocellular and pancreatic cancers.[5] This is due to alternative splicing of the 5'-noncoding exons, which in humans generates at least three different types of transcripts, referred to as type 1, type 2, and type 3.[5]

The aim of the present study was to shed more light on the role of HIP/PAP in hepatoma cells, taking into consideration the results obtained by Itoh *et al.*[5] Our first step was to examine, by reverse transcription-polymerase chain reaction (RT-PCR), the HIP/PAP transcripts present in human hepatoma cell lines of different origins and with different grades of differentiation and genetic profiles. We also used DNA sequencing analysis to investigate the structure of the HIP/PAP gene.

MATERIAL AND METHODS

Cell Cultures. Four different human hepatoma cell lines (HepG2, HuH-6, HuH-7, and HA22T/VGH) were used in this study. All cells were maintained in MEM (Sigma, Milan, Italy) supplemented with 10% heat-inactivated fetal calf serum (HyClone Europe), 1% L-glutamine, 1 mM sodium pyruvate, and 1% penicillin/streptomycin solution (all from Sigma, Milan, Italy). Cells were grown as adherent cells in a humidified atmosphere at 37°C in 5% CO_2. They were subcultured after trypsinization (with 0.05% trypsin/0.02% EDTA in phosphate-buffered saline solution from HyClone Europe) for 5 minutes at 37°C, washing, and resuspension in complete medium. Cells having a narrow range of passage number were used for all experiments.

Extraction of Cellular RNA and Reverse-Transcription-Polymerase Chain Reaction (RT-PCR). Total RNA was extracted from all cell lines by the guanidinium-thiocyanate method according to Chomczynski and Sacchi.[6] Both cDNA synthesis and PCR were then performed using the SUPERSCRIPT One-Step RT-PCR method (Invitrogen, Milan, Italy).

First-strand cDNAs were obtained after 30 minutes at 48°C. Following inactivation at 94°C for 2 minutes, PCR amplification was performed under the following reaction conditions: 94°C for 30 seconds, 50°C for 30 seconds, 72°C for 45 seconds with a total of 40 cycles, and a final extension at 72°C for 10 minutes. All PCR products (10 µl) were analyzed by electrophoresis on 3% agarose gel stained with ethidium bromide, and photographed.

The HIP/PAP primers were designed according to the sequence reported in the EMBL database under accession No. D30715. The sequences of primers used in the RT-PCR were as follows:

S(sense)1 5'-CCACCAGAGAGTGACTC-3',
S2 5'-CCACTGACCACGCTTTCTT-3',
S3 5'-CCCACCAGAGAGTCGCA-3',
A(antisense)1 5'-ATGAGTAGCTGTTACCAATG-3'.

To sequence the HIP/PAP coding region the following primers were used:

S4 5'-GCCTCCTCAAGTCGCAGACA-3' and
A2 5'-ACAGGCTGCTGACTTCCCTC-3'.

Sequence of RT-PCR Products. The RT-PCR products were purified by chromatography and sequenced using the dye terminator cycle sequencing kit (Perkin

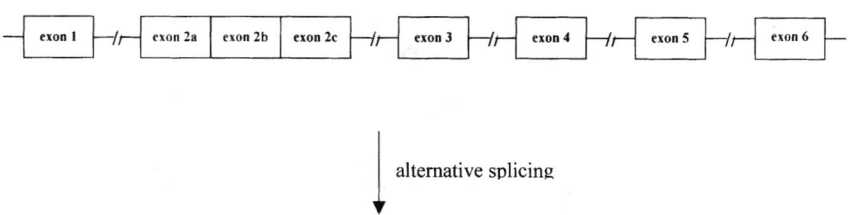
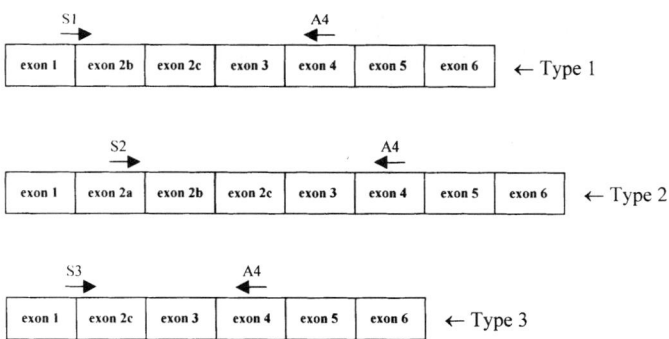

FIGURE 1. Schematic representation of HIP/PAP gene and mRNA transcripts generated through alternative splicing. Number inside the box indicates number of exons. Position of primers S1, S2, S3, and A4 are indicated.

Elmer, Foster City, CA, USA) and an ABI 373 sequencer (Perkin Elmer). Analysis of the nucleotide sequences was performed with Chromas version 1.6 software (Technelysium Pty Ltd, Halensvale, Australia).

RESULTS

In this study we analyzed HIP/PAP mRNA expression in human hepatoma cells. To characterize the types of HIP/PAP transcripts expressed by the cell lines we first isolated total cell RNA and then analyzed the expression of HIP/PAP mRNA by a specific RT-PCR procedure. We used three forward primers developed from the 5'-untranslated region of HIP/PAP mRNA and a reverse primer corresponding to a sequence within the coding region (FIG. 1).

As shown in FIGURE 2, by using primers S1/A1 we detected in all cell lines an HIP/PAP amplification product of 351 bp, which corresponds to the type-1 transcript. The type-2 transcript (358 bp) was found only in HuH-6 cells. By using prim-

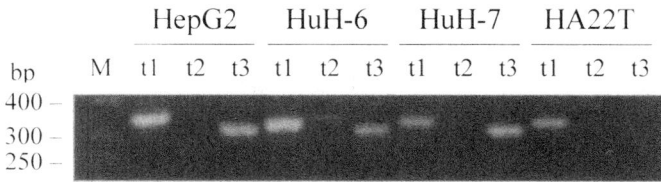

FIGURE 2. RT-PCR analysis of HIP/PAP mRNA in human hepatoma cells. mRNA was isolated and RT-PCR was performed as indicated in **Material and Methods** using specific primers for type-1 (t1), type-2 (t2), and type-3 (t3) transcripts. M = 50-bp marker.

ers S3/A1, the type-3 transcript (324 bp) was observed only in three (HepG2, HuH-6, and HuH-7) of the four cell lines.

To amplify the entire coding region of HIP/PAP mRNA, we used a sense oligonucleotide primer developed from positions 39-58 of the HIP/PAP gene, whereas the anti-sense primer was developed from positions 594-613. DNA sequencing analyses confirmed the identity of the amplification products. The nucleotide sequences were in complete agreement with the sequence reported by Dusetti et al.[7] (data not shown), demonstrating that there were no differences in the coding regions, and therefore in the protein products, in the various cell lines analyzed.

DISCUSSION

In this study we used four different hepatoma-derived cell lines known to have different differentiation grades and origins. HuH-7, a well-differentiated cell line, is derived from an HBV-negative hepatocellular carcinoma. HA22T/VGH is a poorly differentiated hepatoma cell line, which contains HBV integrants. HuH-6 and HepG2 are two well-differentiated hepatoblastoma-derived cell lines. In addition, the different cell lines have different genetic defects. For example, HuH-7 expresses a mutant form of the p53 tumor suppressor gene.[8] On the other hand, a major oncogenic alteration of both HepG2 and HuH-6 cells is their aberrant expression of β-catenin.[9,10]

Previous studies have shown that at least three different types of HIP/PAP transcripts are expressed in human tissues.[5] However, in a population limited to nine patients, only the type-3 transcript occurred in hepatocellular carcinoma tissue.[5] By contrast, the present study shows that human hepatoma cell lines may express different HIP/PAP transcripts. Among the well-differentiated cell lines, the HuH-6 cell line expressed the type-1, type-2, and type-3 transcripts, whereas the HepG2 and HuH-7 cells expressed both type-1 and type–3, but not type-2, transcripts. The poorly differentiated HA22T/VGH cells expressed only the type-1 transcript. The presence of multiple transcripts in liver cells has not previously been reported. The existence of different transcripts with different 5′-untranslated regions may have some effect on mRNA expression, affecting its transcription and translation rates, its stability, and its subcellular localization.

The fact that in the liver HIP/PAP is not expressed either in adult life or during embryonic development suggests that expression of HIP/PAP in hepatic cancer cells is closely related to liver carcinogenesis. Although the molecular mechanisms controlling HIP/PAP expression in the liver have not been clarified, it has been demonstrated that in pancreatic and colon carcinoma cells some cytokines such as interleukin-6 (IL-6) and gamma interferon (IFN-γ) can activate HIP/PAP gene expression.[11,12]

The function of HIP/PAP, it has been proposed, is to increase pancreatic cell resistance to oxidative stress and TNF-α–induced apoptosis.[4,13] Moreover, HIP/PAP was demonstrated to induce cell proliferation in intestinal cells. HIP/PAP and HIP/PAP-related proteins have also been involved in the regeneration of motor neurons[14] and in the proliferation of pancreatic cells.[15] HIP/PAP also acts as a growth factor on Schwann cells *in vitro*[14] and as a survival factor for motor neurons.[16] HIP/PAP expression in hepatoma cells might be part of a defense mechanism against apoptosis or be involved in hepatocyte proliferation. Further investigation should define the role of HIP/PAP during the development of human hepatocellular carcinoma and ascertain whether the use of different transcripts may help to regulate HIP/PAP expression in transformed liver cells.

ACKNOWLEDGMENT

This study was funded, in part, by Assessorato Sanitá Regione Siciliana-Progetto Finalizzato Oncologia to G.M.

REFERENCES

1. DUSETTI, M.J., G. MONTALTO, E.M. ORTIZ, *et al.* 1996. Mechanism of *PAP I* gene induction during hepatocarcinogenesis: clinical implications. Br. J. Cancer **74:** 1767–1775.
2. MONTALTO, G., J.L. IOVANNA, M. SORESI, *et al.* 1998. Clinical evaluation of pancreatitis-associated protein as a serum marker of hepatocellular carcinoma: comparison with α-fetoprotein. Oncology **55:** 421–425.
3. CHRISTA, L., M.T. SIMON, C. BREZAULT-BONNET, *et al.* 1999. Hepatocarcinoma-intestine-pancreas/pancreatic associated protein (HIP/PAP) is expressed and secreted by proliferating ductules as well as by hepatocarcinoma and cholangiocarcinoma cells. Am. J. Pathol. **155:** 1525–1533.
4. MALKA, D., S. VASSEUR, H. BODEKER, *et al.* 2000. Tumor necrosis factor α triggers antiapoptotic mechanisms in rat pancreatic cells through pancreatic-associated protein I activation. Gastroenterology **119:** 816–828.
5. ITOH, T., N. SAWABU, Y. MOTOO, *et al.* 1995. The human pancreatitis-associated protein (PAP)-encoding gene generates multiple transcripts through alternative use of 5′ exons. Gene **155:** 283–287.
6. CHOMCZYNSKI, P. & N. SACCHI. 1987. Single-step method of RNA isolation by acid guanidinium thiocyanate-phenol-chloroform extraction. Anal. Biochem. **162:** 156–159.
7. DUSETTI, N.J., J.M. FRIGERIO, M.F. FOX, *et al.* 1994. Molecular cloning, genomic organization and chromosomal localization of the human pancreatitis-associated protein (PAP) gene. Genomics **19:** 108–114.
8. HSU, I.C., T. TOKIWA, W. BENNET, *et al.* 1993. p53 gene mutation and integrated hepatitis B viral DNA sequences in human liver cancer cell lines. Carcinogenesis **14:** 987–992.

9. DE LA COSTE, A., B. ROMAGNOLO, P. BILLUART, et al. 1998. Somatic mutations of the β-catenin gene are frequent in mouse and human hepatocellular carcinomas. Proc. Natl. Acad. Sci. USA **95:** 8847–8851.
10. CARRUBA, G., M. CERVELLO, M.D. MICELI, et al. 1999. Truncated form of β-catenin and reduced expression of wild type catenins feature HepG2 human liver cancer cells. Ann. N.Y. Acad. Sci. **886:** 212–216.
11. DUSETTI, N.J., E.M. ORTIZ, G.M. MALLO, et al. 1995. Pancreatitis-associated protein I (PAP I), an acute phase protein induced by cytokines. J. Biol. Chem. **38:** 22417–22421.
12. RECHRECHE, H., G. MONTALTO, G.V. MALLO, et al. 1999. *pap*, *reg* Iα and *reg* Iβ mRNAs are concomitantly up-regulated during human colorectal carcinogenesis. Int. J. Cancer **81:** 688–694.
13. ORTIZ, E.M., N.J. DUSETTI, S. VASSEUR, et al. 1998. The pancreatitis-associated protein is induced by free radicals in AR4-2J cells and confers cell resistance to apoptosis. Gastroenterology **114:** 808–816.
14. LIVESEY, F.J., J.A. O'BRIEN, M. LI, et al. 1997. A Schwann cell mitogen accompanying regeneration of motor neurons. Nature **390:** 614–618.
15. ZENILMAN, M.E., T.H. MAGNUSON, K. SWINSON, et al. 1996. Pancreatic thread protein is mitogenic to pancreatic-derived cells in culture. Gastroenterology **110:** 1208–1214.
16. NISHIMUNE, H., S. VASSEUR, S. WIESE, et al. 2000. Reg-2 is a motoneuron neurotrophic factor and a signalling intermediate in the CNTF survival pathway. Nat. Cell. Biol. **2:** 906-914.

Neuroblastoma: A Challenge for Pediatric Oncology of the Third Millennium

LUISA MASSIMO

Director Emeritus, Department of Pediatric Hematology and Oncology, "G. Gaslini" Scientific Children's Hospital, Genoa, Italy

> ABSTRACT: Neuroblastoma is the only cancer of childhood considered in this conference on hormone-related tumors, because the percentage of deaths in children with this rare type of cancer is still very high. Pediatricians feel the need for help from basic researchers to better understand the biological nature of this disease and to improve protocols and the challenge of cure.
>
> KEYWORDS: neuroblastoma; childhood cancer

As co-Director of the Workshop on "Classical and Nonclassical Issues from Prevention to Treatment of Hormone-Related Tumors," it is a pleasure for me to welcome all of you to Erice. We are honored to meet here and have the opportunity to discuss topics of common interest. Erice is a small medieval Sicilian town built atop a mythical holy mountain, home of gods, well known since prehistoric ages.

Since 1978, I have organized 14 courses on pediatric hematology and oncology, and Prof. Luigi Castagnetta 5 courses on oncology. This is the first time that we have joined our efforts. This International Workshop remained in the planning stages for several months in order to provide optimal continuity with the very successful ones held here previously. Prof. Luigi Castagnetta and his collaborators worked very hard. Now the entire group of high-caliber participants, both invited speakers and audience, from so many different countries are gathered here.

One of our aims is to work together with specialists from all branches involved in oncology, to lay the groundwork for cooperative efforts, with the final goal to identify more focal points of mutual interest for future studies.

The only pediatric section of this workshop is devoted to neuroblastoma, a tumor affecting mostly infants and young children with a high percentage of deaths. Pediatricians strongly feel the need for help for our young patients that only biologists can give us.

Neuroblastoma is the most fascinating and enigmatic of childhood neoplasms from both a clinical and a biological viewpoint. It is a tumor of postganglionic sympathetic neurons, arising from primitive neural crest cells. Its annual incidence is ap-

---

Address for correspondence: Prof. Luisa Massimo, Viale Brigata Bisagno 8, 16129 Genoa, Italy. Voice: +39-010-591788; fax: +39-010-593129.
  luisamassimo@yahoo.it

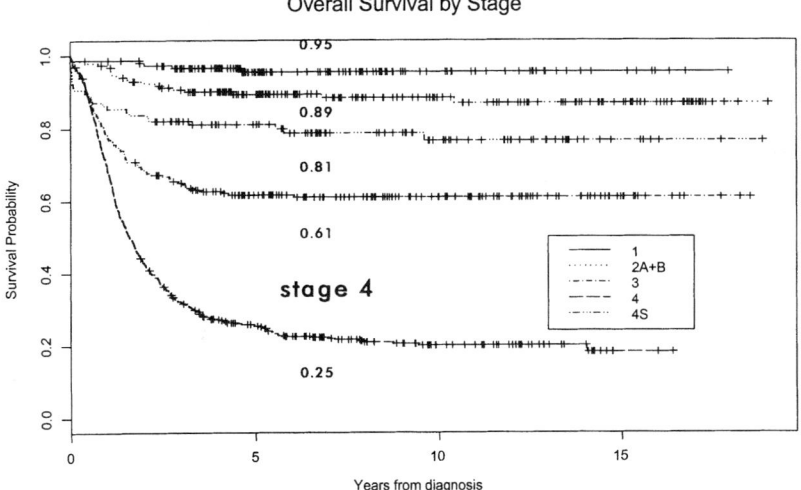

FIGURE 1. Neuroblastoma survival related to extension (stages) of disease.

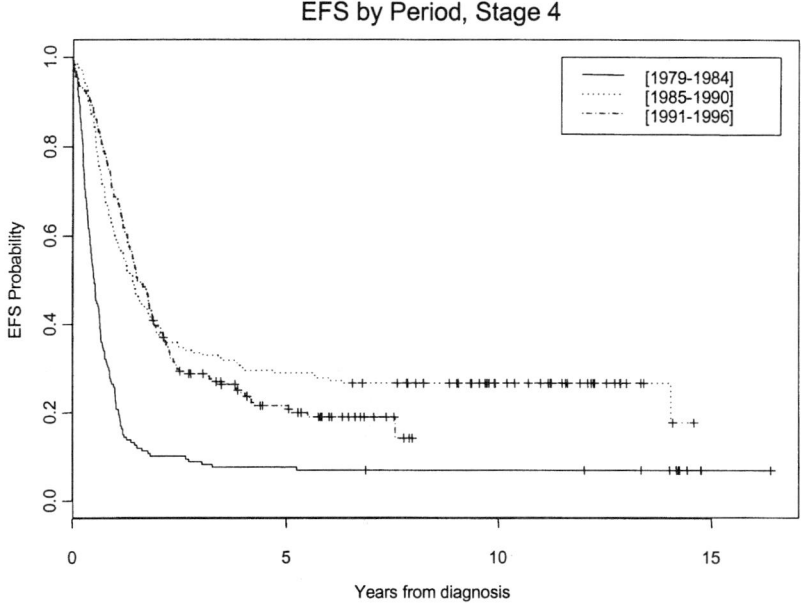

FIGURE 2. Neuroblastoma survival in three consecutive time periods.

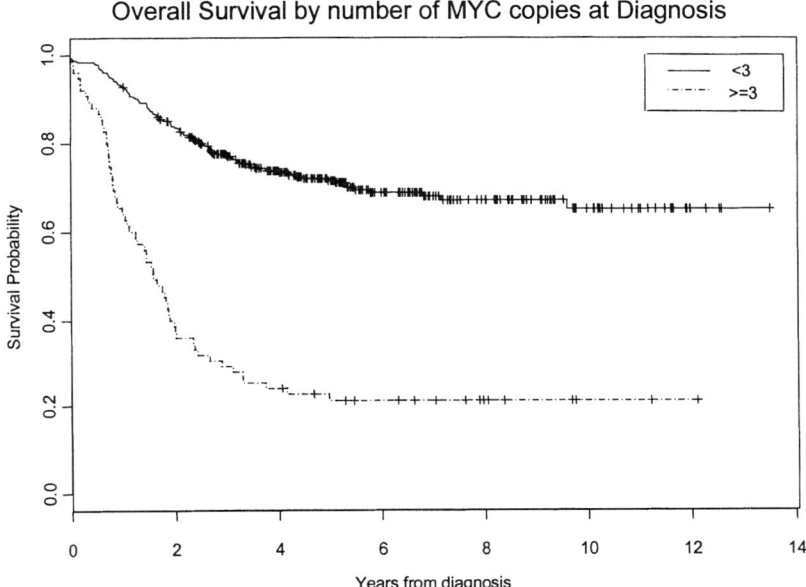

FIGURE 3. Neuroblastoma survival is greatly affected by overexpression of a single gene.

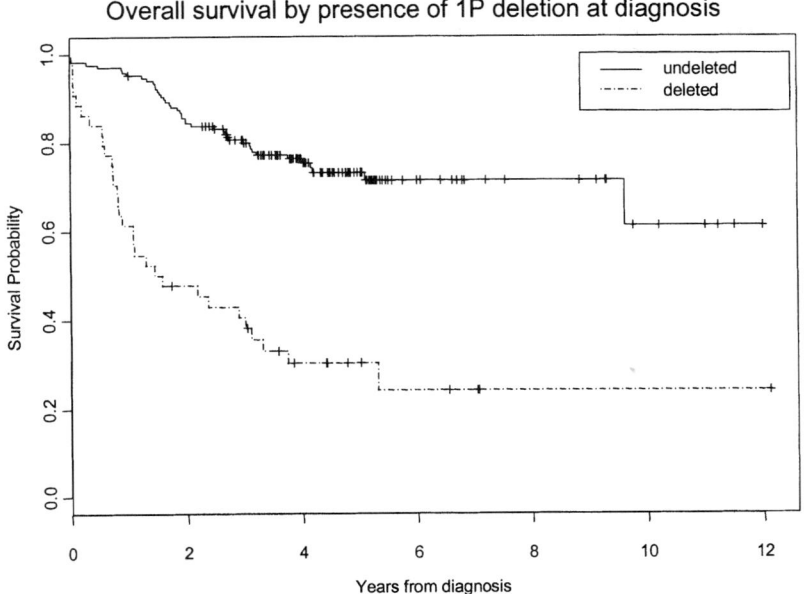

FIGURE 4. Neuroblastoma survival is also affected by the deletion of 1p chromosome.

proximately 10.4 per million children, that is, about 10,000 new cases per year in the world.

It is very important to detect and to take risk and prognostic factors into consideration in order to treat the child with the best protocol available. With this in mind, it is necessary to evaluate the clinical and biological variables. The most important independent variables are age at diagnosis, clinical stage (localized or disseminated), and N-myc amplification. Many other variables, such as site, histology, urinary VMA and HVA, plasmatic levels of LDH, NSE, ferritin, DNA index, and chromosomal abnormalities such as 1p deletion and 17q gain, play a minor role.

Among the major aims of pediatric oncologists is to understand through the biologic characterization of the tumor the aggressive nature of disseminated neuroblastoma (stage 4). Because only a few of you are involved in research on this childhood tumor, I suppose that it could be of help to you to see some survival curves related to widespread neuroblastoma. They derive from the Italian experience, collected by the cooperative Group for Neuroblastoma of the Italian Association of Pediatric Hematology and Oncology (AIEOP) (FIGS. 1–4).

Neuroblastoma is a model for research in oncology in general, for a number of reasons: (1) a multidisciplinary approach; (2) an attempt at early diagnosis of the tumor by urine mass screening program: (3) identification of biological indexes useful for prognosis and treatment (N-myc, 1p deletion, and 17q gain) and for detecting minimal residual disease; (4) efficacy of high dose treatment; (5) targeted delivery of treatment with MIBG and monoclonal antibodies; (6) urgency to evaluate and activate innovative types of therapy (differentiation agents, immunological interventions, etc); and (7) design of international trials.

At the end of this introduction to the pediatric section on neuroblastoma, I would like to express my wish that this meeting fulfill other functions as well, primarily that of encouraging future cooperation and exchange of ideas among the many investigators from the institutions represented here.

Amplified *MYCN* in Human Neuroblastoma

Paradigm for the Translation of Molecular Genetics to Clinical Oncology

MANFRED SCHWAB

Division of Cytogenetics, Deutsches Krebsforschungszentrum, Im Neuenheimer Feld 280, D-69120 Heidelberg, Germany

ABSTRACT: Increase in the dosage of cellular oncogenes by DNA amplification is a frequent genetic alteration of cancer cells. In neuroblastoma, amplification of the gene *MYCN* has been associated with aggressively growing cancers and is an indicator for poor prognosis. *MYCN* amplification is of predictive value in identifying patients with neuroblastoma who require specific therapeutic regimens and those who do not benefit from chemotherapy.

KEYWORDS: *MYCN; MDM2; p53*; chromosomes; FISH; tumorigenesis; pediatric tumors; neuronal tumors; neuroblastoma; gene amplification; oncogenes; genomic instability; translational research; expression profile;oncochip; array

INTRODUCTION

The nervous system is the most common site for the development of solid tumors in children. Neuroblastoma develops as a tumor of the peripheral nervous system from primitive neuroectodermal cells derived from the neural crest.[1] The annual incidence of neuroblastoma is around 9 cases per million children under 15 years of age.[2,3] Different studies have revealed a median age of presentation of less than 2 years. The incidence of neuroblastoma *in situ*, defined as nodules of primitive neuroblastic cells in the adrenal, is much higher, as suggested by random autopsy studies of infants under 3 months of age.[4,5] It is possible that these cells have retained their potential to undergo differentiation, a process that results in regression of *in situ* neuroblastoma. In fact, spontaneous regression is one of the most unusual aspects of neuroblastoma and occurs particularly in infants with a small primary tumor despite extensive liver involvement and the presence of subcutaneous nodules. This group of patients, defined by Evans as stage 4,[6] has a survival rate of 70%. (An excellent picture of the biology of neuroblastoma has been presented by Berthold.[7]) Many ad-

---

N-myc is used alternatively. Here we are following the international nomenclature for human gene symbols.

Address for correspondence: Dr. Manfred Schwab, Division of Cytogenetics, Deutsches Krebsforschungszentrum, Im Neuenheimer Feld 280, D-69120 Heidelberg, Germany. Voice: +6221-42 32 20; fax: +6221-42 32 81.

m.schwab@dkfz.de

vances in understanding the etiology of this tumor have been translated into better clinical management, but little improvement in survival rate has been achieved.

The causes for neuroblastoma development have remained enigmatic, and the higher frequency of neuroblastoma in young, even newborn, children remains unexplained. Although several cases of familial neuroblastoma have been reported[8] that would suggest a hereditary component in a select group of patients, the vast majority of cases of neuroblastoma appear to develop sporadically. It appears, however, that specific changes in the somatic genome contribute to the development of neuroblastoma.[1] This feature aims at presenting the state of the art of our knowledge about the mechanisms by which oncogenes may become amplified, the structural arrangement of amplified oncogenes, and the significance of oncogene amplification for tumorigenesis. From this it will emerge that amplified oncogenes are associated with aggressively growing cancers and can be employed to identify patients that have poor prognosis and require specific therapeutic regimens. Amplification in neuroblastoma was the first oncogene alteration that turned out to be of practical clinical use.

AMPLIFICATION OF ONCOGENES

Cytogenetic analyses have brought to light the frequency of DNA amplification in tumor cells and have provided a starting point to define the contribution for tumorigenesis that comes from an increase in the dosage of cellular oncogenes by amplification.[9] Chromosomal abnormalities associated with DNA amplification are mainly of two types: double minutes (DMs), originally discovered in direct preparations of human neuroblastoma cells, and homogeneously staining chromosomal regions (HSRs), again detected in neuroblastoma cells. By using expression profiling with an "oncochip," the amplification of oncogenes was discovered in human cancer cells carrying DMs or HSRs.[9]

The information that has accrued since this original observation supports the conjecture that DMs and HSRs are indicators of amplified oncogenes in cancer cells, except in some drug-resistant cells that have acquired resistance by gene amplification.[10–12] Amplification of cellular oncogenes ranges usually between five and several hundred copies. Values of less than five copies should be viewed with caution. In particular, tumor surveys by "comparative genomic hybridizations" (CGH) often point to genomic regions with "high level amplification." Such observations should be confirmed by independent experimental approaches.

AMPLIFICATION OF *MYCN* IN NEUROBLASTOMA CELLS

MYCN was originally identified when oncogene expression profiles were established for human neuroblastoma cells showing DMs or HSRs. These surveys quickly established that with few exceptions, cultured neuroblastoma cell lines carry the gene *MYCN* amplified between five and several hundred copies.[13] At the same time, neuroblastoma tumors were also found to carry amplified *MYCN*.[13] Amplification of *MYCN* is less frequent in other types of tumor than in neuroblastoma. Few cases have been reported for medulloblastoma,[14] retinoblastoma,[15] astrocytoma,[16] and small cell lung cancer.[17] Particularly interesting is the setting of small cell lung cancers where, in addition, two other members of the *myc*-gene family have been found amplified, *MYC* and *MYCL* (also referred to as *c-myc* and *L-myc*).[17] It is not clear if differential amplification of various *myc* family genes might define biologically or clinically different subsets of small cell lung cancer. *MYCN* was found to be amplified only in tumors with neuronal qualities as if the function of the *MYCN* gene is normally related to growth control or differentiation of certain neuronal cells.

The oncogenic potential of enhanced expression of *MYCN* as a consequence of amplification was addressed in various experimental systems. Enhanced ectopic expression, resulting after introduction of an *MYCN* expression vector, can assist mutationally activated RAS^H in tumorigenic conversion of primary rat embryo cells,[18] converts established cells of the rat[19] and of humans[20] to tumorigenicity, and rescues primary rat embryo cells from senescence.[21] Furthermore, *MYCN* has frequently been activated by proviral insertion in MULV-induced T-cell lymphomas[22] and is involved in tumorigenesis in transgenic mice.[23,24] These results clearly attest to the capacity of high *MYCN* expression to modulate the growth of cells, and it therefore appears reasonable to suggest that enhanced expression consequent to amplification contributes to tumorigenesis. The available evidence suggests that the nucleotide sequence of *MYCN* in neuroblastoma cells is unaltered compared with that of normal cells. Consistent with this result, the biological activities of *MYCN* derived from normal or neuroblastoma cells have not been found to differ.[18] Studies of the loss of *MYCN* function in transgenic mice have not contributed to an understanding of its role in differentiation, as it results in embryonic lethality.[25]

MECHANISM OF *MYCN* AMPLIFICATION

Although an exact definition of the initial events during DNA amplification cannot be made, a model of amplification has to take into consideration many observations made by cytogenetic and molecular genetic approaches. First, direct preparations of neuroblastoma cells until now have in most instances revealed DMs as cytogenetic evidence of amplified DNA, yet nearly all neuroblastoma cell lines established in long-term culture lack DMs and instead contain HSRs. Second, amplification is associated with transposition of DNA into different chromosomal regions with retention of the single copy gene of *MYCN* at 2p24.[26] HSRs carrying amplified *MYCN* in different neuroblastomas are not located at or near the resistant *MYCN* locus. Third, the size of an HSR is many times that of a single DM. One observation, not independently confirmed, indicates preferential amplification of the paternal allele.[27] It is not clear, however, how this could figure mechanistically in the amplification process.

From all we currently know, amplification of *MYCN* in neuroblastoma appears to be a sporadic event, and there is no obvious reason to invoke external influences. As the initial step of amplification, there are theoretically three possibilities.[9] One is disproportionate DNA replication resulting from second usage of an origin of replication within a single cell cycle. The extra-replicated DNA must be released from the replication structure, joining the extra-replicated DNA segments to yield a head-to-head or head-to-tail circular duplication. In support of this molecular pathway, cytogenetic studies have revealed that the single copy *MYCN* is retained at 2p24 in neuroblastoma cells carrying an HSR.[26] At some stage, the extrachromosomal

MYCN copies can become integrated into a distant chromosomal position, where they appear to re-amplify and to assume a regular head-to-tail repetitive arrangement.[28,29] The other possibility for initial events leading to amplification could be the formation of a DNA loop structure followed by recombination and excision of DNA. This mechanism would inevitably result in deletion of *MYCN* from its native locus at chromosome 2p24,[30] a mechanism that can almost be excluded by our finding of the retention of *MYCN* at its original site.[26] Finally, in some models of amplification associated with cytotoxic drug resistance, it could be shown that multiple gene copies can be formed at the resident site of the corresponding gene, presumably by mechanisms of unequal sister chromatid exchange. HSRs or other alterations have never been observed at 2p24 in neuroblastoma cells; it is therefore unlikely that *MYCN* becomes amplified at its resident site.

NONSYNTENIC AMPLIFICATION OF *MYCN* AND *MDM2* GENES

Until recently *MYCN* was thought to be the only oncogene amplified in human neuroblastoma cells. Through cytogenetic studies we have identified neuroblastoma cell lines that, in addition to amplified *MYCN*, carry "double minutes" (DMs) or "homogeneously staining chromosomal regions" (HSRs) not harboring *MYCN*. In situ hybridization of biotinylated total genomic DNA to normal lymphocytes (reverse genomic hybridization) revealed the amplified DNA to be derived from chromosome 12 band q13-14, and subsequent filter analyses showed 30- to 40-fold amplification of the *MDM2* gene, abundantly expressed, both in some cell lines and in an original tumor, in addition to amplified *MYCN*.[31] Independent high level amplification of the nonsyntenic oncogenes *MYCN* and *MDM2* appears to be a recurrent genetic alteration in human neuroblastoma cells and raises the possibility that the MDM2 protein cooperates with the MYCN protein in a clinically as yet undefined subgroup of neuroblastomas. Because MDM2 can antagonize the function of the p53 tumor suppressor protein by sequestration, it is possible that the enhanced expression of MDM2 acts through the p53 pathway. It is not clear, however, if p53 has a role in many neuroblastomas given the fact that alterations of p53, which are frequent in many human cancers, are at best rare in neuroblastomas.[32] It is definitely possible that *MDM2* can act as an oncogene on its own.

There are two arrangements by which two different oncogenes can persist in tumor cells: either they can be coamplified or their amplification can be nonsyntenic. Coamplification refers to genes that are linked on the same chromosome. In case one gene is amplified, the neighboring gene becomes coamplified by virtue of its location in close vincinity. Coamplification is rather frequent, with the amplification unit on 11q13 in breast cancer being a prominent example.[33] In addition, in some neuroblastoma cell lines and tumors, the *Dead-Box* gene (*DDX1*) has been found coamplified with *MYCN*.[34] By contrast, nonsyntenic amplification involves genes from two different chromosomes and is extremely rare. Obviously two different amplification events must have occurred. The recurrent amplification of the nonsyntenic *MYCN* and *MDM2* genes raises the question of whether neuroblastoma cells have a genetic instability for amplification. Previous studies suggested a correlation between amplification of *MYCN* and deletion at chromosome 1p36,[23,35] which is a frequent alteration in neuroblastoma cells.[35–40] A reciprocal 1:15 translocation could signal the location of a postulated tumor suppressor gene,[41] although it is possible that 1p harbors more than a single such locus.[42,43] Interestingly, both a constitutional translocation[44] and deletion[45] in a neuroblastoma patient also map around this region. We might speculate that altered genetic information at 1p36 is related to instability for gene amplification.

EXPRESSION OF MYCN

MYCN is expressed in a limited spectrum of cell types, in contrast to MYC which is expressed rather ubiquitously.[46] Cells that have amplified MYCN have elevated expression.[47] Neuronal cells generally exhibit MYCN expression.[47,48] By contrast, expression is below the level of deletion in, for instance, epithelial cells or fibroblasts.[46] Expression of MYCN appears to have an important role during brain development, as indicated by high expression during fetal stages; this is in contrast to the adult brain, where MYCN expression is below the level of detection.[49,50] Also, expression of MYCN goes down when in vitro cultivated neuroblastoma cells are forced to differentiate, as by retinoic acid,[51] or during differentiation of mouse teratocarcinoma cells.[52] It appears that regulation of MYCN expression determines the ability of neuroblastoma cells to differentiate.[53] Although some regulatory elements have been described in the MYCN promoter[54] and a down-stream silencer has been reported, the molecular basis for differential expression, for instance, between neuronal cells and fibroblasts is not fully explained.

FUNCTIONS OF THE MYCN PROTEIN

The nucleotide sequence of MYCN shows a high degree of similarity to that of MYC.[55] MYCN encodes two polypeptides of relative molecular masses of 62 and 64 kD that result from alternative use of two translational start codons.[56] The two proteins are localized in the nucleus of the cell, and they are phosphorylated. Under in vitro conditions, casein kinase (CK-II) efficiently carries out phosphorylation in the central region and at serine 367.[57]

Two evolutionary conserved regions of the protein appear particularly suitable to address the question of protein function. One is the carboxy-terminal region containing a helix-loop-helix (HLH) and a leucine zipper motif (Zip), and the other is the N-terminus carrying what has been referred to as "*myc*-boxes."[58]

One cellular function of MYCN appears to be related to apoptosis. Ectopic expression of MYCN, as by experimentally switching on an inducible promoter, sensitizes host cell apoptosis after treatment with gamma interferon or doxorubicin.[59,60] The introduction of an antisense high expression cDNA library from apoptotic cells by transfection can inactivate transcripts functional in apoptosis execution[61] and results in the rescue of cell clones resistant to the drugs. This functional approach, referred to as "technical knockout" (TKO), should be invaluable in isolating and characterizing genes involved in apoptosis and in drug resistance of human neuroblastoma cells.

REGULATION OF MYCN PROTEIN BY INTERACTING PROTEINS

Proteins encoded by the protooncogenes *MYC*, *MYCL*, and *MYCN* contain at their carboxy-terminus a tripartite segment comprising a basic DNA binding region (BR), a helix-loop-helix (HLH), and a leucine zipper motif (Zip) that are believed to be involved in DNA binding and protein-protein interaction. Using two independent approaches, analysis of proteins (1) coprecipitating with N-Myc[62] and (2) binding under *in vitro* conditions,[63] a protein, Max p20/22, was identified to physically interact with N-Myc and Myc. As the associating region, the HLH-Zip domain was identified by site-directed mutagenesis. Recently an alternatively spliced messenger RNA was identified that encodes a form of Max truncated at the C-terminus.[64] This ΔMax protein retained the ability to bind to the CACGTG motif in a complex with MYC, but it lacked the nuclear localization signal. In a *myc-ras* cotransformation assay using rat embryo cells, *max* suppressed, but Δ*max* enhanced, the transformation efficiency. Thus, the *max* gene appears to encode both a negative and a positive regulator of Myc function. It is not clear at this point if Δ*max* is also expressed in human neuroblastoma cells. An important question, therefore, that cannot be answered at this point is how the elevated level of *MYCN*, consequent to *MYCN* gene amplification, might figure into the development of neuroblastoma. Due to overexpression, MYCN could act as a scavenger and eliminate Max and thereby its tumor-suppressing potential. Alternatively, in case Δ*myc* would be expressed, the elevated level of *MYCN* protein could result in a larger number of positive growth-activating complexes. With the identification of two additional proteins, Mad and Mxi1, that both bind to Max,[65,66] the matter has become more complex, and it is clear that Myc proteins are members of a nucleoprotein complex. Even more, the central region of MYCN appears to be a target for interacting proteins as well, as recently demonstrated by the binding of YAF2.[67]

THE *MYC*-BOXES

The *Myc*-boxes were originally defined as two short, roughly 60 and 40, respectively, nucleotides long, in the first coding exon of the *Myc* genes.[13,21] These boxes are highly conserved over a broad evolutionary range from chicken to man. Kato and collaborators[68] were the first to identify the amino terminal portion of the Myc protein as a transcription-activating domain. At least in the MYCN protein this activity could be further mapped to the *Myc*-boxes.[69] It appears that one activity of the Myc-nucleoprotein complex is directed towards regulation of the expression of other, as yet unidentified, genes.

CLINICAL SIGNIFICANCE OF *MYCN* AMPLIFICATION

Important prognostic parameters for neuroblastoma are clinical stage and age of the patient at diagnosis. Patients with neuroblastoma stages I and II have a favorable prognosis: 75–90% can expect to survive at least 2 years. Patients with stage III and IV tumors have a poor prognosis. Significantly different prognoses for patient groups with stage III tumor have been observed in the United States and Germany.

In the United States, the prognosis for stage III tumors is similar to that for stage IV tumors (10–30%), whereas a considerably more favorable prognosis is observed in Germany. The reason for this disagreement is not yet known.[70]

Independent studies by various groups have shown a significant correlation between amplification of *MYCN* and stages III and IV. This correlation was first shown within the framework of a study of 63 neuroblastomas; amplifications were not detected in 15 stage I and stage II tumors, but were observed in 24 of 48 (50%) stage III and stage IV tumors.[71] Subsequent studies by other investigators have confirmed this correlation, although the incidence of amplification was somewhat smaller (between 20 and 30%). The correlation between *MYCN* amplification and poor prognosis is now well established.[72]

A significant correlation between poor prognosis and *MYCN* amplification was also observed when patients over 1 year of age were compared with patients under 1 year. Prognosis for patients over 1 year of age, especially those with stage III and stage IV tumors, is particularly unfavorable.[73] One study showed *MYCN* amplification in more than 50% of the patients older than 1 year; for younger patients, the incidence of amplification was smaller. *MYCN* amplification thus seems to be an independent parameter for evaluating the prognosis of neuroblastoma.

Current therapy protocols for treatment of neuroblastoma depend on the prognosis for survival, which is evaluated on the basis of tumor stage, degree of surgical resectibility, and analysis of genetic alterations. The pilot study of the German Neuroblastoma Study Group recommends treatment according to protocols specific for each of four risk groups. Risk group A includes patients with localized tumors at least 90% of which can be removed surgically (prognosis 90–100%). Risk group B includes patients with localized tumors that extend beyond the organ of origin and that usually cannot be removed completely (prognosis 65–80%). Risk group C includes patients with metastasizing tumors or localized tumors that do not regress after four cycles of chemotherapy (prognosis 20-30%). Risk group D includes only patients with stage IV tumors that frequently show spontaneous regression (prognosis 75–80%).

Patients in risk group C receive the most intensive therapeutic treatment. Amplification of *MYCN* is incompatible with inclusion in risk groups with favorable prognoses, even if the tumor is localized. All patients with amplification are included in risk group C and are submitted to the most intensive therapy. However, this only applies to tumors of stages I–II. In stage IV tumors, no differences in amplification were observed when comparing the patients prognoses. Thus, amplification of *MYCN* is an independent parameter that allows us to classify a patient into a particular risk group and thus to decide on a specific treatment protocol.

Chemotherapy can have serious adverse effects in the patient. Determining the status of *MYCN* can assist in identifying patients for which chemotherapy is not beneficial. This issue is being actively addressed now by various neuroblastoma study groups in Europe as well as in the United States. A rapid approach to identifying amplification and/or high expression of *MYCN* is *in situ* hybridization on sections.[47]

PERSPECTIVES

For many years the amplified *MYCN* gene has served as a paradigm for the translation of molecular biology research into clinical practice. Although determination of MYCN status at this point is still the only genetic parameter sufficiently robust to be employed in clinical practice, it can be envisioned that single gene parameters will be replaced by more complex, and presumably more informative, technologies designed to define individual neuroblastoma tumor phenotypes by their individuial gene expression profiles.[74,75]

ACKNOWLEDGMENT

Work in the authors' laboratory is supported by grants from the Deutsche Krebshilfe.

REFERENCES

1. SCHWAB, M., H. SHIMADA, V. JOSHI, et al. 2000. Neuroblastic tumours of adrenal gland and sympathetic nervous system. In Pathology & Genetics. Tumours of the Nervous System. P. Kleihues & W.K. Cavenee, eds. :153–161. IARC Press. Lyon.
2. KRAMER, S., A.T. MEADOWS, P. JARRETT, et al. 1983. Incidence of childhood cancer: experience of a decade in a population-based registry. J. Natl. Cancer Inst. 70: 49.
3. MICHAELIS, J. & P. KAATSCH. 1986. Cooperative documentation of childhood malignancies in the FRG. System design and five-year results. Monogr. Paediatr. 18: 56–67.
4. BECKWITH, J.B. & E.V. PERRIN. 1963. In situ neuroblastomas: a contribution to the natural history of neural crest tumors. Am. J. Pathol. 43: 1089–1104.
5. HASEGAWA, R., M. TATEMATSU & K. IMAIDA. 1982. Neuroblastoma in situ. Acta Pathol. Jpn 32: 537–541.
6. EVANS, A.E., G.B. D'ANGIO & J. RANDOLPH. 1971. A proposed staging for children with neuroblastoma. Cancer 27: 374–378.
7. BERTHOLD, F. 1990. Overview: biology of neuroblastoma. In Neuroblastoma: Tumor Biology and Therapy. C. Pochedly, Ed. :1–27. CRC Press. Boca Raton.
8. KUSHNER, B.H., F. GILBERT & L. HELSON. 1986. Familial neuroblastoma: case reports, literature review, and etiologic considerations. Cancer 57: 1887–1893.
9. SAVELYEVA, L. & M. SCHWAB. 2001. Amplification of oncogenes revisited: from expression profiling to clinical application. Cancer Letts. 167: 115–123.
10. SCHIMKE, R.T. 1984. Gene amplification in cultured animal cells. Cell 37: 705–713.
11. WINDLE, B., B.W. DRAPER, Y. YIN, et al. 1991. A central role for chromosome breakage in gene amplification, deletion formation, and amplicon integration. Genes & Dev. 5: 160–174.
12. STARK, G.R. 1993. Regulation and mechanisms of mammalian gene amplification. Adv. Cancer Res. 61: 87–113.
13. SCHWAB, M., K. ALITALO, K.H. KLEMPNAUER, et al. 1983. Amplified DNA with limited homology to myc cellular oncogene is shared by human neuroblastoma cell lines and a neuroblastoma tumor. Nature 305: 245–248.
14. FULLER, G. & S. BIGNER. 1992. Amplified cellular oncogenes in neoplasms of the central nervous system. Mut. Res. 276: 299–306.
15. LEE, W.H., A.L. MURPHREE & W.F. BENEDICT. 1984. Expression and amplification of the MYCN gene in primary retinoblastoma. Nature 309: 458–460.
16. GARSON, J.A., P.G. MCINTYRE & J.T. KEMSHEAD. 1985. MYCN amplification in malignant astrocytoma. Lancet 8457: 718–719.
17. NAU, M., B. BROOKS, D. CARNEY, et al. 1986. Human small-cell lung cancers show amplification and expression of the MYCN gene. Proc. Natl. Acad. Sci. USA 83: 1092–1096.
18. SCHWAB, M., H.E. VARMUS & J.M. BISHOP. 1985. Human N-myc gene contributes to neoplastic transformation of mammalian cells in culture. Nature 316: 160–162.

19. SMALL, M.B., N. HAY, M. SCHWAB, et al. 1987. Neoplastic transformation by the human gene *MYCN*. Mol. Cell. Biol. **7:** 1638–1645.
20. SCHWEIGERER, L., S. BREIT, A. WENZEL, et al. 1990. Augmented *MYCN* expression advances the malignant phenotype of human neuroblastoma cells: evidence for induction of autocrine growth factor activity. Cancer Res. **50:** 4411–4416.
21. SCHWAB, M. & J.M. BISHOP. 1988. Sustained expression of the human protooncogene MYCN rescues rat embryo cells from senescene. Proc. Natl. Acad. Sci. USA **85:** 9585–9589.
22. VAN LOHUIZEN, M., M. BREUER & A. BERNS. 1989. N-*myc* is frequently activated by proviral insertion in MuLV-induced T cell lymphomas. EMBO J. **8:** 133–136.
23. CARON, H., P. VAN SLUIS, M. VAN HOEVE, et al. 1993. Allelic loss of chromosome 1p36 in neuroblastoma is of preferential maternal origin and correlates with *MYCN* amplification. Nature Genet. **4:** 187–190.
24. ROSENBAUM, H., E. WEBB, J.M. ADAMS, et al. 1989. N-*myc* transgene promotes B lymphoid proliferation, elicits lymphomas and reveals cross-regulation with c-*myc*. EMBO J. **8:** 749–755.
25. STANTON, B.R., A.S. PERKINS, L. TESSAROLO, et al. 1992. Loss of N-*myc* function results in embryonic lethality and failure of the epithelial component of the embryo to develop. Genes & Dev. **6:** 2235–2247.
26. CORVI, R., L.C. AMLER, L. SAVELYEVA, et al. 1994. *MYCN* is retained in single copy at chromosome 2 band p23-24 during amplification in human neuroblastoma cells. Proc. Natl. Acad. Sci. USA **91:** 5523–5527.
27. CHENG, J.M., J.L. HIEMSTRA, S.S. SCHNEIDER, et al. 1993. Preferential amplification of the paternal allele of the *MYCN* gene in human neuroblastomas. Nature Genet. **4:** 191–194.
28. AMLER, L.C. & M. SCHWAB. 1989. Amplified *MYCN* in human neuroblastoma cells is often arranged as clustered tandem repeats of differently recombined DNA. Molec. Cell. Biol. **9:** 4903–4913.
29. AMLER, L.C. & M. SCHWAB. 1992. Multiple amplicons of discrete sizes encompassing *MYCN* in neuroblastoma cells evolve through differential recombination from a large precursor DNA. Oncogene **7:** 807–809.
30. SCHWAB, M., H.E. VARMUS, J.M. BISHOP, et al. 1984. Chromosome localization in normal human cells and neuroblastomas of a gene related to c-myc. Nature **308:** 288–291.
31. CORVI, R., L. SAVELYEVA, S. BREIT, et al. 1995. Non-syntenic amplification of *MDM2* and *MYCN* in human neuroblastomas. Oncogene **10:** 1081–1086.
32. OHGAKI, H., R.H. EIBL, M. SCHWAB, et al. 1993. Mutations of the *p53* tumor suppressor gene in neoplasms of the human nervous system. Mol. Carcinog. **8:** 74–80.
33. GAUDRAY, P., P. SZEPTOWSKI, C. ESCOT, et al. 1992. DNA amplification at 11q13 in human cancer: from complexity to perplexity. Mutat. Res. **276:** 317–328.
34. SQUIRE, J.A., P.S. THORNER, S. WEITZMAN, et al. 1995. Co-amplification of *MYCN* and a dead box gene (*DDX1*) in primary neuroblastoma. Oncogene **10:** 1417–1422.
35. FONG, C.T., N.C. DRACOPOLI, P.S. WHITE, et al. 1989. Loss of heterozygosity for the short arm of chromosome 1 in human neuroblastomas: correlation with *MYCN* amplification. Proc. Natl. Acad. Sci. USA **86:** 3753–3757.
36. MARTINSSON, T., A. WEITH, C. CZIEPLUCH, et al. 1989. Chromosome 1 deletions in human neuroblastomas: Generation and fine mapping of microclones from the distal 1p region. Genes Chromosomes & Cancer **1:** 67–78.
37. WEITH, A., T. MARTINSSON, C. CZIEPLUCH, et al. 1989. Neuroblastoma consensus deletion maps to chromosome 1p36.1–2. Genes Chromosomes & Cancer **1:** 159–166.
38. SAVELYEVA, L., R. CORVI & M. SCHWAB. 1994. Translocation involving 1p and 17q is a recurrent genetic alteration of human neuroblastoma cells. Am. J. Hum. Genet. **55:** 334–340.
39. TAKAYAMA, H., T. SUZUKI, H. MUGISHIMA, et al. 1992. Deletion mapping of chromosomes 14q and 1p in human neuroblastoma. Oncogene **7:** 1185–1189.
40. CARON, H., P. VAN SLUIS, N. VAN ROY, et al. 1994. Recurrent 1;17 translocations in human neuroblastoma reveal nonhomologous mitotic recombination during the S/G2 phase as a novel mechanism for loss of heterozygosity. Am. J. Hum. Genet. **55:** 341–347.

41. SCHWAB, M. 1991. Is there a neuroblastoma anti-oncogene? *In* Advances in Neuroblastoma Research. A. Evans, G. D'Angio, A. Knudson & R.C. Seeger, eds. Vol. 3: 1. Wiley Liss & Sons, Inc. New York.
42. TAKEDA, O., C. HOMMA, N. MASEKI, *et al.* 1994. There may be two tumor suppressor genes on chromosome arm 1p closely associated with biologically distinct subtypes of neuroblastoma. Genes Chromosomes & Cancer **10**: 30–39.
43. SCHLEIERMACHER, G., M. PETER, J. MICHON, *et al.* 1994. Two distinct deleted regions on the short arm of chromosome 1 in neuroblastoma. Genes Chromosomes & Cancer **10**: 275–281.
44. LAUREYS, G., F. SPELEMAN, G. OPDENAKKER, *et al.* 1990. Constitutional translocation t(1;17)(p36;q12-21) in a patient with neuroblastoma. Genes Chromosomes & Cancer **2**: 252–254.
45. BIEGEL, J.A., P.S. WHITE, H.N. MARSHALL, *et al.* 1993. Constitutional 1p36 deletion in a child with neuroblastoma. Am. J. Hum. Genet. **52**: 176–182.
46. BREIT, S. & M. SCHWAB. 1989. Suppression of *MYC* by high expression of *NMYC* in human neuroblastoma cells. J. Neurosci. Res. **24**: 21–28.
47. SCHWAB, M., J. ELLISON, M. BUSCH, *et al.* 1984. Enhanced expression of the human gene *MYCN* consequent to amplification of DNA may contribute to malignant progression of neuroblastoma. Proc. Natl. Acad. Sci. USA **81**: 4940–4944.
48. KOHL, N.E., C. GEE & F. ALT. 1984. Activated expression of the *NMYC* gene in human neuroblastomas and related tumors. Science **226**: 1335–1338.
49. GRADY-LEOPARDI, E., M. SCHWAB, A.R. ABLIN, *et al.* 1986. Detection of N-*myc* oncogene expression in human neuroblastoma by *in situ* hybridization and blot analysis: relationship to clinical outcome. Cancer Res. **46**: 3196–3199.
50. Grady, E., M. Schwab & W. Rosenau. 1987. Expression of N-*myc* and c-*src* during the development of fetal human brain. Cancer Res. **47**: 2931–2936.
51. THIELE, C.J., C.P. REYNOLDS & M.A. ISRAEL. 1985. Decreased expression of N-*myc* precedes retinoic acid-induced morphological differentiation of human neuroblastoma. Nature **313**: 404–406.
52. JAKOBOVITS, A., M. SCHWAB, J.M. BISHOP, *et al.* 1985. Expression of N-*myc* in teratocarcinoma stem cells and mouse embryos. Nature **318**: 188–191.
53. THIELE, C.J. & M.A. ISRAEL. 1988. Regulation of N-myc expression is a critical event controlling the ability of human neuroblasts to differentiate. Exp. Cell Biol. **56**: 321–333.
54. HILLER, S., S. BREIT, Z.O. WANG, *et al.* 1991. Localization of regulatory elements controlling human *MYCN* expression. Oncogene **6**: 969–977.
55. STANTON, L.W., M. SCHWAB & J.M. BISHOP. 1986. Nucleotide sequence of the human N-*myc* gene. Proc. Natl. Acad. Sci. USA **83**: 1772–1776.
56. MÄKELÄ, T.P., K. SAKSELA & K. ALITALO. 1989. Two *MYCN* polypeptides with distinct amino termini encoded by the second and third exons of the gene. Mol. Cell. Biol. **9**: 1545–1552.
57. HAMANN, U., A. WENZEL, R. FRANK, *et al.* 1991. The *MYCN* protein of human neuroblastoma cells is phosphorylated by casein kinase II in the central region and at serine 367. Oncogene **6**: 1745–1751.
58. SCHWAB, M. 1988. The MYC-box oncogenes. *In* The Oncogene Handbook. E.P. Reddy, A. Skalka & T. Curran, eds. :381–391. Elsevier Science Publishers BV.
59. LUTZ, W., S. FULDA, I. JEREMIAS, *et al.* 1998. MycN and IFNγ cooperate in apoptosis in human neuroblastoma cells. Oncogene **17**: 339–346.
60. FULDA, S., W. LUTZ, M. SCHWAB, *et al.* 1999. MycN sensitizes neuroblastoma cells for drug-induced apoptosis. Oncogene **18**: 1479–1486.
61. WITTKE, I., B. MÄDGE, R. WIEDEMEYER, *et al.* 2001. DAP-5 is involved in MycN/IFNγ-induced apoptosis in human neuroblastoma cells. Cancer Letts. **162**: 237–243.
62. WENZEL, A., C. CZIEPLUCH, U. HAMANN, *et al.* 1991. The *MYCN* oncoprotein is associated *in vivo* with the phosphoprotein Max(p20/22) in human neuroblastoma cells. EMBO J. **10**: 3703–3712.
63. BLACKWOOD, E.M. & R.N. EISENMAN. 1991. Max: a helix-loop-helix zipper protein that forms a sequence-specific DNA-binding complex with Myc. Science **251**: 1211–1217.

64. MÄKELÄ, T.P., P.J. KOSKINEN, I. VÄSTRIK, et al. 1992. Alternative forms of Max as enhancers of suppressors of *myc-ras* cotransformation. Science **256:** 373–377.
65. AYER, D.E., L. KRETZNER & R.N. EISENMAN. 1993. Mad: a heterodimeric partner for Max that antagonizes Myc transcriptional activity. Cell **72:** 211–222.
66. ZERVOS, A.S., J. GYURIS & R. BRENT. 1993. Mxi1, a protein that specifically interacts with Max to bind Myc-Max recognition sites. Cell **72:** 223–232.
67. BANNASCH, D., B. MÄDGE & M. SCHWAB. 2001. Functional interaction of Yaf2 with the central region of MycN. Oncogene **20:** 5913–5919.
68. KATO, G.J., J. BARRETT, M. VILLA-GARCIA, et al. 1990. An amino-terminal c-*myc* domain required for neoplastic transformation activities transcription. Mol. Cell. Biol. **10:** 5914.
69. CZIEPLUCH, C., A. WENZEL, J. SCHÜRMANN, et al. 1993. Activation of gene transcription by the amino terminus of the *MYCN* protein does not require association with the protein encoded by the retinoblastoma suppressor gene *RB1*. Oncogene **8:** 2833–2838.
70. BARTRAM, C.R. & F. BERTHOLD. 1987. Amplification and expression of the *MYCN* gene in neuroblastoma. Eur. J. Pediatr. **146:** 162–165.
71. BRODEUR, G., R.C. SEEGER, M. SCHWAB, et al. 1984. Amplification of *MYCN* in untreated human neuroblastomas correlates with advanced disease stage. Science **224:** 1121–1124.
72. SEEGER, R.C., G.M. BRODEUR, H. SATHER, et al. 1985. Association of multiple copies of the *MYCN* oncogene with rapid progression of neuroblastomas. N. Engl. J. Med. **313:** 1111–1116.
73. NAKAGAWARA, A., K. IKEDA, T. TSUDA, et al. 1988. Biological characteristics of NMYC amplified neuroblastomas in patients over one year of age. Prog. Clin. Biol. Res. **271:** 31–39.
74. BOON, K., H.N. CARON, R. VAN ASPEREN, et al. 2001. N-myc enhances the expression of a large set of genes functioning in ribosome biogenesis and protein synthesis. EMBO J. **20:** 1–11.
75. KHAN, J., J.S. WEI, M. RINGNÉR, et al. 2001. Classification and diagnostic prediction of cancers using gene expression profiling and artificial neural networks. Nature Med. **7:** 673–679.

Linkage Analysis in Families with Recurrent Neuroblastoma

PATRIZIA PERRI,[a] LUCA LONGO,[a] CARMEL McCONVILLE,[b] ROBERTO CUSANO,[c] SALLY A. REES,[b] MARCO SERI,[d] MASSIMO CONTE,[e] GIOVANNI ROMEO,[d] MARCELLA DEVOTO,[f] AND GIAN PAOLO TONINI[g]

[a]*Laboratory of Neuroblastoma Research, Advanced Biotechnology Center, Genoa, Italy*

[b]*Division of Medical Genetics, University of Birmingham, Birmingham, United Kingdom*

[c]*Laboratory of Molecular Genetics, G. Gaslini Children's Hospital, Genoa, Italy*

[d]*Department of Internal Medicine, Cardioangiology and Hepatology, University of Bologna, Bologna, Italy*

[e]*Department of Hematology and Oncology, Gaslini Children's Hospital, Genoa, Italy*

[f]*Department of Oncology, Biology and Genetics, University of Genoa, Genoa, Italy*

[g]*Laboratory of Population Genetics, National Institute for Cancer Research (IST), Genoa, Italy*

ABSTRACT: Neuroblastoma is a neural crest-derived tumor of childhood with a serious prognosis; only 20% of patients with stage 4 disease survive 5 years from diagnosis. Mechanisms involved in neuroblastoma development are unclear, but the engagement of many neuroblastoma-related gene(s) is suggested by specific chromosomal alterations. Most prominent among these is the amplification of the *MYCN* oncogene and the deletion of the 1p36 region. Other genetic aberrations have been discovered over the years such as deletions of 11q and 14q and gain of 17q. Although tumor aggressiveness greatly depends on the most frequent genetic abnormalities, to date no neuroblastoma-related gene has been discovered. Neuroblastoma usually occurs sporadically, but 1.5% of all diagnosed cases show familial recurrence with an autosomal dominant inheritance and incomplete penetrance. A comparison between hereditary and sporadic neuroblastomas led Knudson and Strong to gather that the two-hit hypothesis, proposed for retinoblastoma, could be applied to neuroblastoma. To determine if the 1p36 region harbors a predisposition gene for familial neuroblastoma, we carried out linkage analysis at 1p36 loci in two families with recurrent neuroblastoma. Similarly, we analyzed loci of chromosome 16, where a predisposition locus was recently mapped. We also analyzed markers located close to several candidate genes (*RET*, *NF1*, *GDNF*, *GFRA1*, *EDNRB*, and *EDN3*) involved to a different extent in other neurocristopathies. Our findings indicate that the candidate chromosomal regions and genes analyzed are not in linkage with neuroblastoma.

KEYWORDS: neuroblastoma; MYCN oncogene; 1p36 region; chromosomes; linkage analysis; neural crest cells

Address for correspondence: Dr. Patrizia Perri, Laboratory of Neuroblastoma Research, Advanced Biotechnology Center, Largo R. Benzi, 10, 16132 Genoa, Italy. Voice: +39-010-5737430; fax: +39-010-5737463.
perri@cba.unige.it

STATE OF THE ART

Neuroblastoma (NB) is a childhood embryonic tumor derived from neural crest cells that are destined for the adrenal medulla and the sympathetic nervous system in the normal developmental pathway.

The most relevant genetic defects associated with NB are deletions of the short arm of chromosome 1, consistent with the presence of at least one tumor suppressor gene,[1,2] and the amplification of the *MYCN* oncogene.[3] Other specific chromosomal regions are shown to contain NB-related gene(s), particularly 11q,[4] 14q,[4] and 17q,[5] but other candidate regions have been suggested, supporting the hypothesis that many genes may be involved in the pathogenesis of NB. Although many candidate genes deleted from these chromosomal sites have been suggested, to date the NB-associated gene has not been identified.[6,7]

Neuroblastoma usually occurs as a sporadic form with a frequency of approximately 9.8 per milion children. Among them, however, a few instances of familial clustering have been observed and their recurrence rate is estimated to be 1–1.5%.[8,9] Most pedigrees described are small, spanning three generations at most[10,11] or consisting of multiplex families with affected individuals in the same generation (i.e., cousins), without detection of disease in the intervening relatives.[12] Analyses of reported pedigrees indicate an autosomal dominant mode of inheritance with incomplete penetrance.[12,13]

Linkage analysis has allowed the association between some hereditary cancers and specific tumor suppressor genes (familial retinoblastoma and Wilms' tumor)[14] and genes with dominant mechanism (multiple endocrine neoplasia type 2A and neurofibromatosis type 1).[15,16]

Knudson and Strong[13] suggested that a two-hit hypothesis proposed for retinoblastoma[17] could be applied to NB. A comparison of 29 hereditary neuroblastomas (from 13 families) with 504 unselected sporadic cases[13] led to the following observations: 56% of familial cases versus 26% of sporadic ones were diagnosed in children less than 1 year of age; 23% of familial cases versus 5% of sporadic ones had documentation of multiple primary tumors. Conclusively, a penetrance of 63% was calculated.

The identification of a constitutional deletion in an infant with multifocal neuroblastoma[18] and the somatic deletions found in tumor cells in two siblings with NB at 1p36[19] suggested that the putative 1p tumor suppressor gene could also be involved in familial NB. Notwithstanding this, linkage between a series of 1p36 loci spanning the common region of deletion and familial NB has been excluded in a series of North American families.[20] A recent study by genomewide search for linkage has identified a hereditary neuroblastoma predisposition locus (HNB1) at 16p12-13.[21]

The aim of the present work was to identify chromosome regions that may be candidates for containing the NB predisposition gene(s).

MATERIAL AND METHODS

Two families with recurrent NB were studied by linkage analysis. Genotyping and haplotype reconstruction of patients and family members were performed using polymorphic markers mapped to the regions of interest. The first investigated region was the 1p32-36, frequently deleted in NB. In addition, markers located close to several candidate genes (*RET, NF1, GDNF, GFRA1, EDNRB,* and *EDN3*), reported to be involved in other neurocristopathies,[22–24] were analyzed in one family. Furthermore, we genotyped the two families using markers spanning chromosome 16p12-13, where a locus for NB predisposition was recently mapped.[21]

Genomewide screening was also set up to find new candidate regions.

Family Recruitment

To date, four Italian NB families and an additional three NB families from the UK were recruited. The Italian families were admitted to the Department of Hematology and Oncology of the G. Gaslini Children's Hospital between December 1988 and January 1995. English families were collected at the University of Birmingham, UK. Since constitutional DNAs for all family members were not available, a program of recruitment by clinicians is now dedicated to providing the lacking blood samples.

FIGURES 1 and 2 illustrate the pedigrees of the recruited families. Family IGG-E has three individuals affected by ganglioneuroblastoma (GNB) in the last generation, two first cousins and one second cousin (FIG. 1a). Family UB-NB1 includes in the last generation two half-brothers affected by GNB. One patient was dead with disease (DWD) (FIG. 1b). Family TG-ES consists of two of three siblings affected, one of them DWD, and their affected father (FIG. 2a). Family IGG-MS has a child affected in the last generation and her maternal uncle who was DWD in 1975 (FIG. 2b). Family IGG-M includes two of three siblings affected in the last generation, one of them DWD (FIG. 2c). Family UB-NB4 has two affected individuals, a child in the last generation and his maternal uncle, DWD (FIG. 2d). Family UB-NB3 consists of four affected persons from three generations: a child DWD in the last generation, her father, her grandmother, and her grandmother's brother, DWD (FIG. 2e).

Experimental Procedures

Blood Sample Collections and Nucleic Acid Extraction. Peripheral blood samples from each family member were collected and stored at $-80°C$. Afterwards, DNA was isolated using standard protocols.[25]

Genotyping and Haplotype Reconstruction for Candidate Chromosome Regions. Genotyping by analysis of polymorphic markers was carried out for better characterization of meiotic recombinants and delimitation of target regions for the NB-related gene(s). Genotyping of chromosome 1 (1p32-36) was carried out using 13 dinucleotide repeat markers (D1S243, D1S214, D1S160, D1S228, D1S507, D1S199, D1S234, D1S449, D1S233, D1S201, D1S496, D1S211, and D1S220) in family IGG-E and 6 VNTR/tetranucleotide repeat markers (D1S80, D1S1646, D1S1597, D1S3669, D1S552, and D1S2134) in family UB-NB1. Polymerase chain reaction (PCR) was performed with incorporation of $[\alpha^{33}]$dCTP. All markers were analyzed by electrophoresis through 6–8% denaturing polyacrylamide gel and allele size revealed by autoradiography.

To evaluate the involvement of *RET, GFRA1, GDNF, EDNRB, EDN3,* and *NF1* genes in the pathogenesis of NB, three intragenic polymorphisms (RET-int5, NF1.PCR3-int26, and NF1 53.0-int38) and nine flanking markers (sTCL-2, D5S2025, D5S2101, D10S1773, D10S187, D13S317, D13S170, D20S173, and

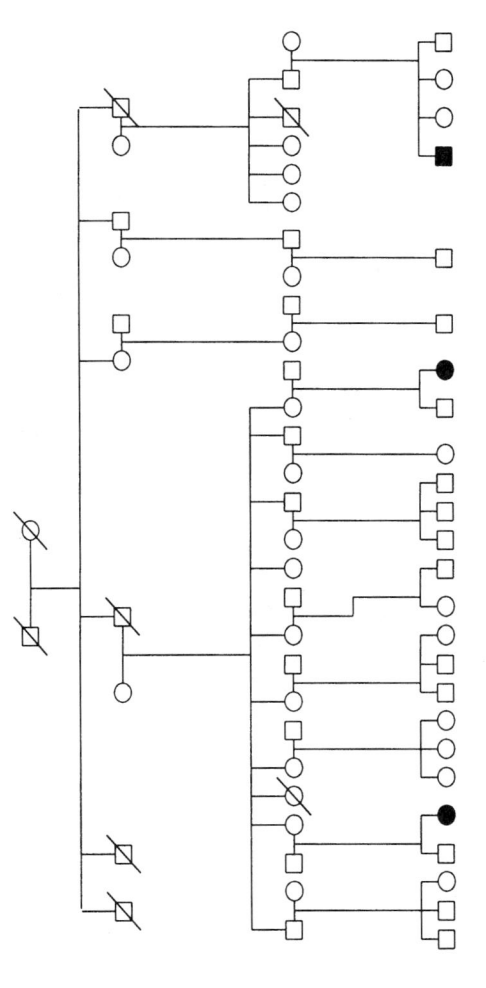
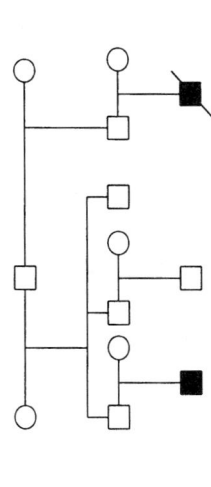

FIGURE 1. Pedigrees of the two investigated families for linkage, family IGG-E (**a**) and family UB-NB1 (**b**).

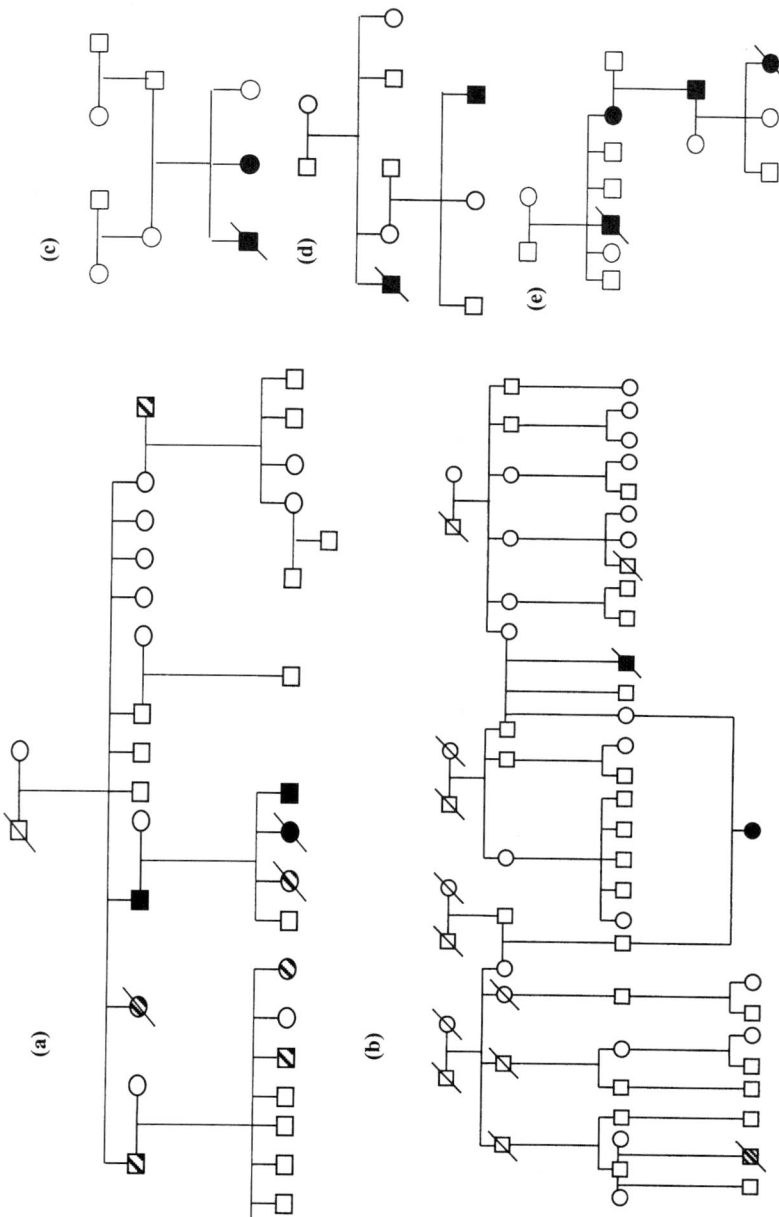

FIGURE 2. Pedigrees of other recruited families: TG-ES (**a**), IGG-MS (**b**), IGG-M (**c**), UB-NB4 (**d**), and UB-NB3 (**e**).

D20S171) were used. Primers were synthesized by an Oligo 1000-M DNA Synthesizer (Beckmann) labeled with FAM fluorescent amidite and purified with OPC columns (PE Biosystems), except for D13S170, D20S173, and D20S171, which were included in the ABI-PRISM Linkage Mapping Set.

For genotype analysis of chromosome 16, the ABI-PRISM Linkage Mapping Set Version 2 was employed.

DNA amplification and electrophoresis were carried out according to the manufacturer's instructions using an ABI 377 automated sequencer, and allele size was defined by GeneScan software.

Genomewide Screening

Genomewide screening was partially performed using the ABI Prism™ Linkage Mapping Set version 2, which includes 400 markers that define a ≈ 10 cM resolution human index map. The loci were selected from the Généthon linkage map, based on chromosomal locations and heterozygosity. The markers are organized into 28 panels. Each panel contains up to 16 fluorescent dye-labeled primer pairs that generate PCR products that can be pooled and detected in a single gel lane.

Linkage Analysis

Classic two-point linkage analysis was carried out in the pedigrees analyzed using the MLINK program included in the LINKAGE package.[26] Analysis was performed modeling NB as a dominant disorder with low penetrance. Additionally, a multipoint linkage analysis was carried out using the GENEHUNTER program.[27]

RESULTS

Genotyping of the 1p32-36 region allowed haplotype reconstruction in both families analyzed. None of the affected children in family IGG-E (IV-5, IV-19, and IV-22) share any haplotype, and even the patient still alive in family UB-NB1 has a different allele combination (FIG. 3). Negative lod score values for all 13 microsatellite markers analyzed provide no evidence for linkage in family IGG-E at the target interval[28] (TABLE 1A). Lod score values for VNTR markers in family UB-NB1 are not informative because of the inadequate pedigree structure.

On the basis of haplotype inspection, the alleles inherited by the three affected individuals, and the negative lod score values obtained in family IGG-E, linkage for *RET*, *GFRA1*, *GDNF*, *EDNRB*, *EDN3,* and *NF1* was also excluded (data not shown).[28]

Microsatellite analysis of chromosome 16 shows no shared haplotype in the affected individuals of family IGG-E (FIG. 3). Moreover, in family UB-NB1, individual II-1 transmits to affected son III-1 the haplotype he inherited from his mother, excluding the possibility that this chromosomal region can be shared by the two affected children (III-1 and III-3). In particular, patient IV-22 in family IGG-E has a different haplotype from the other affected children (IV-5 and IV-19) at those loci (D16S3075, D16S3103, and D16S3046), which have been reported to give a lod score of 7.06 by Maris *et al.*[21] Negative lod score values led to the exclusion of linkage hypothesis in family IGG-E[28] (TABLE 1B). Lod scores of family UB-NB1 are not reported, because of the low informativeness of this pedigree.

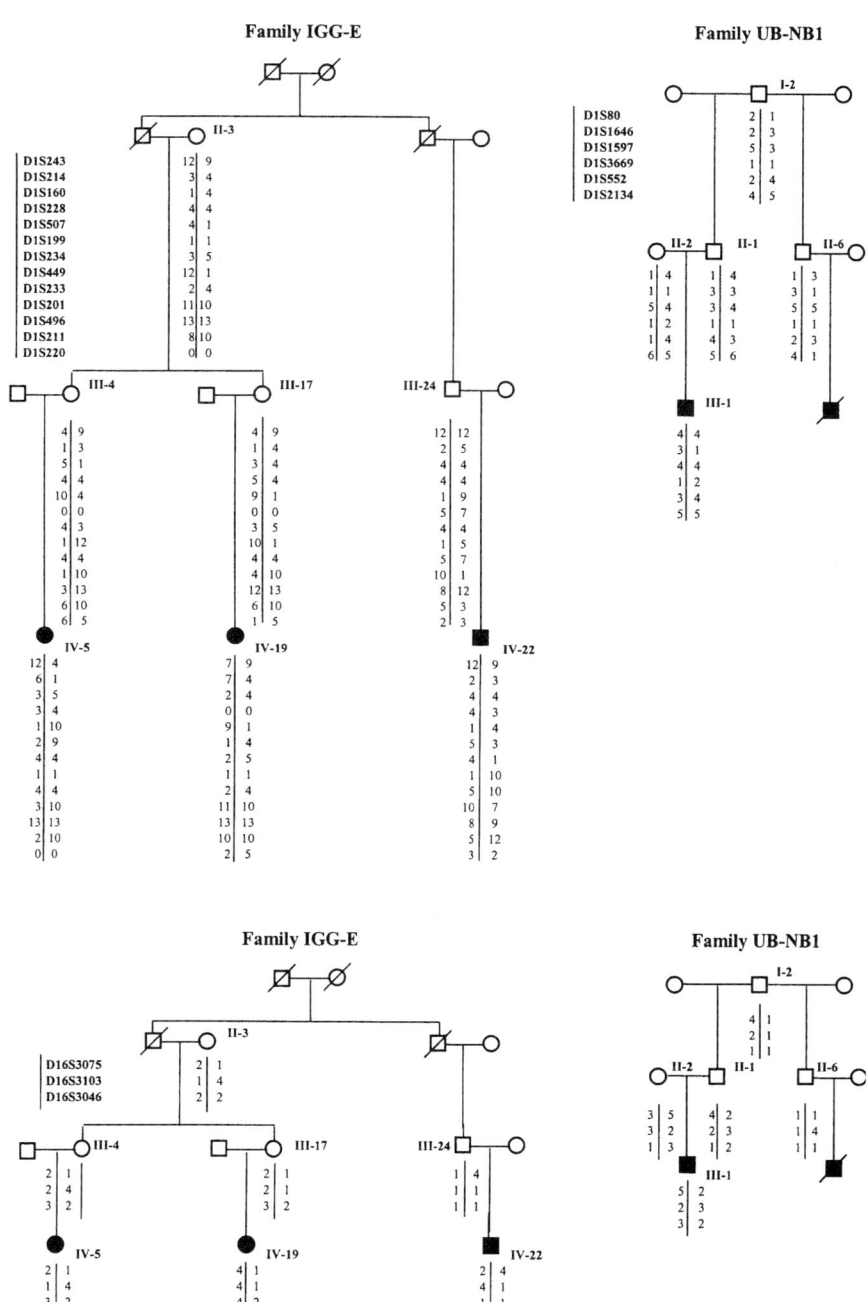

FIGURE 3. Haplotype reconstruction for markers at chromosome 1p32-36 (**a**) and markers at 16p12-13 (**b**) in families IGG-E and UB-NB1.

TABLE 1. Lod score values for markers mapping to candidate chromosomal regions: (A) All analyzed 1p32-36 markers show negative lod score values in family IGG-E. These do not support the hypothesis of linkage at 1p32-36

	θ Values						
Locus	0.0	0.01	0.05	0.1	0.2	0.3	0.4
D1S243	−5.29	−2.44	−1.16	−0.66	−0.26	−0.1	−0.02
D1S214	−5.29	−2.48	−1.16	−0.64	−0.21	−0.04	0.01
D1S160	−5.29	−3.80	−2.04	−1.24	−0.52	−0.20	−0.04
D1S228	−2.41	−1.23	−0.59	−0.35	−0.14	−0.06	−0.01
D1S507	−5.29	−2.38	−1.07	−0.57	−0.16	−0.02	0.02
D1S199	−2.37	−1.40	−0.63	−0.28	0.01	0.09	0.07
D1S449	−2.22	−2.07	−1.18	−0.69	−0.25	−0.07	0.01
D1S233	−2.31	−1.07	−0.44	−0.20	−0.02	0.03	0.03
D1S201	−1.89	−1.91	−1.96	−1.82	−1.11	−0.58	−0.24
D1S496	−2.20	−2.20	−2.21	−1.98	−1.19	−0.64	−0.27
D1S211	−1.89	−1.91	−1.84	−1.44	−0.77	−0.39	−0.15
D1S220	−2.30	−1.11	−0.49	−0.26	−0.09	−0.02	0.00

(B) Markers mapped to chromosome 16 show negative lod score values in family IGG-E. These results lead to the exclusion of linkage

Locus	θ Value = 0
D16S423	−1.895132
D16S404	−1.895080
D16S3075	−2.440647
D16S3103	−5.293050
D16S3046	−2.593520
D16S3136	−2.624985
D16S415	−5.293141
D16S503	−2.320533
D16S515	−3.028488
D16S516	−0.051825
D16S3091	−2.206515
D16S520	−0.344337

DISCUSSION

Cases of familial NB are rare, and transmission of the disease is compatible with autosomal dominant inheritance with incomplete penetrance. Knudson and Strong[13] estimate that 22% of sporadic NB may result from a germinal mutation involving different genes. This high percentage does not fit with the low incidence observed in familial NB, but it can be explained by spontaneous regression of a certain number of NBs in the first months of life and by regression of the so-called NB *in situ*, which are also described.[29]

The high frequency of chromosome 1p36 deletions in sporadic NB suggests that one or more tumor suppressor genes can be located in this region and that NB may develop according to the two-hit model.[30] The results of the present work exclude linkage between NB and loci on 1p32-36 in our two families, with three and two affected children, respectively, which agrees with reported data.[20] This suggests that familial NB predisposition gene(s) may be distinct from the 1p36 putative tumor suppressor gene.

Hirschsprung's disease and neurofibromatosis type 1 are sometimes associated with NB.[22-24] On the basis of different haplotypes in the affected individuals and negative lod score values obtained from the IGG-E family, *RET, GFRA1, GDNF, EDNRB, EDN3,* and *NF1* genes, involved in these neurocristopathies, were also excluded to be in linkage with NB.

Linkage analysis also excludes the involvement of chromosomal region 16p12-13 in the two families studied. This genomic interval of 28 cM, flanked by markers D16S748 and D16S769, was recently identified by a genomewide search to harbor the HNB1 for familial NB.[21] In 3 of 10 families the hypothesis of linkage was accepted with a maximum lod score of 7.06 for markers D16S3075, D16S3103, and D16S3046 by multipoint linkage analysis.[21] On the contrary, our data from the IGG-E and UB-NB1 families revealed for the same markers a negative lod score of −2.44; −5.29 and −2.59, respectively. According to these results, we speculate that different NB predisposition genes are involved in our families. For this reason, a genomewide screening has been set up to find novel candidate regions.

Current findings in familial NB suggest that other predisposition loci might be involved in the disease, and additional linkage studies are required to map them. The low penetrance and the presence of additional genetic and epigenetic factors may explain why NB occurs in only a few family members.

ACKNOWLEDGMENTS

This work was supported by the Associazione Italiana per la Lotta al Neuroblastoma, Project CNR-MURST, Research "Finalizzata 2000," Children Nationwide Medical Research Fund (UK), The Royal Society–The UK Academy of Science, and the Association for International Cancer Research (UK). The TIGEM laboratory is gratefully acknowledged for providing fluorescent markers. We thank the Surgery Department, the Pathology Division of the G. Gaslini Children's Hospital, and the clinicians and surgeons of the Associazione Italiana Ematologia/Oncologia Pediatrica (AIEOP).

REFERENCES

1. MARTINSSON, T., R.M. SJÖBERG, F. HEDBORG, *et al.* 1997. Delimitation of a critical tumour suppressor region at distal 1p in neuroblastoma tumours. Eur. J. Cancer **33:** 1997–2001.

2. WHITE, P.S., J.M. MARIS, C. BELTINGER, et al. 1995. A region of consistent deletion in neuroblastoma within human chromosome 1p36.2–36.3. Proc. Natl. Acad. Sci. USA **92:** 5520–5524.
3. BRODEUR, G.M., R.C. SEEGER, M. SCHWAB, et al. 1984. Amplification of N–MYC in untreated human neuroblastomas correlates with advanced disease stage. Science **224:** 1121–1124.
4. SRIVATSAN, E.S., K.L. YING & R.C. SEEGER. 1993. Deletion of chromosome 11 and of 14q sequences in neuroblastoma. Genes Chromosomes Cancer **7:** 32–37.
5. SAVELYEVA, L., R. CORVI & M. SCHWAB. 1994. Translocation involving 1p and 17q is a recurrent genetic alteration of human neuroblastoma cells. Am. J. Hum. Genet. **55:** 334–340.
6. BRODEUR, G.M., J.M. MARIS, D.J. YAMASHIRO, et al. 1997. Biology and genetics of human neuroblastomas. J. Pediatr. Hematol. Oncol. **19:** 93–101.
7. MARIS, J.M. & K.K. MATTHAY. 1999. Molecular biology of neuroblastoma. J. Clin. Oncol. **17:** 2264–2279.
8. BERTHOLD, F. 1990. Overview: biology of neuroblastoma. In Neuroblastoma: Tumor Biology and Therapy. C. Pochedly, ed. :1–27. CRC. Boca Raton.
9. CHATTEN, J. & M.L. VOORHESS. 1967. Familial neuroblastoma. Report of a kindred with multiple disorders, including neuroblastomas in four siblings. N. Engl. J. Med. **277:** 1230–1236.
10. MARIS, J.M., J. CHATTEN, A.T. MEADOWS, et al. 1997. Familial neuroblastoma: a three-generation pedigree and a further association with Hirschsprung disease. Med. Pediatr. Oncol. **28:** 1–5.
11. ROBERTSON, C.M., J.C. TYRRELL & J. PRITCHARD. 1991. Familial neural crest tumours. Eur. J. Pediatr. **150:** 789–792.
12. KUSHNER, B.H., F. GILBERT & L. HELSON. 1986. Familial neuroblastoma. Case reports, literature review, and etiologic considerations. Cancer **57:** 1887–1893.
13. KNUDSON, A.G. & L.C. STRONG. 1972. Mutation and cancer: neuroblastoma and pheochromocytoma. Am. J. Hum. Genet. **24:** 514–532.
14. CAVENEE, W.K., B. PONDER & E. SOLOMON. 1991. Genetics and cancer. Eur. J. Cancer **27:**1 706–1707.
15. EASTON, D.F., M.A. PONDER, S.M. HUSON & B.A. PONDER. 1993. An analysis of variation in expression of neurofibromatosis (NF) type 1 (NF1): evidence for modifying genes. Am. J. Hum. Genet. **53:** 305–313.
16. MATHEW, C.G., D.F. EASTON, Y. NAKAMURA & B.A. PONDER. 1991. Presymptomatic screening for multiple endocrine neoplasia type 2A with linked DNA markers. The MEN 2A International Collaborative Group. Lancet **337:** 7–11.
17. FRIEND, S.H., R. BERNARDS, S. ROGELJ, et al. 1986. A human DNA segment with properties of the gene that predisposes to retinoblastoma and osteosarcoma. Nature **323:** 643–646.
18. BIEGEL, J.A., P.S. WHITE, H.N. MARSHALL, et al. 1993. Constitutional 1p36 deletion in a child with neuroblastoma. Am. J. Hum. Genet. **52:** 176–182.
19. LO CUNSOLO, C., A. IOLASCON, A. CAVAZZANA, et al. 1999. Neuroblatoma in two siblings supports the role of chromosome 1p36 in tumor development. Cancer Genet. Cytogenet. **109**: 126–130.
20. MARIS, J.M., S.M. KYEMBA, T.R. REBBECK, et al. 1996. Familial predisposition to neuroblastoma does not map to chromosome band 1p36. Cancer Res. **56:** 3421–3425.
21. WEISS, M.J., C. GUO, S. SHUSTERMAN, et al. 2000. Localization of a hereditary neuroblastoma predisposition gene to 16p12-p13. Med. Pediatr. Oncol. **35:** 526–530.
22. GAISE, G., K. SANG OH, et al. 1979. Coexistent neuroblastoma and Hirschsprung's disease. Another manifestation of the neurocristopathy? Pediatr. Radiol. **8:** 161–163.
23. KNUDSON, A.G., JR. & G.D. AMROMIN. 1966. Neuroblastoma and ganglioneuroma in a child with multiple neurofibromatosis. Implications for the mutational origin of neuroblastoma. Cancer **19:** 1032–1037.
24. CLAUSEN, N., P. ANDERSSON & N. TOMMERUP. 1989. Familial occurrence of neuroblastoma, von Recklinghausen's neurofibromatosis, Hirschsprung's agangliosis and jaw-winking syndrome. Acta Paediatr. Scand. **78:** 736–741.
25. SAMBROOK, J., E.F. FRITSCH & T. MANIATIS. 1989. Molecular cloning. a laboratory manual. Cold Spring Harbor Laboratory Press. New York.

26. OTT, J. 1992. Analysis of Human Genetic Linkage. The Johns Hopkins University Press. Baltimore.
27. KRUGLYAK, L., M.J. DALY, M.P. REEVE-DALY, et al. 1996. Lander parametric and non-parametric linkage analysis: a unified multipoint approach. Am. J. Hum. Genet. **58:** 1347–1363.
28. TONINI, G.P., C. MCCONVILLE, R. CUSANO, et al. 2001. Exclusion of candidate genes and chromosomal regions in familial neuroblastoma. Int. J. Mol. Med. **7:** 85–89.
29. BECKWITH, J.B. & E.V. PERRIN. 1963. In situ neuroblastoma: a contribution to the natural history of neural crest tumors. Am. J. Pathol. **43:** 1089–1104.
30. KNUDSON, A.G., JR. 1971. Mutation and cancer: statistical study of retinoblastoma. Proc. Natl. Acad. Sci. USA **68:** 820–823.

Breast Cancer Registry in Palermo and Its Province

Incidence in 1999

A. TRAINA,[a] R. CUSIMANO,[b] M. LIQUORI,[a] V. FERRIGNO,[a] A. GUTTADAURO,[a] B. RAVAZZOLO,[a] A.M. GIAMMANCO,[a] AND L. CASTAGNETTA[c,d]

[a]*Cancer Registry, and* [c]*Unit of Experimental Oncology & Palermo Branch of IST-GE, Department of Clinical Oncology, "M. Ascoli" Cancer Centre Hospital, A.R.N.A.S., Civico, Palermo, Italy*

[b]*Department of Epidemiology, A.U.S.L. 6, Palermo, Italy*

[d]*Department of Experimental Oncology and Clinical Application, University Medical School, Palermo, Italy*

ABSTRACT: The incidence of breast cancer in the city of Palermo and its Province was investigated. The cancer rate was higher in the city of Palermo (100.8/100,000/year), a great southern urban area, than in the 81 municipalities of the Province (79.2/100,000/year). Rates were also compared with those in other geographic areas of Italy, showing a smaller than expected negative north-south gradient in incidence, especially in the young age group, as shown by the cumulative risk observed in the 0–54-year-old group. These findings confirm the role of recent life style changes in the cancer risk distribution.

KEYWORDS: breast cancer; Cancer Registry in Palermo

INTRODUCTION

Breast cancer is the most prevalent neoplasm affecting women in Western countries.[1] In recent years, the age-adjusted incidence of breast cancer has shown an increase in the European areas covered by Cancer Registries, and this pattern has been observed in several areas in the United States and Great Britain as well.[1–3]

The incidence of breast cancer varies greatly among different geographic areas, but also between regions of the same country. It is widely accepted that the incidence of breast cancer is lower in the south of Italy, even though this information is confined to the Province of Ragusa, a small area in the southeastern part of Sicily with 280,000 inhabitants,[4,10] with data on great urban areas being unavailable. To fill this gap, the objective of our study was to measure the incidence of breast cancer in 1999 in the city of Palermo and its Province (overall 1,250,000 inhabitants, half of whom live in the city of Palermo).

Address for correspondence: Dr. Adele Traina, Cancer Registry, Department of Clinical Oncology, Via Parlavecchio 139, 96127 Palermo, Italy. Voice: +39 091 666-4287; fax: 091 666-4352.

lucashbl@unipa.it

Ann. N.Y. Acad. Sci. 963: 85–90 (2002). © 2002 New York Academy of Sciences.

MATERIAL AND METHODS

Cases of breast cancer were collected by means of an information system based on records organized according to the International Agency for Research on Cancer (IARC) guidelines.[6] Each record contains 36 items related to cancer characterization (such as localization, histology, stage, and prognostic factors), social and demographic variables, and disease management, including therapy and follow-up procedures, as proposed in the EUROCARE project.[7] We included all cases of invasive breast cancer (/3 code according to ICDO morphology classification)[8] diagnosed in women residents in the city of Palermo and its Province. Standard sources of cases (clinical records, hospital discharge forms, hospital archives, and death certificates) were considered according to IARC guidelines. Linkage was done by the regional archive of hospital discharge forms relating to patients who resided in Palermo Province and were treated in Sicily or elsewhere. The death certificate archive was used to compute mortality/incidence (M/I) ratio.

We computed the following indicators:

- age-specific incidence rates resulting from the ratio between the number of cases in a 5-year age group and the resident population in January 1, 1999 in the corresponding group from data supplied by Istituto Nazionale di Statistica (ISTAT);
- the truncated rate limited to the 35–64–year age interval;
- the cumulative hazard of 0–54, 0–64, and 0–74 years;
- age-standardized incidence rate obtained by a direct method using the 1991 Italian population as standard; and
- mortality/incidence ratio resulting from the number of 1999 incident cases over the number of women dead from breast cancer in 1999, having 174.0–174.9 codices in the death certificate archive.[8]

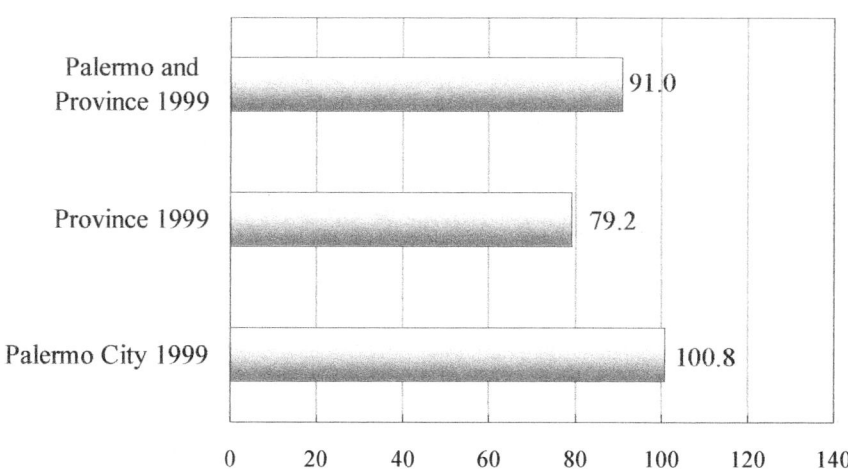

FIGURE 1. Age-standardized rates (Italian female population census -/100,000/year).

TABLE 1. Age-specific incidence rates (/100,000/year)

Age	Total	Palermo City	Palermo Province
25–29	8.7	4.1	13.8
30–34	35.3	49.7	18.2
35–39	67.4	72.9	60.1
40–44	146.1	186.7	89.9
45–49	157.1	174.2	132.9
50–54	131.1	116.0	153.3
55–59	156.9	164.5	146.8
60–64	189.5	197.0	180.4
65–69	214.1	252.5	169.0
70–74	219.2	198.7	241.9
≥ 75	178.6	223.2	132.0

TABLE 2. Distribution by stage

	Frequency	Percent
T1 N0 M0	154	27.6
T2-3 N0 M0	79	14.2
T1-3 N+ M0	173	31.1
T4	66	11.8
M1	13	2.3
Stage not available	72	12.9
	557	100.0

RESULTS

We collected 579 records of breast cancer: 22 were excluded because the cancer was not invasive (in situ). The linkage between the different sources allowed us to identify 557 cases of invasive breast cancer in residents of the city of Palermo and its Province. The overall standardized incidence was 91.0/100,000. If we separate data relevant to the city of Palermo and Palermo Province, the rates were 100.8 and 79.2, respectively (FIG. 1). The age-specific rates are shown in TABLE 1.

The truncated 35–64-year rate was 140.2/100,000. The cumulative risks 0-54, 0-64, 0-74 years were, respectively, 2.7, 4.4, and 6.4/100 M/I ratio was 0.36 (201/557).

The quality of the collected data is supported by the availability of pathological report in 93% of cases, the staging in 87% (TABLE 2) and the surgical treatment in 99% (TABLE 3).

TABLE 3. Distribution by surgical treatment

	Frequency	Percent
Biopsy	4	0.7
Lumpectomy	26	4.7
Quadrantectomy	22	3.9
Mastectomy	22	3.9
Mastectomy Patey	105	18.9
Mastectomy Madden	116	20.8
Mastectomy Halsted	6	1.1
No surgery	6	1.1
	557	100.0

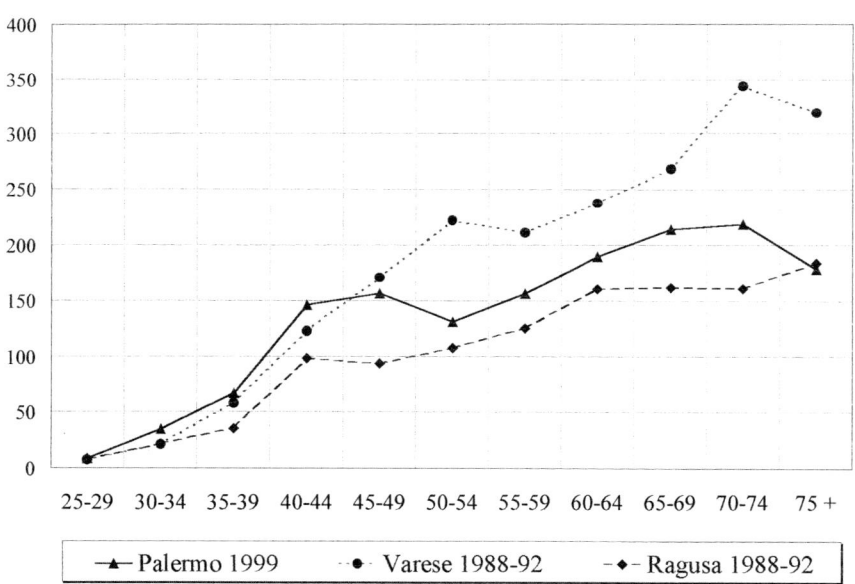

FIGURE 2. Age-specific incidence (/100,000/year).

DISCUSSION

The standardized incidence of breast cancer in the city of Palermo and its Province in 1999 (91.0/100,000) is lower than that reported for Varese (119.8), a small town in northwestern Italy, but this difference is smaller if we consider only the incidence of Palermo city (100.8). Evidence of a different breast cancer incidence in the city of Palermo and the other small municipalities of Palermo Province (79.2)

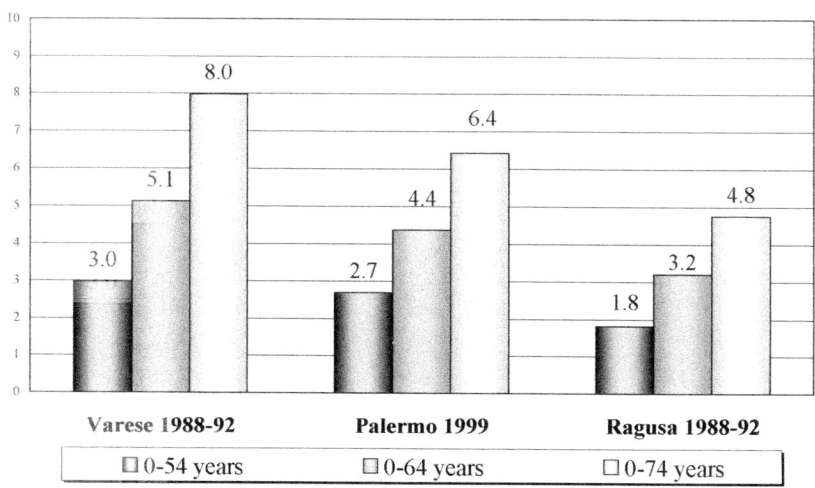

FIGURE 3. Cumulative risk (×100).

suggests a different cancer risk distribution, probably related to differences in life style. This may explain the apparent discrepancy between the present data and those of the Ragusa Registry. Even if the comparison is influenced by the different period of the survey (Palermo 1999 versus Ragusa 1988-1992), the rise in incidence of breast cancer in Europe could not explain such a divergence (91.0 versus 71.0/100,000). Data on the 1993-1998 observation period in Ragusa confirm the previous incidence rates (unpublished data).

Furthermore, the distribution of age-specific rates shows the typical difference between high and low risk areas, the former having rising rates throughout the life span, the latter with a flattening curve after the age of 50. Before 50 the curve for Palermo is equivalent to that of Varese (1988-1992), even though the standardized incidence rate is lower (91.0 versus 119.8), whereas the Ragusa age-specific curve resembles a typical low risk one (FIG. 2).

The observation that the 0–54 cumulative risk in Palermo in 1999 (2.7) is close to that of Varese (3.0) confirms that the risk in young women is similar for Palermo and Varese and is markedly different between Palermo and Ragusa (FIG. 3).

Evidence of a higher incidence of breast cancer in Palermo might also be useful to optimize the resources devoted to this pathology, also taking into account the intracounty (Sicily) differences in incidence.

ACKNOWLEDGMENTS

We wish to thank all of the institutions, physicians, and personnel who have contributed to achieving a deeper knowledge of breast cancer epidemiology in our county.

REFERENCES

1. PARKIN, D.M., S.L. WHELAN, et al. 1997. Cancer Incidence in Five Continents. Vol VII. IARC Scientific Publication No. 143. International Agency for Research on Cancer. Lyon.
2. PACI, E. 2000. The changing pattern of breast cancer and the role of risk factors. Eur. J. Cancer **36**: suppl 5: 16–17.
3. MUIR, C.S., J.A.H. WATERHOUSE, et al. 1992. Cancer Incidence in Five Continents. Vol VI. IARC Scientific Publication No. 120. International Agency for Research on Cancer. Lyon.
4. ZANETTI, R., P. CROSIGNANI, et al. 1997. Cancer in Italy, Incidence Data from Cancer Registries 1988–1992. Il Pensiero Scientifico Editore.
5. ZANETTI, R. & P. CROSIGNANI. 1992. Cancer in Italy: Incidence Data from Cancer Registries 1983–1987. Torino.
6. JENSEN, O.M., D.M. PARKIN, et al. 1991. IARC Cancer Registration: Principles and Methods. IARC Scientific Publication No. 95. International Agency for Research on Cancer. Lyon.
7. BERRINO, F., M. SANT, et al. 1995. Survival of cancer patients in Europe. The EUROCARE Study. IARC Scientific Publication No. 132. International Agency for Research on Cancer. Lyon.
8. PERCY, C., V. VAN HOLTEN, et al. 1990. International Classification of Disease in Oncology. 2nd Ed. WHO Library. Geneva.
9. CUSIMANO, R., A. TRAINA, et al. 1996. Breast cancer incidence in Palermo City (Italy). In Basis for Cancer Management. Ann. N.Y. Acad. Sci. **784**: 467–471.
10. BERRINO, F. 1998. L'incidenza del cancro in Italia. Epidemiol. Prev. **22**: 116–120.

New Approaches to Breast Cancer

Oxaliplatin Combined with 5-Fluorouracil and Folinic Acid in Pretreated Advanced Breast Cancer Patients: Preliminary Reports

V. LEONARDI, G. SAVIO, A. LAUDANI, L. BLASI, AND B. AGOSTARA

Division of Medical Oncology, "M. Ascoli" Oncologic Hospital - ARNAS Civico, Palermo, Italy

ABSTRACT: Oxaliplatin is a platinum compound that inhibits DNA synthesis. This drug has a broad spectrum of antineoplastic activity, and its results in breast cancer are promising. We began a phase II study in pretreated advanced breast cancer patients using oxaliplatin together with 5-fluorouracil and folinic acid, a combination based on the efficacy of both drugs in breast cancer and their different toxicity profiles. Seventeen patients with advanced breast cancer were treated with oxaliplatin, 5-fluorouracil, and folinic acid, and preliminary data were analyzed. The mean number of courses per patient was 2.82 (range 1-8). The main toxicity was gastrointestinal, with nausea and vomiting G2-3 in 53% of the patients. Hematologic toxicity was moderate with neutropenia G2-3 in 13% of the patients. Among 10 evaluable patients we obtained partial response in one and stabilized the disease in two patients. No data on survival were evaluated. The small number of enrolled and evaluable patients does not permit any conclusions to be drawn. The study is ongoing.

KEYWORDS: breast cancer; oxaliplatin; 5-fluorouracil; folinic acid

INTRODUCTION

Metastatic breast cancer poses a challenging therapeutic dilemma and represents one of the most controversial areas for medical oncologists. Conventional treatment has no curative impact on advanced disease, with a median survival of 12–24 months after evidence of metastases. Treatment of advanced breast cancer is still complex and partly controversial, as there is still no universally accepted therapy.[1] Anthracyclines and, more recently, taxanes and vinorelbine are the most active agents in this disease and are now commonly used as frontline therapy. Some new experimental approaches, such as high-dose chemotherapy, have not demonstrated a clear advantage over conventional treatment in terms of survival. To date, the main objective in this field is to improve the response rate, with the aim of offering patients good quality of life and good palliation of their symptoms of disease. Therefore, discovery

---

Address for correspondence: Vita Leonardi, p.zza Sturzo, 4 Palermo, Italy. Voice: +39 091-6664459; fax: +39 091 6664447.
vitaleonardi@iol.it

of new active drugs as well as exploration of new combinations and schedules of drugs with proven efficacy is clearly needed.

Oxaliplatinum (L-OHP) is a new agent of the diaminocyclohexane platinum family, and although its mechanism of action is similar to that of cisplatinum/carboplatin, its activity against tumor models is different from that of other platinum derivates. L-OHP demonstrates a broad spectrum of activity in colorectal, ovarian, and lung carcinoma and promising results in breast cancer.[2–5]

5-Fluorouracil (5-FU) is active in breast cancer. Folinic acid (FA) can increase its therapeutic activity. This cofactor is essential for stabilization of the link between the 5-FU metabolite (FdUMP) and its target enzyme, thymidylate synthase.[6–8] A major determinant of the action of 5-FU is considered the duration of drug exposure to the cancer cell. Prolonged infusions achieved higher response rates with a simultaneous reduction in side effects.[9–11] A number of investigators have reported positive results with the combination of 5-FU/FA in either pretreated or untreated patients with breast cancer with tolerable side effects.[12–14]

With this background, we began a phase II study in pretreated advanced breast cancer patients using L-OHP together with 5-FU and FA, a combination based on the efficacy of both drugs in breast cancer, the low burden of subjective side effects associated with their use, and their different toxicity profiles.

MATERIAL AND METHODS

To enter the study, patients had to fulfill the following criteria: histologic diagnosis of breast carcinoma, age ≤75 years, performance status according to ECOG index 0–2, life expectancy >3 months, adequate bone marrow function (WBC ≤4,000/mm^3, platelet ≥120,000/mm^3), serum bilirubin ≤1.2 mg/dl, blood urea nitrogen ≤50 mg/dl, no second malignant neoplasm except *in situ* carcinoma of the cervix and cutaneous basal cell carcinoma, and no severe and/or uncontrolled concomitant cardiovascular, respiratory, metabolic, or neurolologic disease. Informed consent was required from all patients. Before starting chemotherapy all patients were extensively staged with physical examination, medical history, chest x-ray, abdominal sonogram, 99Tc bone scan, hematologic and routine chemistry tests, ECG, and CT scan of the involved sites. Most of the aforementioned procedures were used to define the objective response at restaging.

Patients were evaluated for toxicity every cycle and for response after a minimum of 2 cycles according to WHO criteria. Briefly, complete response (CR) was defined as the complete disappearance of all signs of disease; partial response (PR) as a >50% reduction in the sum of the products of the major perpendicular diameters of all measurable lesions without the appearance of any new lesions; no change (NC) as a <50% reduction or >25% increase in the size of the tumor; and progression of disease (PD) as the appearance of a new lesion or a ≥25% increase in the size of pre-existing lesions. Response duration was defined as the time from treatment commencement to the documented data of progression (PR, NC) or the time from the date of response to the documented date of progression (CR) for responding patients.

The treatment regimen in eligible patients was as follows: oxaliplatin 130 mg/m^2 2 hours i.v. d1, 5-fluorouracil 400 mg/m^2 i.v., folinic acid 100 mg/m^2 2 hours i.v.,

TABLE 1. Patient characteristics

	n	Percent
Enrolled patients (n)	17	100
Evaluable patients for response (n)	10	58.8
Evaluable patients for toxicity (n)	15	88.2
ECOG	0–2	
Mean age (yr)	54 (range 31–73)	
Histology		
Ductal infiltrating carcinoma	11	64.7
Lobular infiltrating carcinoma	2	11.7
Ductal and lobular infiltrating carcinoma	1	5.8
Other	3	17.6
Previous therapy		
Surgery	16	94
Radiotherapy	13	76.4
Hormonotherapy	14	82
Adjuvant chemotherapy	14	82
Neoadjuvant chemotherapy	4	23
Advanced chemotherapy	17	100
I line	17	100
II line	13	76
≥ III line	8	47
Sites of disease		
Nodes	11	64
Liver	8	47
Lung	8	47
Bone	6	35
Skin	5	29
Breast	4	23
Soft tissue	3	17
Pleura	2	11
Ovary	1	5
Involved sites (n)		
< 3	7	41.2
≥ 3	10	58.8

and 5-fluorouracil 600 mg/m^2 22 hours of infusion d1 and 2. Cycles wee repeated every 3 weeks.

Patients one and two were treated with oxaliplatin 130 mg/m^2 for 2 hours i.v. on infusion d1 in combination with 5-fluorouracil 375 mg/m^2 i.v. and folinic acid 100 mg/m^2 i.v. d1–5. This schedule was modified because of grade 4 hematologic toxicity.

5Ht3 antagonists were employed as antiemetic therapy. Subcutaneous G-colony stimulating factor (GCSF) was given to patients with severe neutropenia when needed. If neutropenia and/or thrombocytopenia occurred on the day of planned chemotherapy, administration was delayed until recovery.

TABLE 2. Objective responses

	Patients (n)	Mean duration (range)
Evaluable patients (n = 10, 58%)		
Partial response	1 (6%)	9+
No change	2 (13%)	6.5+ (6–7)
Progressive disease	7 (46%)	

RESULTS

Seventeen patients with advanced breast cancer were enrolled in this study. Their main characteristics are shown in TABLE 1. All patients but 1 underwent surgery, 13 (76.4%) had radiotherapy, and 14 (82%) had hormone therapy. At entry all patients had progressive disease during previous frontline chemotherapy, and eight patients (47%) had received three or more lines of treatment for advanced disease. All patients had previously received a doxorubicin- and/or taxanes-containing regimen for adjuvant or advanced neoplasm. Sites of disease included the liver, lung, lymph nodes, skin, bone, breast, soft tissue, and others; 10 patients (58.8%) had three or more sites of disease. The type and duration of objective response are shown in TABLE 2. One patient (6%) had a partial response, two patients (13%) experienced stable disease, and seven patients (46%) had disease progression. The remaining seven patients were not evaluable for the following reasons: too early, three patients; toxicity, two patients; and lost to follow-up after first cycle, two patients. Subjective improvement in tumor-related symptoms was reported by responding patients, but the small number of responsive patients does not allow evaluation of these data. Because of the small number of enrolled and evaluable patients, survival has still not been evaluated.

Fifteen patients were evaluated for toxicity (in two it was too early). Grade 2–3 neutropenia was occurred in two patients (13%), grade 4 thrombocytopenia in one patient (6%), and grade 3–4 anemia in two patients (13%). N/V G2-3 was noted in eight patients (53%), G2–3 diarrhea in two patients (13%). Peripheral neurosensorial toxicity did not not exceed grade 2 and was always reversible. One patient (6%) experienced an allergic reaction to oxaliplatin. No patients had alopecia, and no cases of toxic death were recorded (TABLE 3).

DISCUSSION

Platinum analogues, widely employed antitumor agents, were long considered to be ineffective in breast cancer due to the very poor results obtained in heavily pretreated patients; moreover, the role of cisplatin (CDDP) has been revised on the basis of the results when employed in frontline treatment with an overall mean response rate of 9% in pretreated patients and 50% in previously untreated patients.[15,16] Oxaliplatin (L-OHP) is a third-generation platinum compound with broad-spectrum *in vitro* antiproliferative activity against a variety of murine and human tumor cell lines. In human cell lines, oxaliplatin is active against breast cancer cells and has

TABLE 3. Toxicity

Patients	Grade	Number	Percent
Evaluable for toxicity (n)		15	88.2
Cycles (n)		48	
Mean		2.82 (1–8)	
WBC (neutrophiis)	G1	3	20
	G2-3	2	13
Hb	G1	1	6
	G3-4	2	13
PTL	G1	1	6
	G4	1	6
N/V	G2-3	8	53
Mucositis	G2	3	20
Diarrhea	G1	1	6
	G2-3	2	13
Neurotoxicity	G1	1	6
	G2	4	26
Allergy	G3	1	6

greater activity than cisplatin in approximately 40% of the human cell lines tested.[4,5] A difference between cisplatin and oxaliplatin was also detected by the U.S. National Cancer Institute (NCI) COMPARE computer program. The studies indicated that L-OHP can be identified as a separate family, differing from cisplatin and carboplatin in cellular target, mechanism of action, and resistance.[17,18]

Results obtained with oxaliplatin in patients with advanced breast cancer during phase I and II trials, the efficacy of 5-fluorouracil, and the synergism observed between L-OHP and 5-FU in colon cancer prompted us to design these trials in which heavily pretreated advanced breast cancer patients were treated with L-OPH in combination with 5-FU/FA. Preliminary data showed a 6% partial response and a 13% no-change response in this selected population considered refractory or resistant to anthracyclines and taxanes and treated with a different regimen of chemotherapy for advanced disease. The results obtained confirm the good toxicity profile of this combination, but the assessment of neurotoxicity was clearly inadequate due to the relatively limited number of courses delivered (mean being 2.82).

Among the trials recently reported, Cottu et al.[19] used L-OHP 130 mg/m^2 with 5-fluorouracil given by continuous infusion in 61 women with advanced breast cancer pretreated with doxyrubicin and/or taxanes. They obtained a 25% response rate with a median duration of 7.5 months. In other trials, L-OHP was used alone[20] or in combination with docetaxel,[21] with an interesting response rate of 21 and 24%, respectively.

Although our efficacy data are worse than data of other studies, the number of enrolled and evaluable patients in our study is small, but data are still accruing. Moreover, patients enrolled in our trial are heavily pretreated (47% ≥III line of chemotherapy) unlike those in the aforementioned studies.

In conclusion, the preliminary data of our trial seem to show promising activity of L-OHP in combination with 5-FU/FA with moderate toxicity, but the small number of enrolled patients does not permit any conclusions to be drawn. The sudy is ongoing.

REFERENCES

1. HORTOBAGY, G.N. 1998. Treatment of breast cancer. N. Engl. J. Med. **339:** 974–984.
2. RAYMOND, E. & C. GESPACH. 1997. *In vitro* and *in vivo* antitumor activity of oxaliplatin in combination with 5FU and other cytotoxic agents in human colorectal, ovarian and breast cancer cell lines. Montpellier (France): Sanofi Recherche. 1995 Sept. 15. Internal Report. (Raymond, E., C. Buquet-Fagot, S. Djelloul, *et al.* 1997. Antitumor activity of oxaliplatin in combination with 5fluorouracil and thymidylate synthase inhibitor AG337 in human colon, breast and ovarian cancer. Anti-Cancer Drugs **8:** 876–885.)
3. FUKUDA, M., Y. OHE, F. KANZAWA, *et al.* 1995. Evaluation of novel platinum complexes, inhibitors of topoisomerase I and II in non small cell lung cancer (NSCLC) sublines resistant to cisplatin. Anticancer Res. **15:** 393–398.
4. FINK, D., S. NEBEL, S. AEBI, *et al.* 1996. The role of DNA mismatch repair in platinum drug resistance. Cancer Res. **56:** 4881–4886.
5. RIXE, O., W. ORTUZAR, A. ALVAREZ, *et al.* 1996. Oxaliplatin, tetraplatin, cisplatin and carboplatin: spectrum of activity in drug-resistant cell lines and in the cell lines of the National Cancer Institute's Anticancer Drug Screen panel. Biochem. Pharmacol. **52:** 1855–1865.
6. MADAJEWICZ, S., N. PETRELLI, Y.M. RUSTUM, *et al.* 1984. Phase I-II trial of high dose calcium leucovorin and 5fluorouracil in advanced colorectal cancer. Cancer Res. **44:** 4667–4669.
7. POGOLOTTI, A.R., K.M. IVANETICH, H. SOMMER, *et al.* 1976. Thymidylate synthetase: studies on the peptide containing covalently bound 5-fluoro-2'-deoxyuridylate and 5-10-methylene tetraydrofolate. Biochem. Biophys. Res. Commun. **59:** 972–978.
8. DANENBERG, P.V. & K.D. DANENMBERG. 1978. Effect of 5-10-methylene tetrahydrofolate on the dissociation of 5-fluoro-2-deoxyuridylate from thymidylate synthetase: evidence for an ordered mechanism. Biochemistry **17:** 4018–4024.
9. LOKICH, J.J., J.D. AHLGREN, J.J. GULLO, *et al.* 1989. Prospective randomized comparison of continuous infusion fluorouracil with a conventional bolus schedule in metastatic colorectal carcinoma: a Mid-Atlantic Oncology Program Study. J. Clin. Oncol. **7:** 425–432.
10. HOUGHTON, J.A., J.G. WILLIAMS, S.S.N. DEGRAAF, *et al.* 1990. Relationship between dose rate of (6RS)-leucovorin administration, plasma concentration of reduced folates, and pools of 5,10-methylenetetrahydrofolates and tetrahydrofolates in human colon adenocarcinoma xenografts. Cancer Res. **50:** 3493–3502.
11. MELI, M., S. PALMERI, V. LEONARDI, *et al.* 1994. A short term infusion regimen of cisplatin, 5fluorouracil and l-folinic acid in advanced head and neck carcinoma. Oncol. Rep. **1:** 1133–1138.
12. MARINI, G., E. SIMONCINI, A. ZANIBONI, *et al.* 1987. 5Fluorouracil and high dose folinic acid as salvage treatment of advanced breast cancer: an update. Oncology **44:** 336–340.
13. SWAIN, S.M., M.E. LIPPMAN, E.F. EGAN, *et al.* 1989. Fluorouracil and high-dose leucovorin in previously treated patients with metastatic breast cancer. J. Clin. Oncol. **7:** 890–899.
14. LOPRINZI, C.L., J.N. INGLE, D.J. SCHAID, *et al.* 1991. 5-Fluorouracil plus leucovorin in women with metastatic breast cancer. Am. J. Clin. Oncol. **14:** 30–32.
15. HWEE-YONG, Y., P. SALEM & G.N. HORTOBAGY. 1978. Phase II study of cis-dichlorodiamminoplatinum in advanced breast cancer. Cancer Treat. Rep. **62:** 405–408.
16. SLEDGE, G.W. 1992. Cisplatinum and platinum analogues in breast cancer. Sem. Oncol. **19** (1 suppl 2): 78–82.

17. PAULL, K.D., R.H. SHOEMAKER, L. HODES, et al. 1989. Display and analysis of patterns of differential activity of drugs against human tumor cell lines: development of mean graph and COMPARE algorithm. J. Natl. Cancer Inst. **81:** 1088–1092.
18. PAULL, K.D., C.M. LIN, L. MALSPEIS, et al. 1992. Identification of novel antimitotic agents acting at the tubulin level by computer-assisted evaluation of differential cytoxicity data. Cancer Res. **52:** 3892–3900.
19. COTTU, P.H., L. ZELEK, J. VANNETZEL, et al. 2000. A phase II study of oxaliplatin (Oxa) and 5fluorouracil (Fu) in advanced/metastatic breast carcinoma (Abc) patients previously treated with taxane (T): preliminary results [abstr]. Proc. Am. Soc. Clin. Oncol. **19:** 609G.
20. GARUFI, C., C. NISTICÒ, S. BRIENZA, et al. 2001. Single agent oxaliplatin in pretreated breast cancer patients: a phase II study. Ann. Oncol. **12:** 179–182.
21. AGELAKI, S., C. KOUROUSSIS, D. MAVROUDIS, et al. 2000. A phase I study of docetaxel (D) and oxaliplatin (L-OHP) as front line treatment in metastatic breast cancer (MBC) and non-small-cell lung cancer [abstr]. Proc. Am. Soc. Clin. Oncol. **19:** 443.

Ligand Binding and Cytochemical Analysis of Estrogen and Progesterone Receptors in Relation to Follow-Up in Patients with Breast Cancer

L. CASTAGNETTA,[a,b] A. TRAINA,[c] B. AGOSTARA,[d] M. MIELE,[a] I. CAMPISI,[a] M. CALABRÒ,[a] L. MARASÀ,[a] AND G. CARRUBA[b]

[a]*Unit of Experimental Oncology & Palermo Branch of IST-GE,* [c]*Cancer Registry, and* [d]*Unit of Medical Oncology, Department of Clinical Oncology, "M. Ascoli" Cancer Hospital Centre, A.R.N.A.S., Civico, Palermo, Italy*
[b]*Department of Experimental Oncology and Clinical Application, University Medical School, Palermo, Italy*

ABSTRACT: Soluble and nuclear estrogen receptor (ER) content was measured by ligand binding assay, and estrogen and progesterone receptors by immunohistochemical assays (ER-ICA and PR-ICA) in 214 patients with breast cancer recruited at the "M. Ascoli" Cancer Hospital Centre in Palermo, Sicily, to assess the discriminant and predictive value of these parameters. On follow-up, data from both ER-ICA and PR-ICA showed a statistically significant difference, PR-positive patients having longer disease-free (DSF) and overall (OS) survival than PR-negative ones. Conversely, ER status did not correlate significantly with both DFS ($P = 0.6$) and OS ($P = 0.2$). In particular, PR-positive patients had 59 ± 18 months DFS and 67 ± 12 months OS, compared to 51 ± 22 months DFS and 57 ± 17 months OS of PR-negative cases. The present evidence implies that a PR-negative status identifies breast cancer patients with early relapse, as also suggested by previous studies. It also agrees with the results of ligand binding assay of ER, where ER status is a good discriminant and predictor of response to endocrine treatment, but is unable to anticipate early relapse in breast cancer patients. Evidence that PR status is a statistically significant prognostic indicator deserves further study to ascertain whether or not PR should be regarded as an ER-dependent parameter or be related to other biological variables such as growth factor (e.g., EGF), oncogene (e.g., Her2/Neu), or tumor suppressor gene (e.g., p53) products.

KEYWORDS: ligand binding; cytochemical analysis; estrogen receptors; progesterone receptors; breast cancer

Address for correspondence: Prof. Luigi Castagnetta, Experimental Oncology, Department of Clinical Oncology, "M. Ascoli" Cancer Hospital Centre, Via Parlavecchio 139, 90127 Palermo, Italy. Voice: +39 091 666-4346; fax: +39 091 666-4352.
lucashbl@unipa.it

INTRODUCTION

In recent years, steroid receptor analysis has been widely used to classify breast cancer patients so that more pertinent individual therapeutic strategies can be designed.[1] The use of the ligand binding assay to identify high affinity–low capacity binding sites of estrogen (ER) in both soluble and nuclear cell fractions, often coupled with that of progestin receptors (PgR), has proved to be a helpful predictor of patients' responses to endocrine treatment and to have some prognostic value.[2] For years, however, limits inherent in this approach have emerged, especially among specific subgroups of patients; in addition, the potential value of newly identified tools was recently realized. The introduction of the immunocytochemical assay (ICA) has allowed the estimation of ER and PgR on tissue sections, thus eliminating the need for the large amount of tissue required in the ligand binding assay.[3–5]

Although cytochemical assay is being used increasingly, the resulting data are often inconsistent, and comparisons with data obtained by other methods are scarce. In the present work, we measured soluble and nuclear ER content using the ligand binding assay as well as ER and PgR by immunohistochemistry in 214 patients with breast cancer who were recruited at the "M. Ascoli" Cancer Hospital Center in Palermo, Sicily, to assess the discriminant and predictive value of these parameters on the basis of clinical features and follow-up of patients.

MATERIAL AND METHODS

Immunocytochemistry of Estrogen and Progestin Receptors. The presence of both ER and PgR was investigated using a modification of the ER-ICA and PgR-ICA methods, as described elsewhere.[6] Briefly, tissue sections were incubated with the primary rat monoclonal anti-ER or anti-PgR antibody. Control slides were incubated with normal rat immunoglobulin G under identical conditions. All slides were incubated with the bridging antibody (goat anti-rat), and exposed to the rat peroxidase antiperoxidase (PAP) complex after addition of chromogen substrate (DAB), and counterstained with ethyl green. Receptor staining was analyzed using the CAS200 Image Analyzer, which measures the percentage of positive nuclei and stain intensity. Cells were defined as ER and PgR positive or negative on the basis of a cut-off value of 10% stained cells.

Ligand Binding Assay of Estrogen Receptors. Ligand binding assay procedures for assaying both estrogen and androgen receptors have been extensively described elsewhere.[7,8] Briefly, fragments (20–50 mg/ml) of tissue were homogenized in buffer (Hepes 10 mM, EDTA 1.5 mM, dithiothreitol 0.5 mM, sodium molybdate 10 mM, and glycerol 30% v/v) using a glass/glass homogenizer. The homogenate was spun at $3,600 \times g$ for 5 minutes to separate the particulate (nuclear) from the supernatant (soluble) fraction. Aliquots (150 ml) of each fraction were incubated overnight at 4°C with increasing concentrations (0.1–5 nM) of the radioligand estradiol. A 100-fold excess of cold diethylstilbestrol was also used for competition studies. Receptor data were processed using Scatchard analysis and a modification of a least-square fit routine,[9] yielding both a dissociation constant (Kd) and concentration values. A positive ER status is defined by the concurrent presence of receptor in both soluble (S)

TABLE 1. Clinical features of breast cancer patients

	n	%
T 1	110	51.4
T 2	82	38.3
T 3	8	3,7
T 4	13	6.1
T x	1	0.5
N 0	96	44.9
N 1	112	52.3
N 2	5	2.3
N x	1	0.5
M 0	214	100.0
G 1	31	14.5
G 2	101	47.2
G 3	73	34.1
G x	9	4.2
PreM	73	34.1
PostM < 10	64	29.9
PostM > 10	77	36.0

NOTATION: T = tumor size; N = nodal status; M = metastasis; G = grading.

and nuclear (N) cell fractions, whereas the absence of ER from one or both fractions identifies a negative receptor status.

RESULTS

At presentation, the patients had a median age of 58 years (range 27–84) and a mean postmenopausal age of 13 ± 8 years. The median follow-up time was 63 months, ranging from 48–72 months. All patients underwent radical mastectomy or quadrantectomy and received adjuvant therapy according to their menopausal status, the presence of metastatic axillary nodes, and the ER status of the primary tumors. As reported in TABLE 1, a prevalence of postmenopausal patients (66%) and T1 tumors (51%) was observed. Nodal status was distributed between N0 (44.9%) and N+ (54.6%) patients, whereas Nx patients represented <1% of the total. Data from both ER-ICA and PgR-ICA assays are reported in TABLES 2 and 3, respectively. As can be seen, a different receptor distribution according to menopausal status of patients was observed; the PostM>10 was mostly receptor positive (ER, 69%; PgR, 63%), whereas the PreM was less ER positive (ER, 43%). The ligand binding assay of ER (TABLE 4) revealed that PostM>10 patients had a prevalence (64%) of ER positive (+/+) tumors, whereas ER-positive and ER-negative cases were almost equally distributed in both PreM and PostM<10 patients. As for follow-up, a statistically sig-

TABLE 2. ER-ICA in relation to menopausal status of breast cancer patients

	ER-ICA status ($n = 214$)	
	Positive	Negative
PreM	32 (43%)	41 (57%)
PostM ≤ 10	33 (51%)	31 (49%)
PostM > 10	53 (69%)	24 (31%)

TABLE 3. PgR-ICA in relation to menopausal status of breast cancer patients

	PgR-ICA status ($n = 172$)	
	Positive	Negative
PreM	40 (62%)	25 (38%)
PostM ≤ 10	20 (44%)	25 (56%)
PostM > 10	39 (63%)	23 (37%)

TABLE 4. Distribution of estrogen receptor status in breast tumor tissues

	ER (S/N) status ($n = 214$)			
	+/+	0/+	+/0	0/0
PreM	39 (53%)	18 (25%)	3 (4%)	13 (18%)
PostM ≤ 10	31 (48%)	19 (30%)	—	14 (22%)
PostM > 10	49 (64%)	12 (16%)	1 (1%)	15 (19%)

nificant difference emerged, PgR-positive patients having longer disease-free and overall survival than PgR-negative ones (FIGS. 1 and 2). Conversely, the ER status of these patients was not significantly associated with both disease-free survival ($p = 0.6$) and overall survival ($p = 0.2$). In particular, PgR-positive patients had a disease-free survival of 59 ± 18 months and an overall survival of 67 ± 12 months; conversely, PgR-negative patients had a disease-free survival of 51 ± 22 months and an overall survival of 57 ± 17 months.

CONCLUSIONS

Our evidence indicates that a PgR-negative status identifies breast cancer patients at high risk of early relapse, as also suggested by previous studies.[10] It is also in accordance with the results of our studies on ligand binding assay of ER, where ER status behaves as a good discriminant and predictor of the response to endocrine treatment, but its value in anticipating early relapse in breast cancer patients is limited.[11] Peculiarly, although PostM>10 patients exhibited nearly equivalent percentages of ER and PgR positivity, PreM patients showed a greater frequency (62%) of PgR-positive tumors. This may be ascribed to inappropriate cut-off values, leading to overestimation of the PgR content.

Concerning follow-up, results of both disease-free and overall survival curves were independent of the patient's nodal and menopausal status (not shown). Evi-

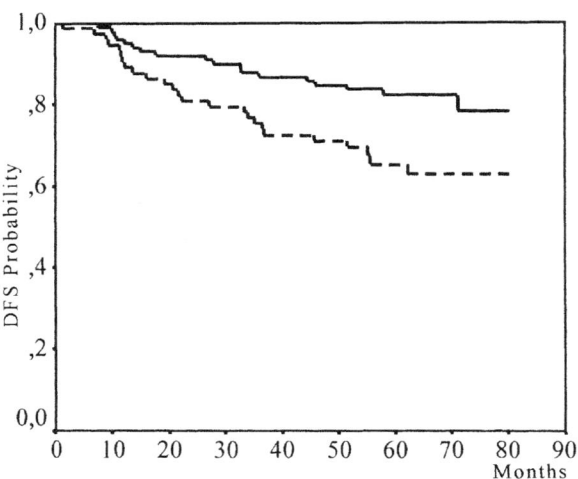

FIGURE 1. Disease-free survival of patients with breast cancer according to the PgR-ICA status of primary tumors. —, PgR-ICA positive; ----, PgR-ICA negative. Statistical analysis: $p = 0.012$.

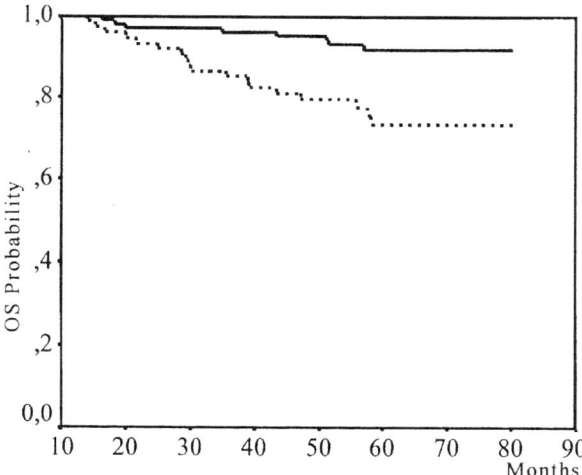

FIGURE 2. Overall survival of patients with breast cancer according to the PgR-ICA status of primary tumors. —, PgR-ICA positive; ----, PgR-ICA negative. Statistical analysis: $p = 0.0018$.

dence that PgR status is a statistically significant prognostic indicator deserves further study to ascertain whether PgR should be regarded as an ER-dependent parameter or, rather, should also be related to other biologic variables, such as growth factors (e.g., EGF), oncogene (e.g., Her2/Neu), or tumor suppressor gene (e.g., p53) products. We are currently investigating the potential relation of ER and PgR status in human breast tumor tissues with specific biomolecular markers and also their relation to the histopathologic features and clinical outcome of the disease.

REFERENCES

1. JENSEN, E.V. 1996. Steroid hormones, receptor, and antagonist. Ann. N.Y. Acad. Sci. **784:** 1–17.
2. CASTAGNETTA, L. et al. 1992. The prognosis of the breast cancer patients in relation to the oestrogen receptor status of both primary disease and involved nodes. Br. J. Cancer **65:** 167–170.
3. CASTAGNETTA, L. et al. 1999. Quantitative image analysis of estrogen and progesterone receptor as prognostic tool for selection of breast cancer patients. Anal. Quant. Cytol. Histol. **21:** 59–62.
4. HARVEY, J.M. et al. 1999. Estrogen receptor status by immunohistochemistry is superior to the ligand-binding assay for predicting response to adjuvant endocrine therapy in breast cancer. J. Clin. Oncol. **17:** 1474–1481.
5. BARNES, D.M. et al. 1998. Increased use of immunohistochemistry for oestrogen receptor measurement in mammary carcinoma: the need for quality assurance. Eur. J. Cancer **34:** 1677–1682.
6. HUANG, S.A. et al. 1991. Growth modulation by epidermal growth factor (EGF) in human colonic carcinoma cells: constitutive expression of the human EGF gene. J. Cell Physiol. **48:** 220–227.
7. CASTAGNETTA, L. et al. 1989. Do multiple ER assays give significant additional information for the management of breast cancer? Br. J. Cancer **59:** 636–638.
8. CUTOLO, M. et al. 1992. Evidence for the presence of androgen receptors in the synovial tissue of rheumatoid arthritis patients and healthy controls. Arthritis Rheum. **35:** 1007–1015.
9. LEAKE, R.E. et al. 1987. In Steroid Hormones: A Practical Approach. B. Green & R.E. Leake, eds. :93–97. IRL Press. Oxford.
10. PICHON, M.F. et al. 1992. Prognostic value of progesterone receptor after long-term follow-up in primary breast cancer. Eur. J. Cancer Clin. Oncol. **28A:** 1676–1680.
11. TRAINA, A. et al. 1996. Recent postmenopause but non ER status identifies a subset of primary breast cancer patients with an higher risk of relapse. Ann. N.Y. Acad. Sci. **784:** 491–495.

Modulation of Epidermal Growth Factor Receptor in Endocrine-Resistant, Estrogen-Receptor–Positive Breast Cancer

R.I. NICHOLSON,[a] I.R. HUTCHESON,[a] M.E. HARPER,[a] J.M. KNOWLDEN,[a] D. BARROW,[a] R.A. McCLELLAND,[a] H.E. JONES,[a] A.E. WAKELING,[b] AND J.M.W. GEE[a]

[a]*Tenovus Centre for Cancer Research, Welsh School of Pharmacy, Cardiff, Wales*
[b]*AstraZeneca, Macclesfield, United Kingdom*

ABSTRACT: An increasing body of evidence demonstrates that growth factor networks are highly interactive with estrogen receptor signaling in the control of breast cancer growth. As such, tumor responses to antihormones are likely to be a composite of the estrogen receptor and growth factor inhibitory activity of these agents. The modulation of growth factor networks during endocrine response is examined, and *in vitro* and clinical evidence is presented that epidermal growth factor receptor signaling, maintained in either an estrogen receptor-dependent or a receptor-independent manner, is critical to antihormone-resistant breast cancer cell growth. The considerable potential of the epidermal growth factor receptor-selective tyrosine kinase inhibitor Iressa (ZD 1839) to efficiently treat, and perhaps even prevent, endocrine-resistant breast cancer is highlighted.

KEYWORDS: breast cancer; estrogen receptor; tyrosine kinase inhibitor; ZD 1839

INTRODUCTION

Until relatively recently endocrine response pathways in breast cancer were described solely in terms of the intracellular pathways used by estrogens and the subsequent disruptive effects exerted by antihormonal treatment on estrogen receptor (ER) signaling.[1] Thus, it was frequently proposed that estrogens promoted tumor growth by binding to ERs, which then acted as nuclear transcription factors regulating the expression of genes involved in proliferation and survival mechanisms. By contrast, antihormones, acting to either reduce the amount of estrogens available to the tumor cells or bind the ER to antagonize the cellular actions of estrogens, prevented this flow of information to promote tumor remission.[1,2]

Address for correspondence: Prof. Robert I. Nicholson, Tenovus Centre for Cancer Research, Welsh School of Pharmacy, Cardiff University, Redwood Building, King Edward VII Ave., Cardiff CF10 3XF, Wales. Voice: +44 (0)29 2087 4922; fax: +44 (0)29 2087 5152.
nicholsonri@cardiff.ac.uk

A more modern view of endocrine response pathways, however, retains the concept that estrogens acting through ERs are central to the development of breast cancer, but also recognizes that it is naïve to consider ER signaling in isolation from the remainder of the cancer cell biology.[3] Indeed, an increasing number of elements within the breast cancer phenotype, notably including peptide growth factors, have now been identified that modify and can be modified by ER signaling.[3] As such, they have the capacity to significantly influence the sensitivity of breast cancer cells to estrogens. Importantly, however, these factors are also likely to be critical in the mechanism of response to antihormonal drugs. Moreover, they may be integral in the escape from antihormone control of growth that occurs on disease relapse.

Within this context, the current article outlines concepts regarding the interplay between ER and growth factor signaling in hormone-sensitive breast cancer. In particular, although antihormones suppress both ER and insulin-like growth factor (IGF) signaling during response, paradoxically they promote the expression of epidermal growth factor receptor (EGFR) and c-erbB2, receptors employed by epidermal growth factor (EGF)-like ligands.[4-10] Our recent experimental data demonstrate that increased expression of EGFR and c-erbB2 can occur *in vitro* after challenge with several antihormonal drugs.[11-13] Importantly, although such increases are redundant in antihormonal response, we have shown that the EGFR/c-erbB2 signaling network is ultimately harnessed by the cells, enabling re-establishment of their growth in an ER-dependent or ER-independent manner. These events thus appear to be critical in the generation of several forms of acquired endocrine resistance and insensitivity. Excitingly, examination of the phenotypic characteristics of breast tumors from patients with hormone-resistant disease in many ways parallels these experimental data.[14-19] Furthermore, our *in vitro* data also show that such endocrine-resistant or endocrine-insensitive cells are highly sensitive to the EGFR-selective tyrosine kinase inhibitor Iressa (ZD 1839). The compound obliterates EGFR signaling and effectively blocks antihormonal resistant tumor cell growth in the presence or absence of exogenous ligands for the EGFR. Because the antitumor effects are long lasting and synergistic with antihormones, the data highlight the considerable potential of such inhibition to efficiently treat endocrine-resistant and endocrine-insensitive breast cancer.

ESTROGEN RECEPTOR SIGNALING AND GROWTH FACTORS IN HORMONE-SENSITIVE BREAST CANCER

The concept that peptide growth factors can act as mediators in the growth of hormone-sensitive breast cancer is not a new one. It originated in the late 1980s, when it was first recognized that estrogens were able to stimulate expression of growth factor regulatory elements (e.g., transforming growth factor-alpha [TGF-α] and IGF-II) in hormone-sensitive human breast cancer cell lines.[20,21] Such actions significantly supplemented the cellular mitogenic responses and gene expression directly primed by estrogens.[22,23] Importantly, this concept, although not repudiated in recent years, has now been substantially modified to incorporate a further fascinating dimension. The intracellular signaling pathways associated with estrogen and growth factor action are more highly networked and interactive than was originally thought. Indeed, it is unlikely that mitogenic signaling arising from either of the pathways can operate efficiently in the absence of the other.[3] Moreover, this is perceived not only to be a function of their ability to co-regulate the expression of genes involved in proliferation and cell survival, but also, in part, to be due to a physical overlapping and common use of their signaling elements.[3,24–27] For example, numerous studies have shown that key receptors in such pathways (for example, ER and IGF-1 receptor [IGF-1R]) are subject to activation by both estrogens and peptide growth factors.[28–30] The important pharmacologic significance of such convergence in hormone-sensitive breast cancer cells is that antihormonal drugs possess not only antiestrogenic activity through their ability to block ER signaling, but also antigrowth factor actions by virtue of their ability to disrupt the intimate cross talk between estrogen and growth factor signaling.[4,5] Indeed, the increasing body of experimental data, supplemented by recent clinical studies examining the phenotypic profile during the tamoxifen-responsive phase of the disease, indicates that a combination of these antiestrogenic and antigrowth factor actions is most likely responsible for tumor remissions after antihormonal challenge of breast cancer patients.[31]

At this juncture, it is noteworthy that experimental and clinical data imply that not all growth factors are used equally to drive the growth of estrogen-sensitive breast cancer cells, a phenomenon governed, at least in part, by the cellular availability of growth factor receptors. Thus, estrogens appear to "favor" synergistic growth interactions with IGFs, with estrogens inducing expression of the IGF-1R. Not surprisingly, therefore, many ER-positive breast cancer cells *in vitro* and *in vivo* co-express considerable levels of IGF-1R, with an apparent strong correlation between IGF-1R and ER levels in the clinic.[6,32–34]

In marked contrast, estrogens appear to disfavor growth interactions with EGF and TGF-α. Expression of the EGFR protein (and mRNA), as well as its favored heterodimerization partner c-erbB2, is suppressed by long-term therapy with estrogens *in vitro*.[7–10,35] By contrast to IGFs, EGFR ligands are poor growth inducers of hormone-sensitive cells, where, at best, they promote growth responses that are additive (but not synergistic) with estradiol. Finally, inverse associations obviously exist between these tyrosine kinase receptors and ER expression in clinical and experimental samples.[14,15,17,18,36,37] In parallel, there is merely low expression of the EGFR ligand TGF-α, with activation of the important downstream signaling target for EGFR, MAP kinase, also minimal in ER-positive disease both in the clinic and *in vitro*.[11,16,19] In total, these data convincingly demonstrate that hormone-sensitive breast cancer cells possess potent mechanisms to limit EGFR/c-erbB2-mediated signaling.

This concept has significant clinical implications. Several studies have demonstrated that although antihormones disrupt favored ER-growth factor interactions to inhibit breast cancer cell growth (e.g., via diminishing activation/expression of IGF-1R), there is parallel de-repression of disfavored pathways. Indeed, we and others have observed time-dependent increases in expression of EGFR/c-erbB2 during antihormonal challenge of MCF-7 human breast cancer cells *in vitro* and within clinical material obtained during therapy.[7–10,38] The existence of such cellular mechanisms may offer breast cancer cells the option of using these pathways to (1) initially survive estrogen deprivation and (2) eventually reinstigate endocrine-resistant/insensitive tumor cell growth.[11,39]

Long-Term Effects of Antihormones on the Growth of MCF-7 Breast Cancer Cells

To further monitor the inductive effects of antihormonal drugs on EGFR and c-erbB2 signaling pathways, the interplay with ER signaling, and tumor regrowth during therapy (i.e., endocrine-resistant or endocrine-insensitive growth), we cultured MCF-7 breast cancer cells with various antiestrogens in long-term monolayer culture.[11]

Antiestrogens Induce EGFR and c-erbB2 Signaling and Instigate an EGFR Primed Autocrine Growth Regulatory Loop in Tamoxifen- and Faslodex-Resistant Breast Cancer Cells

MCF-7 cells are estrogen responsive for their growth and are growth inhibited by many antiestrogenic drugs.[40,41] However, their continuous culture in the presence of tamoxifen or Faslodex eventually generates sublines that tolerate the presence of the antiestrogens, regrowing at rates equivalent to those of the original hormone-responsive parental cells.[11] This closely mirrors the clinical scenario, where development of resistance is almost inevitable in patients demonstrating an initial endocrine therapeutic sensitivity.[42]

In our own studies, such antihormonal resistant MCF-7 sublines uniformly express increased amounts of EGFR mRNA and protein.[11] Thus, for example, while EGFR immunostaining of the parental MCF-7 cells demonstrates that they express only extremely modest levels of EGFR, both tamoxifen- and Faslodex-resistant cells contain up to 10-fold higher levels of EGFR membrane staining. We also noted parallel increases in c-erbB2 immunostaining in antiestrogen-resistant cells. Complementary data were previously reported for EGFR by Yarden *et al.*,[39] who showed that in the absence of estrogen, EGF had a much stronger proliferative effect, indicating an increased potential of such cells to use the EGFR for growth. Indeed, treatment of cells with ICI 164,384, a pure antiestrogen that similarly increases EGFR levels, also increased EGF growth responses, again indicating that therapies depriving cells of their estrogenic input increase sensitivity to EGFR ligands. Our phenotypic data monitoring EGFR and c-erbB2 in cell lines are further supported by a battery of *in vitro* gene transfer studies and the expression profiles observed in several additional acquired tamoxifen resistance models.[43–52]

Consistent with the concept that overexpressed EGFR and c-erbB2 may play a role in the development of antiestrogen resistance, we demonstrated by immunoprecipitation studies that these receptors are heterodimerized and fully active in such cells.[13] Because the tamoxifen-resistant variants also express numerous EGFR ligands, each of which can further increase the levels of activated EGFR and c-erbB2 and induce additional growth responses, it is likely that the new growth signal originates from an EGFR-primed autocrine regulatory loop. Significantly, Yarden *et al.* (1997) demonstrated that increased EGFR acts as a survival factor, because blocking this receptor with an EGFR-neutralizing antibody caused a twofold induction of apoptosis.[39]

Further assessment of the importance of EGFR/c-erbB2 signaling in resistant cells was made after we developed an immunohistochemical procedure for localizing the activated (i.e., phosphorylated) forms of erk 1/2 mitogen-activated protein kinases (actMAPK) using a phosphorylation state-specific antibody.[19] These enzymes are pivotal components of the intracellular phosphorylation cascade from the plasma membrane to the nucleus recruited for EGFR/c-erbB2 signal transduction.[53] Using this technique, we found that actMAPK was considerably higher in the antihormonal resistant sublines than in the parental MCF-7 cells and was further inducible by various ligands for the EGFR receptor.[11] Interestingly, complementary associations have previously been reported *in vitro* between acquisition of steroid hormone independence or tamoxifen resistance by ER-positive breast cancer cells and increased erk 1/2 MAPK phosphorylation.[54,52] We confirmed staining specificity in the resistant cells after its reduction by PD 098059, a MEK1 inhibitor previously shown to inhibit the phosphorylation and activation of erk 1/2 MAPK.[55] Importantly, PD 098059 was also a highly effective inhibitor of the growth of the antihormonal resistant cells, arresting cell proliferation.[11] These data in total confirm that this signaling pathway has been harnessed by the resistant cells and is of critical importance in their escape from the growth restraints imposed by antihormonal challenge.

Tamoxifen-Resistant Breast Cancer Cells Express and Use Estrogen Receptor as Part of the EGFR-Regulated Growth Pathway

The tamoxifen-resistant variants, like their clinical counterparts, continue to express ER at an equivalent level to that observed in the parental cell line. Significantly, the ER can be demonstrated to be involved in maintaining the new EGFR-driven growth regulatory loop.[56–58] Exposure of tamoxifen-resistant cells to the pure antiestrogen Faslodex at a dose that obliterates ER protein by increasing sensitivity of the receptor to proteolytic attack and disrupting its nucleocytoplasmic shuttling interestingly leads to a concomitant loss of activation of EGFR and c-erbB2.[1,59,60] There is an equivalent reduction in activation of the EGFR/c-erbB2 downstream signaling components erk 1/2 MAPK. Importantly, a parallel loss of ER and EGFR/c-erbB2 signaling after Faslodex treatment is associated with effective inhibition of the growth of the cells.[13] Because Faslodex does not decrease the total cellular levels of the EGFR, c-erbB2, or erk 1/2 MAPK proteins in such cells, it appears likely that this antiestrogen influences the activity of the growth factor signaling pathway by limiting the availability of one or more of its ligands. Interestingly, our preliminary studies indicate that a ligand targeted by Faslodex in tamoxifen-resistant cells may be TGF-α. Such a concept is reinforced by "add-back" experiments in which exogenous TGF-α or EGF not only activates EGFR, c-erbB2, and erk 1/2 MAPK, but also supports substantial tumor cell growth in the presence of Faslodex. Strengthening the EGFR pathway is thus able to entirely circumvent the catastrophic effects of this antiestrogen on ER protein in such cells. EGFR ligand-treated cells are thus refractory to the growth-inhibitory effects of both tamoxifen and Faslodex (i.e., complete endocrine insensitivity), data certainly implying that the primary growth regulatory role for ER in the tamoxifen-resistant cells is to maintain the efficiency of EGFR signaling.

Faslodex-Resistant Cell Growth Is EGFR Regulated Independent of Estrogen Receptor

In marked contrast to the tamoxifen-resistant subline, cells actively growing in the presence of Faslodex (i.e., Faslodex resistant) showed only very low basal expression of ER protein. Indeed, using our standard H222-ERICA assay, only 2% of such cells were shown to be weakly or very weakly stained for ER, also with lower ER mRNA levels than the parental cell line.[11] Faslodex-resistant cells also failed to express the classically estrogen-regulated gene progesterone receptor (PR) and showed no estrogen-response element (ERE) activity as judged through transient transfection of an ERE-bearing reporter gene plasmid construct into the cells.[11] Results in many aspects comparable with these data were recently reported by Larsen *et al.*[61] These data indicate that the enhanced EGFR signaling observed in Faslodex-resistant cells provides their primary mitogenic stimulus that is not supplemented by ER-mediated input.

EGFR/C-ERBB2 SIGNALING AND ENDOCRINE RESPONSE IN CLINICAL BREAST CANCER

Almost two decades have elapsed since the first report of EGFR in some human breast tumors.[62] Of particular interest was the observation that predominance of the protein was associated with elevated proliferative capacity, disease progression, and extremely poor patient prognosis.[14,15,17,18] Since that time, a universal finding has been that expression of the EGFR protein is highly variable within the breast cancer population. For example, ~50% of operable cases show EGFR membrane immunostaining and several studies have recorded that EGFR positivity is associated with an increased likelihood of failure to respond to endocrine measures *de novo*.[14,15,17,18] A parallel relation between c-erbB2 overexpression, poorer prognosis, and antihormonal resistance has also been observed, but these associations remain controversial.[14,17,18,63,64]

Similarly, we observed that elevated TGF–α expression is correlated with *de novo* endocrine failure in ER-positive disease, where there is also a prominent association with proliferation.[16] In addition, we observed a highly significant association between elevated actMAPK, shortened survival, and poorer quality and shortened duration of antihormonal response.[19] Enhanced actMAPK was observed in ~80% of ER-positive tamoxifen-resistant tumors that also demonstrated evidence of elevated TGF–α/EGFR signaling, with multivariate analysis demonstrating actMAPK to be a significant independent predictor for response duration and patient survival in such patients.[19] In total, these data certainly indicate the existence of an EGFR-driven autocrine growth regulatory loop capable of maintaining tumor cell growth in the presence of antihormonal drugs. Indeed, although few data exist that monitor EGFR/c-erbB2/TGF–α/actMAPK levels in breast cancer specimens obtained during endocrine response and at the time of relapse, our early clinical data employing highly sensitive immunocytochemical procedures have demonstrated small but significant increases in these elements at the time of acquisition of tamoxifen resistance. Moreover, it is feasible that there is cross talk of such signaling with ER in acquired resistant disease, because second-line antihormonal responses and substantial ER expression are commonly noted in such patients.[42,56–58,65]

STUDIES WITH THE EGFR-SELECTIVE TYROSINE KINASE INHIBITOR IRESSA

Inhibition of Tumor Cell Growth and EGFR Signaling

The observation that our tamoxifen- and Faslodex-resistant cells express high levels of EGFR, c-erbB2, and actMAPK and a profile of EGFR ligands led us to evaluate the antitumor effects of Iressa (ZD 1839).[11] This is a small molecule EGFR-selective tyrosine kinase inhibitor that we previously demonstrated to be highly effective in blocking growth of EGFR-positive DU145 and LnCAP prostate carcinoma cells *in vitro*.[66,67] The compound is a nonpeptide anilinoquinazoline currently demonstrating considerable promise in preclinical and clinical studies examining cancer types enriched for EGFR positivity.[68–70] It inhibits EGFR tyrosine kinase at concentrations at least 100-fold lower than those of many other kinases tested, notably including c-erbB2.[71,72] In line with its action as a competitive inhibitor of ATP binding to EGFR, Iressa was shown to prevent autophosphorylation of EGFR in cultured tumor cell lines, resulting in inhibition of the activation of key downstream signaling molecules.[68]

Significantly, in our breast cancer models of tamoxifen and Faslodex resistance, 1 µM Iressa efficiently blocked EGFR autophosphorylation and activation of erk 1/2 MAPK under both basal and EGFR-primed conditions.[13] In each instance, cell growth was markedly inhibited, contrasting the relative lack of effect of this drug with the growth of the parental endocrine-responsive MCF-7 cells.[11] Importantly, the growth inhibitory effects of Iressa were long lasting, indicating that the autocrine EGFR loop is critical for the growth of these antihormonal resistant cells and that no other mitogenic network is readily available when EGFR signaling is blocked. The increase in cellular expression of EGFR generated by antihormones thus appears to provide a promising molecular target for effective treatment of endocrine-resistant and endocrine-insensitive phases of the disease. Because parallel analysis of EGFR expression profiles in resistant breast tumor specimens indicates that this concept could prove applicable to clinical disease, trial data with Iressa in such breast cancer patients are eagerly awaited.[14,15,17,18]

Combination of Antiestrogen and anti-EGFR Treatment Efficiently Blocks Development of Resistance in Parental Antihormone-Sensitive Breast Cancer Cells

As just described, in our breast cancer cell lines the upregulation of EGFR proved to be consistently critical in the development of antihormone resistance. In anticipation of their switch to this essential EGFR pathway used in resistance, we undertook experiments in which the parental antihormone-responsive MCF-7 cells were treated with Iressa alone or in combination with tamoxifen or Faslodex. Importantly, although Iressa was largely without additive growth inhibitory effect with the antihormones during the first month of therapy, the agents thereafter show synergistic growth inhibitory activity, fully blocking the development of antihormone resistance (J.M.W. Gee & R.I. Nicholson, in preparation). Indeed, during this period, not only did Iressa substantially suppress proliferative activity within the dually-treated cells, but also its presence led to massive loss of cell numbers because of marked increases in the rate of apoptosis. This finding is highly supportive of the concept that combination therapies that simultaneously target estrogen and growth factor signaling may be more effective than the sequential use of such drugs. Moreover, these exciting experimental studies indicate that Iressa may prevent the development of the endocrine-resistant state.

Herceptin Challenge Reveals an Important Role for c-erbB2 in Directing the Growth of Tamoxifen-Resistant Cells

Although the data with Iressa that we have presented clearly demonstrate a central role for EGFR in the development of antihormone resistance, it is equally evident that phosphorylation of c-erbB2, the favored heterodimerization partner of the EGFR, is also relevant.[35] We have thus examined the role of c-erbB2 in antihormone-resistant cell growth using Herceptin, a c-erbB2-directed antibody therapy that inhibits the growth of many c-erbB2-positive cancer cell lines and promotes tumor remission in breast cancers overexpressing c-erbB2 by gene amplification.[73–75] We have noted that Herceptin is highly effective in inhibiting the growth of the tamoxifen-resistant variants, in marked contrast to its lack of effect on the parental hormone-responsive cell line. Complementary data have been obtained by Kurokawa *et al.*[52] who report efficacy of a small molecule inhibitor of this receptor in their MCF-7 model of tamoxifen resistance derived by stable transfection of c-erbB2 cDNA.[52] Our data indicate that (1) the role of c-erbB2 in growth regulation is extremely limited in parental antihormone-sensitive cells, and (2) autocrine activation of EGFR in tamoxifen-resistant cells recruits the c-erbB2 receptor protein as an essential partner directing cell growth.

SUMMARY AND CONCLUSIONS

Antiestrogen therapy is considered by many as the first-line therapeutic option for the management of estrogen receptor-positive breast cancer. Unfortunately, clinical application of such endocrine measures has revealed that responses are remarkably variable and often short-lived. An understanding of the complex mechanisms contributing towards loss of antiestrogen response is an important research goal, because it should allow a rational approach to be taken in the effective treatment, delay, or even prevention of the development of resistance, thereby severely compromising the disease process and improving patient survival.

Significantly, in our current studies we demonstrated that increases in EGFR/c-erbB2/actMAPK signaling can promote tamoxifen and Faslodex resistance in a human breast cancer cell line *in vitro* and that resistant growth can be inhibited in a sustained manner by blocking EGFR signaling using Iressa. Moreover, if Iressa is used to treat hormone-responsive cells in combination with either of the antiestrogens, it increases tumor cell kill to such a degree that resistance to these agents cannot occur. Clinical trials of Iressa are now obviously required to determine if such responses apply as fully to human breast cancer exposed to antihormones *in vivo* as they apparently do *in vitro*. Finally, our model indicates that in order for breast cancer cells to escape the cellular actions of antihormones, they must possess compensatory survival pathways that ultimately allow the development of drug resistance. The strategic targeting of such survival factors could potentially prove a highly complementary addition to the existing pharmacologic armory appropriate to the cancer patient. The identification and exploitation of such pathways in cancer cells treated with antihormones or chemotherapeutic agents are now the primary research goal at the Tenovus Centre for Cancer Research.

REFERENCES

1. SEERY, L.T., J.M.W. GEE, O.L. DEWHURST & R.I. NICHOLSON. 1999. *In* Molecular mechanisms of antioestrogen action. M. Oettel & E. Schillinger, eds. :201–220. Springer-Verlag. Berlin.
2. NICHOLSON, R.I., D.L. MANNING & J.M.W. GEE. 1993. New anti-hormonal approaches to breast cancer therapy. Drugs of Today **29:** 363–372.
3. NICHOLSON, R.I. & J.M.W. GEE. 2000. Oestrogen and growth factor cross-talk and endocrine insensitivity and acquired resistance in breast cancer. Br. J. Cancer **82:** 501–513.
4. FREISS, G., H. Rochefort & F. VIGNON. 1990. Mechanisms of 4-hydroxytamoxifen antigrowth factor activity in breast cancer cells: alterations of growth factor receptor binding sites and tyrosine kinase activity. Biochem. Biophys. Res. Commun. **31:** 919–926.
5. GUVAKOVA, M.A. & E. SURMACZ. 1997. Tamoxifen interferes with the insulin-like growth factor I receptor (IGF-1R) signalling pathway in breast cancer cells. Cancer Res. **57:** 2606–2610.
6. SURMACZ, E. 2000. Function of the IGF-1 receptor in breast cancer. J. Mammary Gland Biol. Neoplasia **5:** 95–105.
7. DATI, C., S. ANTONIOTTI, D. TAVERNA, *et al.* 1990. Inhibition of c-erbB2 oncogene expression by oestrogens in human breast cancer cells. Oncogene **5:** 1001–1006.
8. CHRYSOGELOS, S.A., R.I. YARDEN, A.H. LAUBER & J.M. MURPHY. 1994. Mechanisms of EGF receptor regulation in breast cancer cells. Breast Cancer Res. Treat. **31:** 227–236.
9. YARDEN, R.I., A.H. LAUBER, D. EL-ASHRY & S.A. CHRYSOGELOS. 1996. Bimodal regulation of epidermal growth factor receptor by estrogen in breast cancer cells. Endocrinology **137:** 2739–2747.
10. DEFAZIO, A., Y.E. CHIEW, M. MCEVOY, *et al.* 1997. Antisense estrogen receptor RNA expression increases epidermal growth factor receptor gene expression in breast cancer cells. Cell Growth Differ. **8:** 903–911.
11. MCCLELLAND, R.A., D. Barrow, T.A. MADDEN, *et al.* 2001. Enhanced epidermal growth factor receptor signalling in MCF-7 breast cancer cells after long-term culture in the presence of the pure antioestrogen ICI 182780 (Faslodex). Endocrinology **142:** 2776–2788.
12. JONES, H.E., J. PAMMENT, J.M.W. GEE, *et al.* 2002. Enhanced epidermal growth factor receptor signalling in MCF-7 breast cancer cells following long-term culture in the presence of tamoxifen. Submitted.
13. KNOWLDEN, J.M., I. HUTCHESON, J.M.W. GEE & R.I. NICHOLSON. 2002. Increased EGFR signalling is associated with the development of endocrine resistance in breast cancer cells. Submitted.
14. NICHOLSON, R.I., R.A. McClelland, P. FINLAY, *et al.* 1993. Relationship between EGF-R, c-erbB2 protein expression and Ki67 immunostaining in breast cancer and hormone sensitivity. Eur. J. Cancer **29A:** 1018–1023.
15. NICHOLSON, R.I., R.A. MCCLELLAND, J.M. GEE, *et al.* 1994. Epidermal growth factor receptor expression in breast cancer: association with response to endocrine therapy. Breast Cancer Res. Treat. **29:** 117–125.

16. NICHOLSON, R.I., R.A. MCCLELLAND, J.M. GEE, et al. 1994. Transforming growth factor-alpha and endocrine sensitivity in breast cancer. Cancer Res. **54:** 1684–1689.
17. NICHOLSON, R.I., J.M.W. GEE, M.E. HARPER, et al. 1997. erbB signalling in clinical breast cancer: relationship to endocrine sensitivity. Endocrin. Rel. Cancer **4:** 1–9.
18. NICHOLSON, R.I., J.M.W. GEE, H. JONES, et al. 1997. In erbB Signalling and Endocrine Sensitivity of Human Breast Cancer. R.B. Lichtner & R.N. Harkins, Eds. :105–128. Springer Verlag Publ. Boston.
19. GEE, J.M., J.F. ROBERTSON, I.O. ELLIS & R.I. NICHOLSON. 2001. Phosphorylation of erk 1/2 mitogen-activated protein kinase is associated with poor response to anti-hormonal therapy and decreased patient survival in clinical breast cancer. Int. J. Cancer (Predictive Oncol.) **95:** 247–254.
20. BATES, S.E., N.E. DAVIDSON, E.M. VALVERIUS, et al. 1988. Expression of transforming growth factor alpha and its messenger ribonucleic acid in human breast cancer: its regulation by estrogen and its possible functional significance. Mol. Endocrinol. **2:** 543–555.
21. LEE, A.V., P. DARBRE & R.J. KING. 1994. Processing of insulin-like growth factor-II (IGF-II) by human breast cancer cells. Mol. Cell Endocrinol. **99:** 211–220.
22. CHO, H., S.M. ARONICA & B.S. KATZENELLENBOGEN. 1994. Regulation of progesterone receptor gene expression in MCF-7 breast cancer cells: a comparison of the effects of cyclic adenosine 3′, 5′-monophosphate, estradiol, insulin-like growth factor-I, and serum factors. Endocrinology **134:** 658–664.
23. SMITH, C.L. 1998. Cross-talk between peptide growth factor and estrogen receptor signaling pathways. Biol. Reprod. **58:** 627–632.
24. MUSGROVE, E.A., J.A. HAMILTON, C.S. LEE, et al. 1993. Growth factor, steroid and steroid antagonist regulation of cyclin gene expression associated with changes in T-47D human breast cancer cell cycle progression. Mol. Cell Biol. **13:** 3577–3587.
25. LUKAS, J., J. BARTKOVA & J. BARTEK. 1996. Convergence of mitogenic signalling cascades from diverse classes of receptors at the cyclin D-cyclin-dependent kinase-pRb-controlled G1 checkpoint. Mol. Cell Biol. **16:** 6917–6925.
26. HUANG, Y., S. RAY, J.C. REED, et al. 1997. Estrogen increases intracellular p26Bcl-2 to p21Bax ratios and inhibits taxol-induced apoptosis of human breast cancer MCF-7 cells. Breast Cancer Res. Treat. **42:** 73–81.
27. WANG, Q., P. MALOOF, H. WANG, et al. 1998. Basic fibroblast growth factor downregulates Bcl-2 and promotes apoptosis in MCF-7 human breast cancer cells. Exp. Cell Res. **238:** 177–187.
28. ARONICA, S.M. & B.S. KATZENELLENBOGEN. 1993. Stimulation of estrogen receptor-mediated transcription and alteration in the phosphorylation state of the rat uterine estrogen receptor by estrogen, cyclic adenosinemonophosphate, and insulin-like growth factor-I. Mol. Endocrinol. **7:** 743–752.
29. BUNONE, G., P.A. BRIAND, R.J. MIKSICEK & D. PICARD. 1996. Activation of the unliganded estrogen receptor by EGF involves the MAP kinase pathway and direct phosphorylation. EMBO J. **15:** 2174–2183.
30. RICHARDS, R.G., R.P. DIAUGUSTINE, P. PETRUSZ, et al. 1996. Estradiol stimulates tyrosine phosphorylation of the insulin-like growth factor-1 receptor and insulin receptor substrate-1 in the uterus. Proc. Natl. Acad. Sci. USA **93:** 12002–12007.
31. GEE, J.M.W., T.A. MADDEN, J.F.R. ROBERTSON & R.I. NICHOLSON. 2002. Clinical response and resistance to SERMS. Endocr. Manage. Breast Cancer. In press.
32. DUPONT, J., M. KARAS & D. LEROITH. 2000. The potentiation of estrogen on insulin-like growth factor I action in MCF-7 human breast cancer cells includes cell cycle components. J. Biol. Chem. **275:** 35893–35901.
33. RAILO, M.J., K. VON SMITTEN & F. PEKONEN. 1994. The prognostic value of insulin-like growth factor-I in breast cancer patients. Results of a follow-up study on 126 patients. Eur. J. Cancer **30A:** 307–311.
34. HAPPERFIELD, L.C., D.W. MILES, D.M. BARNES, et al. 1997. The localization of the insulin-like growth factor receptor 1 (IGFR-1) in benign and malignant breast tissue. Pathology **183:** 412–417.
35. MARTINEZ-LACACI, I., C. BIANCO, M. DE SANTIS & D. SALOMON. 1999. In Breast Cancer: Molecular Genetics, Pathogenesis and Therapeutics. A.M. Bowcock, Ed. :1–30. Humana Press. New Jersey.

36. SHARMA, A.K., K. HORGAN, A. DOUGLAS-JONES, et al. 1994. Dual immunocytochemical analysis of oestrogen and epidermal growth factor receptors in human breast cancer. Br. J. Cancer **69:** 1032–1037.
37. SHARMA, A.K., K. HORGAN, R.A. MCCLELLAND, et al. 1994. A dual immunocytochemical assay for oestrogen and epidermal growth factor receptors in tumour cell lines. Histochem. J. **26:** 306–310.
38. WARRI, A.M., A.M. LAINE, K.E. MAJASUO, et al. 1991. Estrogen suppression of erbB2 expression is associated with increased growth rate of ZR-75-1 human breast cancer cells *in vitro* and in nude mice. Int. J. Cancer **49:** 616–623.
39. YARDEN, R.I., M.A. WILSON, M. BARTH & S.A. CHRYSOGELOS. 1997. *In* EGF Receptor in Tumour Growth and Progression. R.B. Lichtner & R.N. Harkins, Eds. :129–154 Springer Verlag Publ. Boston.
40. NICHOLSON, R.I., J.M. GEE, A.B. FRANCIS, et al. 1995. Observations arising from the use of pure antioestrogens on oestrogen-responsive (MCF-7) and oestrogen growth-independent (K3) human breast cancer cells. Endocr.-Related Cancer **2:** 115–121.
41. NICHOLSON, R.I., J.M. GEE, S. BRYANT, et al. 1996. Pure antiestrogens. The most important advance in the endocrine therapy of breast cancer since 1896. Ann. N.Y. Acad. Sci. **30:** 325–335.
42. CHEUNG, K.L., P.C. WILLSHER, S.E. PINDER, et al. 1997. Predictors of response to second-line endocrine therapy for breast cancer. Breast Cancer Res. Treat. **45:** 219–224.
43. VICKERS, P.J., R.B. DICKSON, R. SHOEMAKER & K.H. COWAN. 1988. A multidrug-resistant MCF-7 human breast cancer cell line which exhibits cross-resistance to antiestrogens and hormone-independent tumor growth *in vivo*. Mol. Endocrinol. **2:** 886–892.
44. CLARKE, R., N. BRUNNER, D. KATZ, et al. 1989. The effects of a constitutive expression of transforming growth factor-alpha on the growth of MCF-7 human breast cancer cells *in vitro* and *in vivo*. Mol. Endocrinol. **3:** 372–380.
45. VALVERIUS, E.M., T. VELU, V. SHANKAR, et al. 1990. Over-expression of the epidermal growth factor receptor in human breast cancer cells fails to induce an estrogen-independent phenotype. Int. J. Cancer **46:** 712–718.
46. VAN AGTHOVEN, T., T.L. VAN AGTHOVEN, H. PORTENGEN, et al. 1992. Ectopic expression of epidermal growth factor receptors induces hormone independence in ZR-75-1 human breast cancer cells. Cancer Res. **52:** 5082–5088.
47. VAN AGTHOVEN, T., T.L. VAN AGTHOVEN, A. DEKKER, et al. 1994. Induction of estrogen independence of ZR-75-1 human breast cancer cells by epigenetic alterations. Mol. Endocrinol. **8:** 1474–1483.
48. BENZ, C.C., G.K. SCOTT, J.C. SARUP, et al. 1993. Estrogen-dependent, tamoxifen-resistant tumorigenic growth of MCF-7 cells transfected with HER2/neu. Breast Cancer Res. Treat. **24:** 85–95.
49. MILLER, D.L. D. EL-ASHRY, A.L. CHEVILLE, et al. 1994. Emergence of MCF-7 cells over-expressing a transfected epidermal growth factor receptor (EGFR) under estrogen-depleted conditions: evidence for a role of EGFR in breast cancer growth and progression. Cell Growth Differ. **5:** 1263–1274.
50. PIETRAS, R.J. J. ARBOLEDA, D.M. REESE, et al. 1995. HER-2 tyrosine kinase pathway targets estrogen receptor and promotes hormone-independent growth in human breast cancer cells. Oncogene **10:** 2435–2446.
51. VAN DEN BERG, H.W., D. CLAFFIE, M. BOYLAN, et al. 1996. Expression of receptors for epidermal growth factor and insulin-like growth factor I by ZR-75-1 human breast cancer cell variants is inversely related: the effect of steroid hormones on insulin-like growth factor I receptor expression. Br. J. Cancer **73:** 477–481.
52. KUROKAWA, H., A.E.G. LENFERINK, J.F. SIMPSON, et al. 2000. Inhibition of HER/neu (erbB-2) and mitogen-activated protein kinases enhances tamoxifen action against HER2-over-expressing, tamoxifen resistant breast cancer cells. Cancer Res. **60:** 5887–5894.
53. ENGLISH, J., G. PEARSON, J. WILSBACHER, et al. 1999. New insights into the control of MAP kinase pathways. Exp. Cell Res. **253:** 255–270.
54. COUTTS, A.S. & L. MURPHY. 1998. Elevated mitogen-activated protein kinase activity in estrogen-nonresponsive human breast cancer cells. Cancer Res. **58:** 4071–4074.

55. ALESSI, D.R., A. CUENDA, P. COHEN, et al. 1995. PD 098059 is a specific inhibitor of the activation of mitogen-activated protein kinase kinase in vitro and in vivo. J. Biol. Chem. **270:** 27489–27494.
56. ROBERTSON, J.F., I.O. ELLIS, R.I. NICHOLSON, et al. 1992. Cellular effects of tamoxifen in primary breast cancer. Breast Cancer Res. Treat. **20:** 117–123.
57. NICHOLSON, R.I. & J.M.W. Gee. 1996. In Hormones and Cancer. W.V. Vedeckis, Ed. :227–261. Birkhauser. Boston.
58. JOHNSTON, S.R., B. LU & M. DOWSETT, 1997. Comparison of estrogen receptor DNA binding in untreated and acquired antiestrogen-resistant human breast tumors. Cancer Res. **57:** 3723–3727.
59. GIBSON, M.K., L.A. NEMMERS, W.C. BECKMAN, et al. 1991. The mechanism of ICI 164,384 antiestrogenicity involves rapid loss of estrogen receptor in uterine tissue. Endocrinology **129:** 2000–2010.
60. DAUVOIS, S., P.S. DANIELIAN, R. WHITE & M.G. PARKER. 1992. Antiestrogen ICI 164384 reduces cellular estrogen receptor content by increasing its turnover. Proc Natl Acad Sci. **89:** 4037–4041.
61. LARSEN, S.S., M.W. MADSEN, B.L. JENSEN & A.E. LYKKESFELDT. 1997. Resistance of human breast cancer cells to the pure steroidal anti-estrogen ICI 182780 is not associated with a general loss of estrogen receptor expression or lack of estrogen responsiveness. Int. J. Cancer **72:** 1129–1136.
62. SAINSBURY, J.R.C., J.R. FARNDON, A.L. HARRIS & G.V. SHERBET. 1985. Epidermal growth factor receptors on human breast cancers. Br. J. Surg. **72:** 186–188.
63. ELLEDGE, R.M., S. GREEN, D. CIOCCA, et al. 1998. HER-2 expression and response to tamoxifen in estrogen receptor-positive breast cancer: a Southwest Oncology Group Study. Clin. Cancer Res. **4:** 7–12.
64. HOUSTON, S.J., T.A. PLUNKETT, D.M. BARNES, et al. 1999. Over-expression of c-erbB2 is an independent marker of resistance to endocrine therapy in advanced breast cancer. Br. J. Cancer. **79:** 1220–1226.
65. ROBERTSON, J.F.R. 1996. Oestrogen receptor: a stable phenotype in breast cancer. Br. J. Cancer **73:** 5–12.
66. JONES, H.E., C.M. DUTKOWSKI, D. BARROW, et al. 1997. New EGF-R selective tyrosine kinase inhibitor reveals variable growth responses in prostate carcinoma cell lines PC-3 and DU-145. Int. J. Cancer **71:** 1010–1018.
67. JONES, H.E., D. BARROW, C.M. DUTKOWSKI, et al. 2001. Effect of an EGF-R selective tyrosine kinase inhibitor and an anti-androgen on LNCaP cells: identification of divergent growth regulatory pathways. Prostate **49:** 38–47.
68. BASELGA, J. & S.D. AVERBUCH. 2000. ZD1839 ("Iressa") as an anticancer agent. Drugs **60**(Suppl. 1): 33–40.
69. CIARDIELLO, F., R. CAPUTO, R. BIANCO, et al. 2000. Antitumour effect and potentiation of cytotoxic drugs activity in human cancer cells by ZD-1839 (Iressa), an epidermal growth factor receptor-selective tyrosine kinase inhibitor. Clin. Cancer Res. **6:** 2053–2063.
70. MERIC, J.B., S. FAIVRE, C. MONNERAT, et al. 2000. ZD 1839 Iressa. Bull. Cancer **87:** 873–876.
71. WAKELING, A.E., A.J. BARKER, D.H. DAVIES, et al. 1994. Inhibition of EGF receptor tyrosine kinase activity by 4-aniloquinazolines. Br. J. Cancer **69:** 18.
72. WAKELING, A.E., A.J.BARKER, D.H. DAVIES, et al. 1996. Specific inhibition of epidermal growth factor receptor tyrosine kinase by 4-aniloquinazolines. Breast Cancer Res. Treat. **38:** 67–73.
73. SLIWKOWSKI, M.X., J.A. LOFGREN, G.D. LEWIS, et al. 1999. Nonclinical studies addressing the mechanism of action of trastuzumab (Herceptin). Semin. Oncol. **26** (Suppl 12): 60–70.
74. BASELGA, J. 2001. Clinical trials of Herceptin (trastuzumab). Eur. J. Cancer **37** (Suppl 1): S18–24.
75. SLAMON, D.J. B. LEYLAND-JONES, S. SHAK, et al. 2001. Use of chemotherapy plus a monoclonal antibody against HER2 for metastatic breast cancer that overexpresses HER2. N. Engl. J. Med. **344:** 783–792.

Molecular Mechanisms of RET Activation in Human Cancer

MASSIMO SANTORO, ROSA MARINA MELILLO, FRANCESCA CARLOMAGNO, ALFREDO FUSCO, AND GIANCARLO VECCHIO

Centro di Endocrinologia ed Oncologia Sperimentale del CNR c/o Dipartimento di Biologia e Patologia Cellulare e Molecolare, Facoltà di Medicina e Chirurgia, Università di Napoli "Federico II," 80131 Naples, Italy

ABSTRACT: Mutations that produce oncogenes with dominant gain of function target receptor protein tyrosine kinases (PTKs) in cancer and confer uncontrolled proliferation, impaired differentiation, or unrestrained survival to the cancer cell. However, insufficient PTK signaling may be responsible for developmental diseases. Gain of function of the RET receptor PTK is associated with human cancer. At the germline level, point mutations of RET are responsible for multiple endocrine neoplasia type 2 (MEN2A, MEN2B, and FMTC). Mutations of extracellular cysteines are found in MEN2A patients, and a Met918Thr mutation is responsible for most MEN2B cases. At the somatic level, gene rearrangements juxtaposing the tyrosine kinase domain of RET to heterologous gene partners are found in papillary carcinomas of the thyroid. These rearrangements generate the chimeric RET/PTC oncogenes. Both MEN2 mutations and PTC gene rearrangements potentiate the intrinsic tyrosine kinase activity of RET and, ultimately, the RET downstream signaling events. A multidocking site of the C-tail of RET is essential for both mitogenic and survival RET signaling. Such a site is involved in the recruitment of several intracellular molecules, such as the Shc, FRS2, IRS1, Gab1/2, and Enigma. The different activating mutations not only potentiate the enzymatic activity of the RET kinase but also may alter qualitatively RET signaling properties by: (1) altering RET autophosphorylation (in the case of the MEN2B mutation), (2) modifying the subcellular distribution of the active kinase, and (3) providing the active kinase with a scaffold for novel protein-protein interactions (as in the case of RET/PTC oncoproteins). This review describes the molecular mechanisms by which the different genetic alterations cause the conversion of RET into a dominant transforming oncogene.

KEYWORDS: kinase; oncogene; thyroid; endocrine; receptor; carcinoma; papillary; chromosome

Address for correspondence: Giancarlo Vecchio, Dipartimento di Biologia e Patologia Cellulare e Molecolare, Facoltà di Medicina e Chirurgia, Università di Napoli "Federico II," via S. Pansini 5, 80131 Naples, Italy. Voice: 39.081.7463324; fax: 39.081.7463037.
vecchio@unina.it

STRUCTURE-FUNCTION OF THE RET KINASE

RET encodes an evolutionary conserved transmembrane receptor of the protein tyrosine kinase family.[1] RET protein is composed by three domains, an extracellular domain, which contains the signal peptide and cadherin-like and cysteine-rich regions, a transmembrane domain, and an intracellular portion containing the tyrosine kinase domain (TK) split by the insertion of 27 amino acids. RET is the receptor of growth factors belonging to the glial cell line-derived neurotrophic factor (GDNF) family. This family is comprised of the GDNF, neurturin (NTN), persephin (PSP), and artemin, which all have trophic influences on a variety of neuronal populations.[2] These ligands interact with multimeric receptors composed of high-affinity glycosyl-phosphatidylinositol (GPI)-linked receptors and the RET kinase. Four GPI-linked coreceptors have been isolated and designated GFRα1, 2, 3, and 4. A preferential, in some cases exclusive, interaction of GDNF, NTN, artemin, and PSP with GFRα1, 2, 3, and 4, respectively, has been demonstrated. In turn, the ligand-coreceptor complex interacts with RET and induces dimerization and activation of the kinase and signal transduction. Ligand-dependent RET activation can promote neuronal cell survival and differentiation.[2] Moreover, RET plays an essential role in kidney development. Accordingly, RET- and coreceptor-*null* mice show severe defects of the innervation of the hindgut and branching of the ureteric bud.

RET IN PAPILLARY CARCINOMAS OF THE THYROID GLAND

Thyroid tumors are the most prevalent malignancies of the endocrine system. They are comprised of differentiated (papillary and follicular), poorly differentiated (insular), and de-differentiated (anaplastic) carcinomas. Papillary thyroid carcinomas are frequently associated with specific alterations affecting the RET gene.[3] These rearrangements led to the fusion of the RET TK-encoding domain to the 5′-terminal regions of heterologous genes, generating chimeric oncogenes designated as RET/PTC. As illustrated in FIGURE 1, several RET fusion partners have been isolated so far, including the H4, RIα, and RFG genes in the case of RET/PTC1, 2, and 3.[4–6] RET, H4, and RFG genes map on the long arm of chromosome 10, and their fusion is generated by chromosome inversions; RET/PTC2 is generated by a balanced translocation between chromosomes 10 and 17.[3]

Among the different subtypes of thyroid tumor,[7] RET/PTC oncogenes are found with variable frequency (from 2.5–40%) in the papillary subgroup.[8] More recently, RET rearrangements have been reported in Hürthle cell tumors and trabecular adenomas, suggesting that these tumor variants are genetically linked to papillary carcinoma. A high frequency of RET rearrangements is found in thyroid microcarcinomas, which are papillary tumors with low growing and invading tendency.[9] Ionizing radiation can induce RET/PTC rearrangements, and thyroid cancer is the most common solid neoplasm associated with radiation exposure.[10] Accordingly, a dramatic increase in the incidence of pediatric papillary carcinoma has been reported after the Chernobyl nuclear accident, which released 50–200 million curies of radiation.[11] RET/PTC rearrangements are highly prevalent in these carcinomas.[12] RET/PTCs are transforming oncogenes. They have been isolated by virtue of their

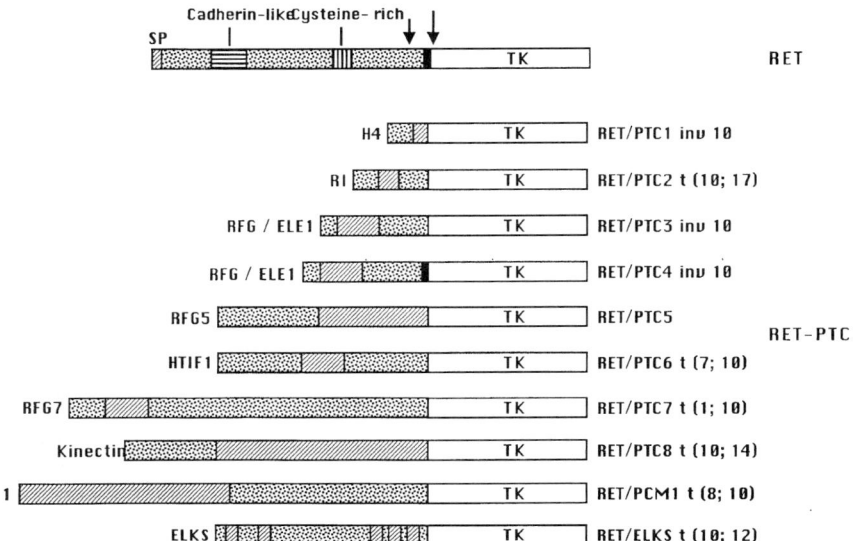

FIGURE 1. RET/PTC oncogenes, which are found in papillary thyroid carcinomas, are chimeric genes generated by the fusion of the RET tyrosine-kinase (TK)-encoding domain to different heterologous genes. *Arrows* indicate breakpoints in papillary thyroid cancer. Chromosomal aberrations leading to the formation of RET rearrangements are indicated. SP, signal peptide. Coiled-coild motifs in RERT fusion partners are indicated as *dashed boxes*.

ability to transform NIH 3T3 fibroblasts, and they transform epithelial thyroid cells[13] and induce papillary thyroid carcinoma in transgenic mice.[14,15]

RET/PTC rearrangements activate the transforming potential of RET by multiple mechanisms. First, by substituting its transcriptional promoter with those of the fusion partners, they allow the expression of RET in the thyroid cells, where it is normally transcriptionally silent. On the other hand, the rearrangements generate constitutively active chimeric oncoproteins, which are distributed in the cytosolic compartment of the cell. At this time, it is still unknown which functional consequence, if any, may derive from the altered localization (from the plasma membrane to the cytosol) of the RET kinase. Finally, activation of the RET kinase is mediated by fusion to domains that are capable of dimerization. RET fusion partners contain coiled-coil domains, which are well-known protein-protein interaction motifs.

RET IN MEN2 SYNDROMES

Germline point mutations of RET are responsible for the inheritance of MEN2 familial cancer syndromes; somatic RET mutations are found in a fraction of sporadic medullary thyroid carcinomas and, rarely, pheochromocytomas. MEN2 are divided into three different clinical varieties: MEN2A, characterized by the presence of medullary thyroid carcinoma, pheocromocytoma, and parathyroid hyperplasia;

FMTC, in which medullary thyroid carcinoma is the only phenotype; MEN2B, characterized by medullary thyroid carcinoma associated with pheochromocytoma, enteric ganglioneuroma, and skeletal and ocular abnormalities.[16] These clinical varieties are caused by different RET mutations falling into two main groups: those affecting the extracellular and those of the TK domain. MEN2A mutations cause the substitution of extracellular cysteines (609, 611, 618, 620, 630, and 634) with several other residues. Most MEN2A patients have a mutation of Cys634, this mutation being highly predictive of pheochromocytoma and parathyroid hyperplasia. Alternative mutations have been described.[16] FMTC mutations can be of the extracellular or the TK type. Extracellular FMTC mutations are similar to those causing MEN2A, but are more homogeneously distributed on cysteines 618, 620, and 634. Mutations of residues 768, 790, 791, 804, 844, or 891 of the RET TK domain have also been found in FMTC patients. Finally, MEN2B is caused by the highly specific Met918Thr (95%) or the Ala883Phe (3%) mutations. The Met918Thr substitution is the most frequently found mutation in sporadic medullary thyroid carcinomas.[16]

All these point mutations have a "gain of function" effect: A constitutive dimerization is the molecular mechanism of the activation of RET molecules carrying mutations affecting extracellular cysteines.[17] Although the three-dimensional structure of the RET extracellular domain is still unknown, these cysteines likely form intramolecular disulfide bonds in the wild-type receptor, and the mutation results in an unpaired cysteine, which forms an activating intermolecular bridge. A different intensity in the induction of the dimerization is a reasonable explanation for the phenotypes caused by mutations of the different cysteines. Indeed, RET mutants associated with FMTC have low dimerization and maturation efficiencies, and this can explain why their kinase and oncogenic activities are lower than those of the classic MEN2A mutant.

MEN2B mutations cause constitutive activation of the RET transforming potential. However, in addition to "quantitative" changes of the basal kinase activity, the most frequent MEN2B mutation (Met918Thr) has been proposed to affect also the "quality" of RET-generated intracellular signals. The residue corresponding to RET methionine 918 is conserved in all receptor tyrosine kinases (RTKs), whereas cytoplasmic protein tyrosine kinases (PTKs) show a threonine in that position. This residue maps in the pocket of the kinase involved in substrate binding, and, thus, it is predicted to alter the substrate selection.[17] Thus, the molecular mechanism by which the Met918Thr mutation alters RET function is probably multiple. On one side, this mutation leads to ligand-independent activation of the kinase without causing a constitutive dimerization of the RET molecules. On the other side, the Met918Thr substitution modifies RET substrate specificity. This may result in an alteration of RET autophosphorylation sites as well as of the pattern of intracellular phosphorylated proteins. MEN2B kinase activity can be further enhanced by the ligand, and this probably results in a stimulation that is stronger than that caused by the MEN2A mutation.

CONCLUSIONS

Somatic rearrangements, which, at the same time, substitute RET transcriptional promoter and cause activation of the kinase are selected in carcinoma derived from follicular thyroid cells, where RET is normally transcriptionally silent. The chronic activation of intracellular pathways downstream RET tyrosine kinase may specifically cause the papillary tumoral phenotype. On the other side, RET is normally expressed in tissues which are affected by the MEN2 syndromes. Alternative point mutations cause the different MEN2 phenotypes. MEN2B disease is the most aggressive form of MEN2; its severe phenotype is probably explained by a combination of mechanisms including constitutive activation of the kinase, susceptibility to further stimulation by the ligand, and change of the signaling specificity. Several aspects of the molecular mechanisms of RET activation deserve further investigation. The role played by the RET fusion partners and by delocalization of the kinase as well as the reason for the restriction of RET/PTC rearrangements to the thyroid gland still need to be clarified. A polyclonal hyperplasia of thyroid C-cells is the first result of the inheritance of a MEN2-type RET mutant, and it is reasonable to think that further genetic events are required to induce the tumor phenotype. Whether RET has prevalently mitogenic, transforming, or survival effects in its *in vivo* cell targets has yet to be ascertained; moreover, at this time, the intracellular signal transducers involved in these biological responses can only be hypothesized. It is already possible to identify MEN2 carriers through the analysis of germline DNA and on the basis of the genotype-phenotype correlation to program a differentiated treatment. Moreover, the identification of RET/PTC rearrangements may be of help in the differential diagnosis of follicular thyroid tumoral diseases. Finally, understanding the molecular basis of RET signaling will help in attempting novel therapeutic strategies aimed at interfering with these pathways.

ACKNOWLEDGMENTS

This study was supported by the Associazione Italiana per la Ricerca sul Cancro (AIRC), the Progetto Biotecnologie "5%" of the Consiglio Nazionale delle Ricerche (C.N.R.), and Progetto M.U.R.S.T. "Terapie antineoplastiche innovative."

REFERENCES

1. TAKAHASHI, M., Y. BUMA, T. IWAMOTO, *et al.* 1988. Cloning and expression of the ret protooncogene encoding a tyrosine kinase with two potential transmembrane domains. Oncogene **3:** 571–578.
2. ROBERTSON, K. & I. MASON. 1997. The GDNF-RET signalling partnership. Trends Genet. **13:** 1–3.
3. PIEROTTI, M.A., I. BONGARZONE, M.G. BORELLO, *et al.* 1996. Cytogenetics and molecular genetics of carcinomas arising from thyroid epithelial follicular cells. Genes Chrom. Cancer **16:** 1–8.
4. GRIECO, M., M. SANTORO, M.T. BERLINGIERI, *et al.* 1990. PTC is a novel rearranged form of the ret proto-oncogene and is frequently detected *in vivo* in human thyroid papillary carcinomas. Cell **60:** 557–563.
5. SANTORO, M., N.A. DATHAN, M.T. BERLINGIERI, *et al.* 1994. Molecular characterization of RET/PTC3: a novel rearranged version of the RET proto-oncogene in a human thyroid papillary carcinoma. Oncogene **9:** 509–516.
6. BONGARZONE, I., N. MONZINI, M.G. BORRELLO, *et al.* 1993. Molecular characterization of a thyroid tumor-specific transforming sequence formed by the fusion of ret tyrosine kinase and the regulatory subunit RI alpha of cyclic AMP-dependent protein kinase A. Mol. Cell. Biol. **13:** 358–366.

7. HEDINGER, C., E.D. WILLIAMS & L.H. SOBIN. 1989. The WHO histological classification of thyroid tumors: a commentary on the second edition. Cancer **63:** 908–911.
8. TALLINI, G., M. SANTORO, M. HELIE, et al. 1998. RET/PTC oncogene activation defines a subset of papillary thyroid carcinomas lacking evidence of progression to poorly differentiated or undifferentiated tumor phenotypes. Clin. Cancer Res. **4:** 287–294.
9. VIGLIETTO, G., G. CHIAPPETTA, F.J. MARTINEZ-TELLO, et al. 1995. RET/PTC oncogene activation is an early event in thyroid carcinogenesis. Oncogene **11:** 1207–1210.
10. WILLIAMS, E.D. 1993. Radiation-induced thyroid cancer. Histopathology **23:** 387–393.
11. JACOB, P., G. GOULKO, W.F. HEIDENREICH, et al. 1998. Thyroid cancer risk to children calculated. Nature **392:** 31–32.
12. FUGAZZOLA, L., S. PILOTTI, A. PINCHERA, et al. 1995. Oncogenic rearrangements of the RET proto-oncogene in papillary thyroid carcinomas from children exposed to the Chernobyl nuclear accident. Cancer Res. **55:** 5617–5620.
13. SANTORO, M., R.M. MELILLO, M. GRIECO, et al. 1993. The TRK and RET tyrosine kinase oncogenes cooperate with ras in the neoplastic transformation of a rat thyroid epithelial cell line. Cell Growth Differ. **4:** 77–84.
14. JHIANG, S.M., J.E. SAGARTZ, Q. TONG, et al. 1996. Targeted expression of the ret/PTC1 oncogene induces papillary thyroid carcinomas. Endocrinology **137:** 375–378.
15. SANTORO, M., G. CHIAPPETTA, A. CERRATO, et al. 1996. Development of thyroid papillary carcinomas secondary to tissue-specific expression of the RET/PTC1 oncogene in transgenic mice. Oncogene **12:** 1821–1826.
16. PASINI, B., I. CECCHERINI & G. ROMEO. 1996. RET mutations in human disease. Trends Genet. **12:** 138–144.
17. SANTORO M., F. CARLOMAGNO, A. ROMANO, et al. 1995. Germ–line mutations of MEN2A and MEN2B activate RET as a dominant transforming gene by different molecular mechanisms. Science **267:** 381–386.

Proteomic Patterns of Cultured Breast Cancer Cells and Epithelial Mammary Cells

IDA PUCCI-MINAFRA,[a] SIMONA FONTANA, PATRIZIA CANCEMI, GIUSEPPINA ALAIMO, AND SALVATORE MINAFRA

University of Palermo, Center of Experimental Oncobiology, Department of Cell Biology and Development, Institute of Histology and Embryology, Palermo, Italy

ABSTRACT: Breast cancer is one of the leading causes of death from cancer among women in western countries. The different types of breast cancer are grouped into invasive and noninvasive forms. Among the invasive types, ductal infiltrating carcinoma (DIC) is the most common and aggressive form. Using an *in vitro* model consisting of a DIC-derived cell line (8701-BC) and a nontumoral mammary epithelial cell line (HB2), we used the proteomics approach to search for homology and differences in protein expression patterns between tumoral and nontumoral phenotypes. Within an analysis window comprising 1,750 discernible spots we have currently catalogued 140 protein spots of potential interest. Fifty-eight of them were identified by gel matching with reference maps, immunodetection, or N-terminal microsequencing and classified into four functional groups. Twelve proteins were found differentially expressed in two cell lines: four were uniquely present in the neoplastic cell proteome and eight in epithelial cells. In addition, 53 proteins displayed different relative expression levels between the two cell lines, that is, 44 were more elevated in cancer cells and 9 in HB2 cells. Among proteins with greater relative abundance in cancer cells we identified glycolytic enzymes (or their isoforms), which may indicate that the known metabolic dysregulation in cancer can reflect oncogenic-related defects of glycolytic gene expression.

KEYWORDS: proteomics; breast cancer; ductal infiltrating carcinoma

INTRODUCTION

Cancer of the mammary gland is still one of the leading causes of death from tumor among women in western countries. However, breast cancer is not a single disease but includes several different forms grouped as invasive and noninvasive types. Among the invasive histotypes, ductal infiltrating carcinoma (DIC) is the most common and aggressive form of breast cancer.[1] It usually has a poor prognosis and represents the standard histotype with which the other less frequent subtypes (i.e., papillary, mucinous-colloid, tubular, medullary carcinomas) are compared. Carcinomas are potentially malignant tumors of epithelial origin, which, once genetically

---

Address for correspondence: Prof. Ida Pucci Minafra, Center of Experimental Oncobiology, University of Palermo, Viale delle Scienze, 90128 Palermo, Italy. Voice/fax: 39 91 424903.
idapucci@unipa.it

"initiated," grow, progress, invade, and spread in the body with a common phenomenology regardless of their individual derivation.

The major cellular changes involved in the conversion of a normal to a malignant breast are the progressive loss of the stationary epithelial phenotype (consisting of polarized morphology and specific cell-cell and cell-matrix adhesion systems) and the acquisition of a mesenchymal-like phenotype, correlated with the ability to migrate and invade surrounding and distant tissues, even under conditions of a low oxygen supply. These aspects are related to multiple gene defects, whose functional network is hard to understand from a global point of view.

According to recent estimation, the human genome encodes at least 30,000–40,000 structural genes.[2,3] However, due to posttranscriptional and posttranslational modifications, the number of proteins expressed by cells may be several times higher. In addition, posttranslational modifications may be instrumental in altering or adding functions to certain proteins and their oligomeric forms. Therefore, detecting protein profiles, directed towards knowledge of both the identity and the relative quantity of proteins (and their isoforms) in tumors, is the challenge of the postgenomic era. Comparative profiling of paired tumoral and normal counterparts may provide substantial information on qualitative and quantitative modifications of cancer-associated gene expression, which in turn can be fundamental in understanding molecular mechanisms involved in cancer development. The proteomic strategy, based on a high-resolution two-dimensional immobilized pH gradient (2D-IPG) and related techniques (computer-assisted image analysis, microsequencing, and immune detection), is a powerful tool for the separation, detection, and analysis of a large number of proteins on the same preparation, without prior knowledge of their identity.

The study of protein expression in primary human breast cancer (as for most solid tumors), however, is difficult because breast tumors may contain several different cell types, other than carcinoma cells, such as additional epithelial cell types, stromal cells, and infiltrating lymphocytes. On the other hand, laser-capture microdissected sections[4] may contain large amounts of proteins resident in the extracellular interstitium as albumin, globulins, and other serum proteins. Therefore, several laboratories, including ours, have developed an appropriate *in vitro* model of normal and neoplastic mammary cells for biological and molecular assays[5–8] including the recent approach on cDNA microarray[9] and proteomics.[10]

Among the breast cancer cell lines described to date in the literature, 8701-BC[5] deserves particular interest, because it was established from a primary DIC, that is, before clonal selection of the metastatic process. As a nontumoral reference cell line, we used HB2 cells[7] that maintain in culture the lumenal mammary phenotype, which represents the most common target of mammary cancer.

On protein separation by 2D-IPG and computer processing of the 2D gels, we searched for qualitative (presence/absence) and quantitative (relative abundance) differences in protein profiles to identify relevant differences and homologies between the two representative cell lines.

Within an analysis window comprising about 1,750 discernible spots, we have currently catalogued 140 proteins of potential interest, 58 of which were identified by gel matching, immunodetection, or N-terminal microsequencing. Twelve proteins were differentially expressed in the two cell lines: four were expressed uniquely by neoplastic cells and eight by epithelial cells. In addition, 53 proteins of 140 selected in the map displayed different relative quantities, namely, 44 proteins were more elevated in cancer cells and 9 in HB2 cells.

Interestingly, among proteins with higher relative expression levels in cancer cells (at least 1.5- to 3-fold) we identified several glycolytic enzymes and their isoforms. This finding is of interest, because the "Warburg effect" (enhanced anaerobic metabolism in cancer) has long been known, but this is the first report of increased levels of these enzymes in cancer cells at the proteomic level. Therefore, due to their easy detection on the 2D map, the present approach could have great clinical application.

MATERIAL AND METHODS

Cell Culture

Cells were grown in the appropriate culture medium supplemented with 10% fetal calf serum (FCS; GIBCO) and antibiotics (100 units/ml penicillin and 100 μg/ml streptomycin) in a humidified incubator with 3% CO_2 in air at 37°C. The culture medium was RPMI 1640 for the 8701-BC[5] and Dulbecco's modified Eagle's medium (DMEM) supplemented with hydrocortisone (5 μg/ml) and insulin (10 μg/ml) for the HB2 human mammary epithelial cell line.[7]

Sample Preparations

Cells were grown to confluence and then incubated with three changes of serum-free medium. After washing with ice-cold phosphate-buffered saline solution, they were carefully scraped and incubated in ice for 30 minutes with RIPA buffer (50 mM Tris pH 7.5, 0.1% nonidet P-40, 0.1% deoxycholate, 150 mM NaCl, 4 mM EDTA, and a mixture of protease inhibitors, 0.01% aprotinin, 10 mM sodium pyrophosphate, 2 mM sodium orthovanadate, and 1 mM PMSF). The total cellular lysate was centrifuged at 14,000 rpm for 8 minutes to clear cell debris, and the supernatant was dialyzed against ultrapure distilled water, lyophilized, and stored at −80°C until analysis. Protein concentration in the cellular extracts was determined using the Breadford method.

Two-Dimensional Gel Electrophoresis

Aliquots of dried cell lysate were solubilized in buffer containing 8 M urea, 4% CHAPS, 40 mM Tris, 65 mM DTE (1,4-dithioerythritol), and trace amounts of bromophenol blue.

The first dimensional separation was performed at 20°C on commercial sigmoidal immobilized pH gradient strips (IPG) 18 cm long, pH 3.5–10 (Pharmacia), essentially as described by Görg et al.[11] and Bjellqvist et al.[12] Strips were rehydrated in 8 M urea, 2% CHAPS, 10 mM DTE, and 0.5% carrier ampholytes (resolyte 3.5–10). Aliquots of 45 μg (analytical gels) or 1.5 mg (preparative gels) total proteins were applied to the gel strip. Isoelectrofocusing was carried out by linearly increasing voltage from 200–3,500 V during the first 4.5 hours, after which focusing was continued at 8,000 V for 8 hours. After the run, the IPG strips were equilibrated with a solution containing 6 M urea, 30% glycerol, 2% SDS, 0.05 M Tris-HCl pH 6.8, and 2% DTE for 12 minutes to resolubilze proteins and reduce disulfur bonds. The -SH groups were then blocked by substituting the DTE with 2.5% iodoacetamide in the equilibrating buffer.

The focused proteins were then separated on 9–16% linear gradient polyacrylamide gels (SDS-PAGE) with a constant current of 40 mA/gel at 10°C. Gels were stained with ammoniacal silver nitrate, as described by Hochstrasser et al.[13]

Image Acquisition and Data Analysis

Silver-stained gels were digitized using a computing densitometer and processed with a Melanie 3 computer system (GeneBio). Gel calibration was carried out on the basis of internal standard with the support of the ExPaSy molecular biology server. Quantitative variations of proteins were expressed as volumes of spots (i.e., integration of optical density over the spot area). To correct for differences in gel staining, relative volumes to the sum of the volume of all spots in each gel were calculated with the Melanie system and plotted with the Excel program. For figure presentation, images were transferred to Adobe Photoshop and PowerPoint programs.

Protein Microsequencing

N-terminal microsequencing was performed by automated Edman degradation in an Applied Biosystem protein sequenator (Procise, Perkin-Elmer) on protein samples electrotransferred onto polyvinylidene difluoride membranes (Immobilon-PTM, Millipore). The SWISS-PROT (ScanProsite) and EMBL (Bic 2) databases were used for online sequence similarity search at http://expasy.hcuge.ch/.

RESULTS

The In Vitro Model

As an *in vitro* model for present research, we used two representative cell lines: the 8701-BC, derived from a primary ductal infiltrating carcinoma,[5] which shows invasive behavior both *in vivo* and *in vitro*,[14–16] and the nontumorigenic HB2 cell line, derived from immortalized human lumenal mammary epithelial cells,[7] kindly supplied by Dr. J. Taylor-Papadimitriou (Imperial Cancer Research Fund, London, United Kingdom) and presently cultivated in our laboratory.

FIGURE 1 shows representative phase-contrast micrographs of the two cell cultures at the following time of growth: 24 hours, 48 hours, 72 hours, and 1 week after seeding. As can be observed in the micrographs from A to D, the neoplastic cells display an apolarized morphology with irregular profiles; they spread over the substrate with emission of spikes and once they reach confluence, they overgrow, forming typical domes (FIG. 1D). On the contrary, HB2 cells (FIG. 1E–H) maintain *in vitro* the morphology of epithelial cells, being polarized and responsive to contact inhibition.

Proteomic Profiles of the 8701-BC and HB2 Cell Lines

Each cell culture was grown until confluence, deprived of serum, and then processed for lysis and two-dimensional-IPG separation, as described in **Material and Methods**. FIGURES 2 and 3 show the miniature of two representative 2D maps of the

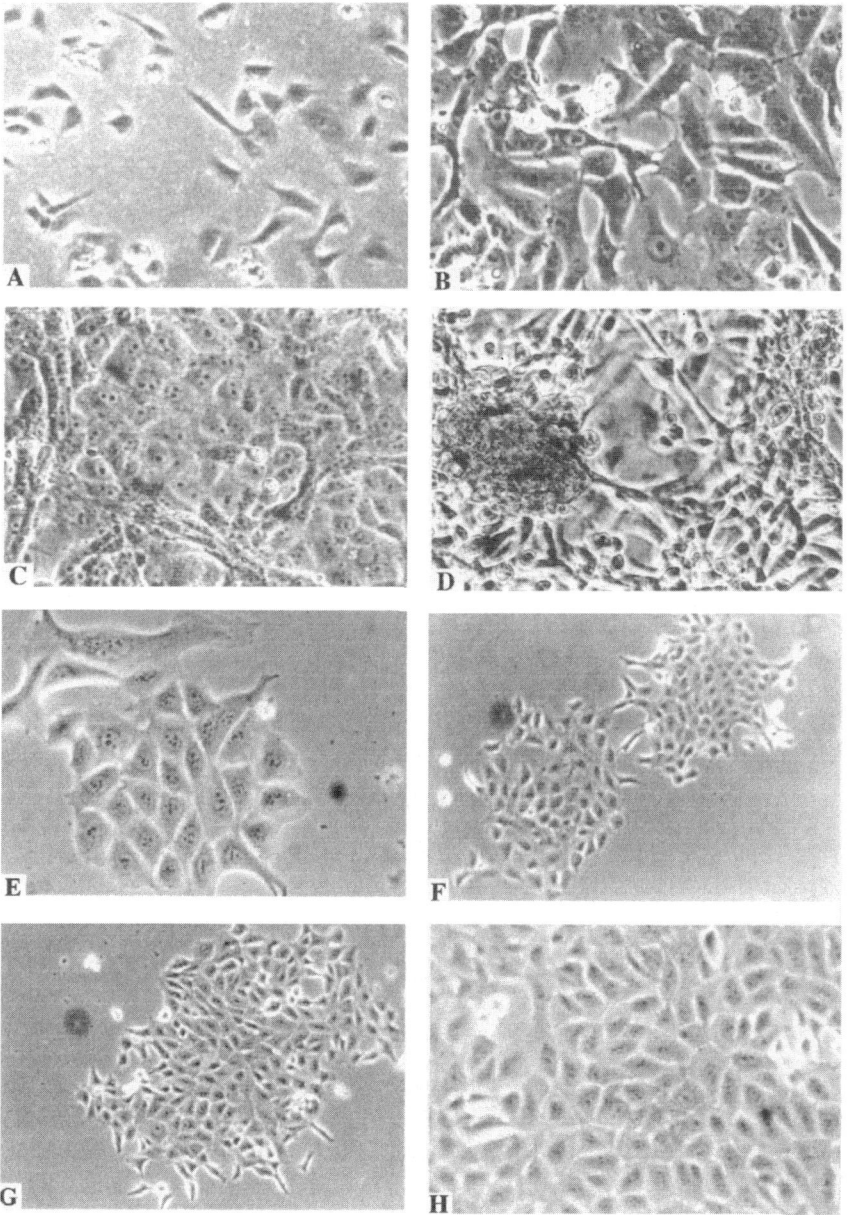

FIGURE 1. Phase contrast micrographs of 8701-BC cells (**A, B, C,** and **D**) and HB2 cells (**E, F, G,** and **H**) at different times from seeding: 24 hours, 48 hours, 72 hours, and 1 week, respectively. Note the different pattern of cell growth and morphology: HB2 cells maintain in culture a polarized morphology and contact inhibition, differently from neoplastic cells, which show apolarized morphology and form multilayered "domes" in the absence of contact inhibition. The two cell lines were confluent at the time of the experiments (600×).

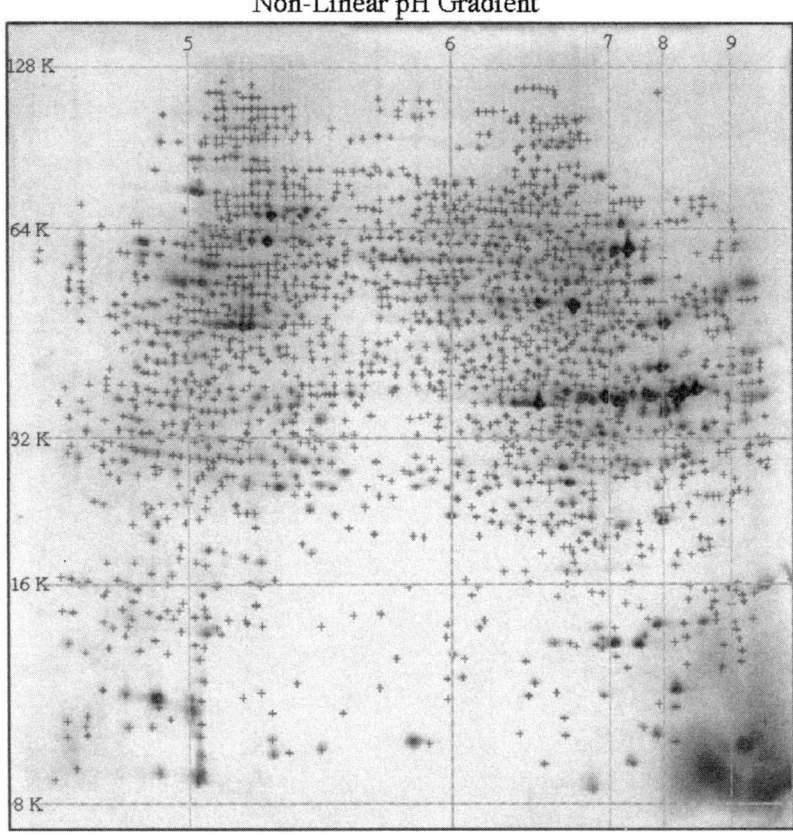

FIGURE 2. Representative two-dimensional electrophoretogram of proteins in 8701-BC cell line. *Crosses* and *grid* indicating p*I* and Mr were automatically assigned by the Melanie system.

8701-BC and HB2 cells, respectively. The crosses on the spots as well as the grid indicating p*I* and Mr were assigned by the Melanie system after cleaning out the background from maps. The number of spots was 1,747 in cancer cells and 1,753 in HB2 cells.

Protein Identification and Clustering in the 8701-BC Map

Protein identification in the 8701-BC map was performed by gel matching, immunodetection, or N-terminal microsequencing, as described in **Material and Methods**. Currently, 58 proteins (including isoforms) were identified in the map and grouped according to their major functions. The first group includes *cytoskeletal proteins*, the second group *folding, chaperons, and heat-shock proteins*, the third

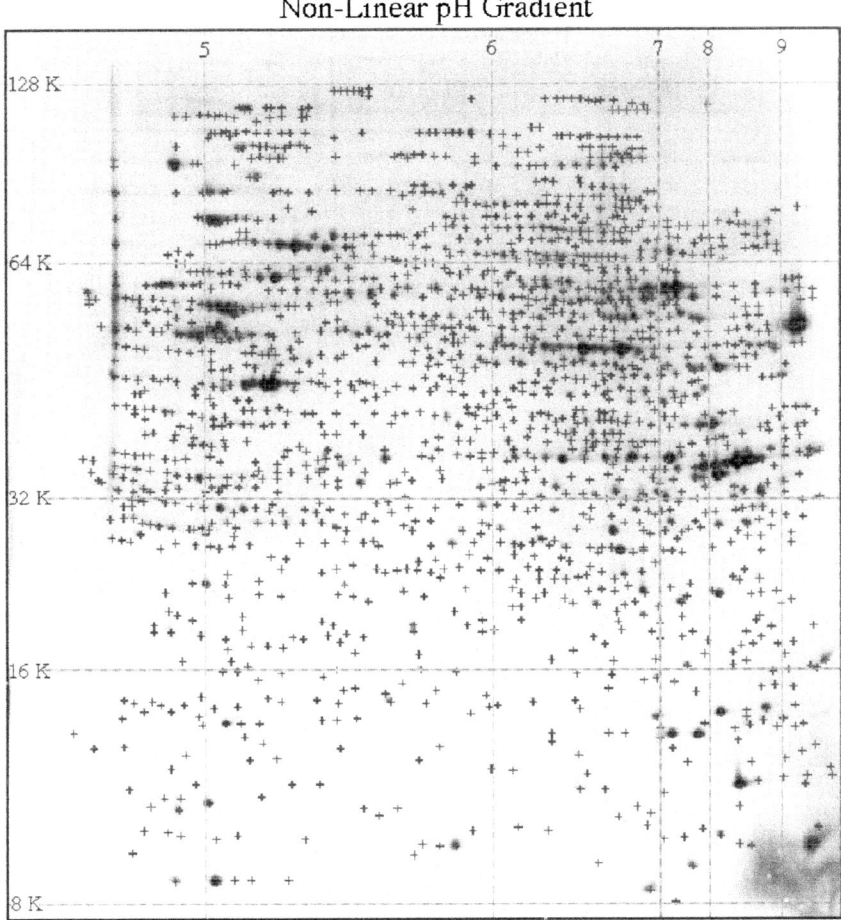

FIGURE 3. Representative two-dimensional electrophoretogram of proteins in the HB2 cell line matched with the 8701-BC profile.

group *proteins involved in metabolism and biosynthesis*, and the fourth group *proteins and enzymes with regulatory functions*. TABLES 1 to 4 list the protein groups, where proteins are indicated by the abbreviations used by the Swiss-Prot database. For each protein the accession number, pI, and Mr and the method of identification are given. When more isoforms of the same protein are present, alphabetical letters are added to the protein name abbreviation .

Proteome Comparison between 8701-BC and HB2 Cells

A representative number of 140 spots was arbitrarily selected to achieve unambiguous gel matching between the two maps. This number represents a significant

TABLE 1. Cytoskeletal proteins

Protein	AC	pI	Mr	ID method
ACTB a	P02570	5.16	42,000	GM
ACTB b	P02570	5.2	42,000	GM
ACTB c	P02570	5.23	42,000	GM
CK 8	P05787	5.09–5.72	42,000–49,830	WB
CK 18	P05783	5.05–5.61	47,074–51,800	WB
EZRI	P15311	6.04	75,194	GM
TBB2	P05217	4.98	49,913	GM

TABLE 2. Folding, chaperones, and heat shock proteins

Protein	AC	pI	Mr	ID method
CBP2 a	P50454	9.23	49,309	GM
CBP2 b	P50454	9.38	49,363	GM
CRTC	P27797	4.52	59,300	GM
CYPH a	P05092	6.66	14,500	GM
CYPH b	P05092	7.07	14,500	GM
CYPH c	P05092	7.51	14,500	GM
ERP60	P30101	5.88	53,600	Nt-Ms
GRP 75 a	P38646	5.24	68,300	GM
GRP 75 b	P38646	5.03	68,300	GM
GRP 78 a	P11021	4.99	73,100	GM
GRP 78 b	P11021	5.02	73,100	GM
GRP 78 c	P11021	5.04	73,100	GM
HSP 60 a	P10809	5.19	59,500	GM
HSP 60 b	P10809	5.21	59,500	GM
HSP 60 c	P10809	5.27	59,500	GM
PDI	P07237	4.84	56,700	GM
TCPZ	P40227	6.2	58,397	GM
TRA	P14625	4.9	91,200	GM

subset of proteins in the proteomic map, corresponding to about 8% of the total amount, and includes the proteins already identified and proteins with unknown identity (U), because they were absent from the data banks or N-terminal blocked. Their identification will be the object of further studies .

Triplicate experiments were performed to ensure reproducible protein separation; to exclude ambiguous spots, synthetic gels of the two cell preparations were constructed by means of the Melanie algorithms. FIGURE 4 shows the synthetic gel of the 8701-BC cell preparation and FIGURE 5 that obtained from HB2 cells. The iden-

TABLE 3. Proteins involved in metabolism and biosynthesis

Protein	AC	pI	Mr	ID method
ALFA a	P04075	7.74	38,100	GM
ALFA b	P04075	7.95	38,100	GM
ENOA a	P06733	6.41	47,074	WB
ENOA b	P06733	6.59	47,074	WB
ENOA c	P06733	6.85	46,635	WB
ENOA tr	...	6.87	41,511	Nt-Ms
G3P2 a	P04406	7.22	34,381	Nt-Ms
G3P2 b	P04406	8.02	35,500	Nt-Ms
G3P2 c	P04406	8.07	35,500	Nt-Ms
G3P2 d	P04406	8.26	35,652	Nt-Ms
G3P2 e	P04406	8.47	35,959	Nt-Ms
G3P2 tr	...	8.38	32,468	Nt-Ms
KPY 1	P14618	7.12	59,300	GM
KPY 2	P17786	7.28	59,300	GM
TPIS a	P00938	6.51	25,000	GM
TPIS b	P00938	6.81	25,000	Nt-Ms
GSTP	P09211	6.01	21,054	Nt-Ms
SODM	P04179	6.96	21,600	GM
ACON	Q99798	6.91	79,190	GM
MDHM	P40926	8.17	33,835	Nt-Ms
MA32	Q07021	4.54	28,600	Nt-Ms
EF1B	P24534	4.62	29,200	GM
EFTU	P49411	6.51	43,300	Nt-Ms
RM12	P52815	5.11	15,820	GM

TABLE 4. Proteins and enzymes with regulatory functions

Protein	AC	pI	Mr	ID method
ANX1	P04083	7.08	32,075	Nt-Ms
ANX1-like	...	7.89	26,932	Nt-Ms
MIF	P14174	7.62	11,900	GM
P53	P04637	6.79	49,039	GM
PSA5	P28066	4.77	25,900	Nt-Ms
TCTP	P13693	4.89	22,100	GM
THIO	P10599	5.02	12,919	Nt-Ms
UBIQ	P02248	6.89	8,700	GM
UBL 1	P09936	5.34	23,940	Nt-Ms

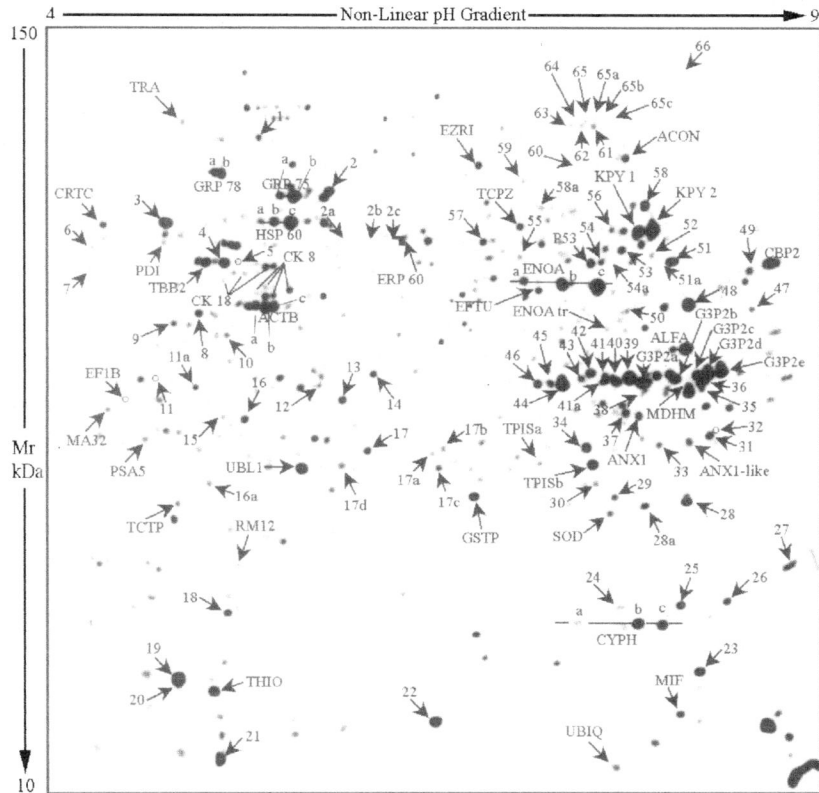

FIGURE 4. Synthetic gel created after elimination of background features from two-dimensional gels of 8701-BC cells. The proteins identified in triplicate gels are indicated with the abbreviations used in the Swiss-Prot database. The letters following the protein names indicate different isoforms. The numbers correspond to protein spots with unknown identity.

tified proteins are indicated with abbreviations used by the Swiss-Prot database; the spots corresponding to proteins with unknown identity are indicated with numbers.

Qualitative differences (presence/absence of spots) were observed within both groups of proteins with known and unknown identity. Proteins present in cancer cells and absent in the HB2 cell map were: the ubiquitin carboxyl-terminal hydrolase isozyme (UBL 1), an isoelectric variant of glutathione S-transferase (GSTP), and two proteins with unknown identity (spot numbers 35 and 36). Conversely, eight spots out of the panel of those selected (namely, 2a, 2b, 2c, 51a, 54, 65a, 65b, and 65c) were uniquely present in the HB2 cell map. (Note that arrows point to corresponding positions of the expected spot, even in the absence of discernible stain.)

After qualitative analysis, we performed comparative quantitation of the comprehensive spectrum of selected protein spots, except the cytokeratins, which were identified by separate western blot analysis (not shown). The comparison was made by

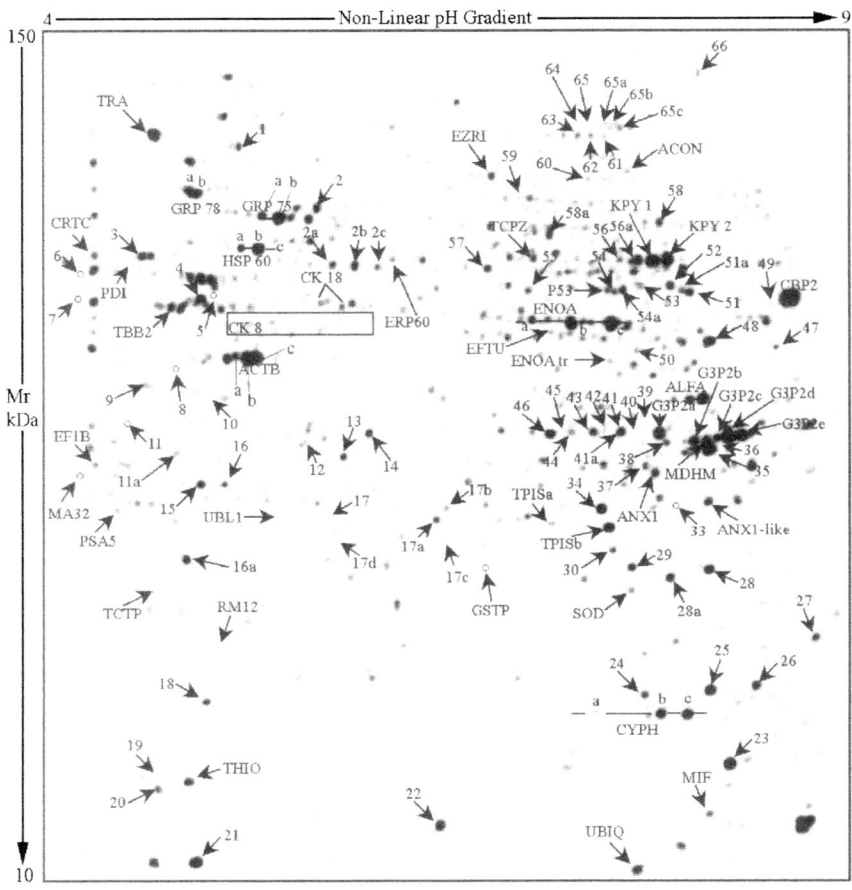

FIGURE 5. Synthetic gel created after elimination of background features from two-dimensional gels of HB2 cells matched to the neoplastic cell profile. Note that in both maps some *arrows* point to corresponding positions of the expected spots, even in the absence of discernible stain.

plotting the relative abundance (%Vol, average of triplicate experiments) of spots from the 8701-BC versus the corresponding spots of the HB2 cell map ordered according to increasing values (graphs 6 and 7) or vice versa (graph 8). The graph in FIGURE 6 shows the comparative profiles of known proteins, and the graphs in FIGURES 7 and 8 those of proteins with unknown identity.

As can be observed in the histograms, the profiles of the sampled protein are notably distinct in the two cell lines, because about 37% of the selected protein spots displayed variable levels of relative abundance in the two proteomes; in particular, 44 were overexpressed in cancer cells and 9 in epithelial cells, whereas the remainder displayed similar levels of expression in both maps.

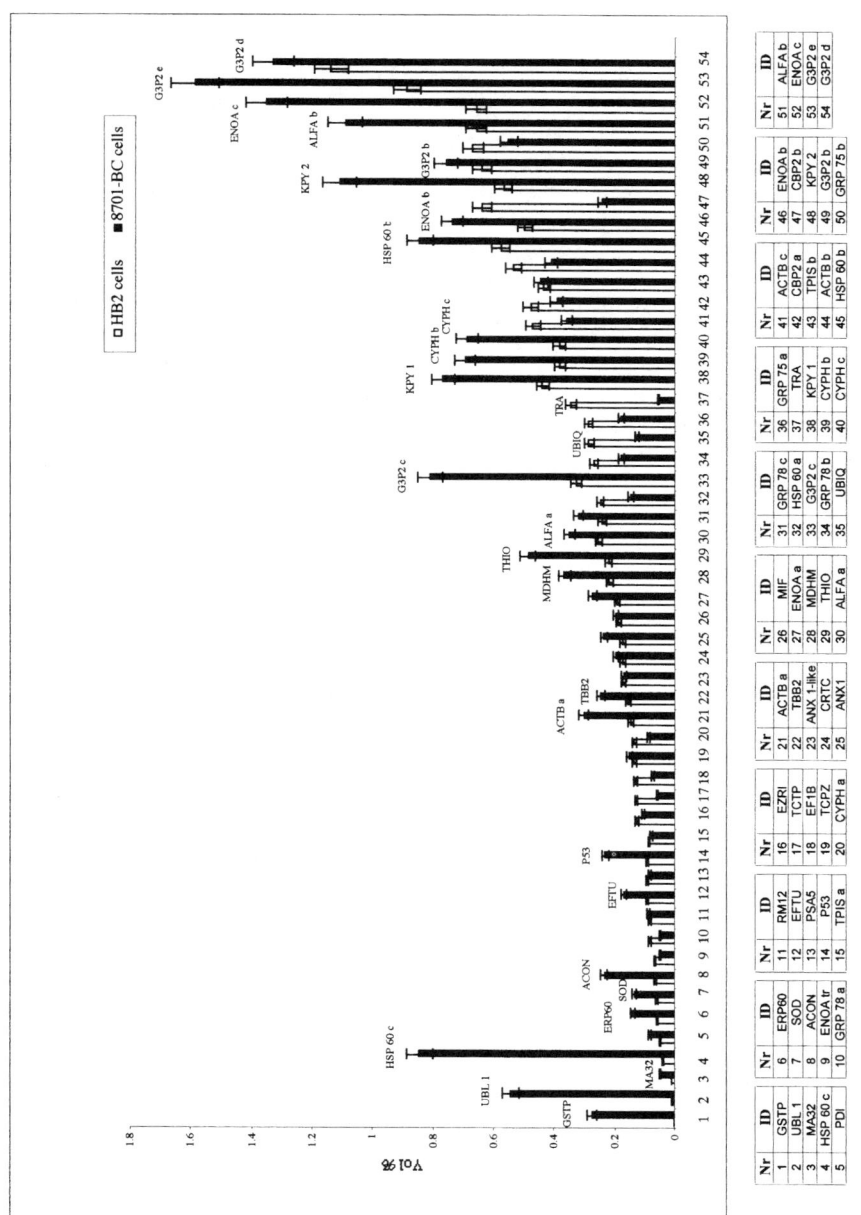

FIGURE 6. See following page for legend.

Proteins that showed higher intensity in cancer cells included glycolytic enzymes, chaperonins, and others with specific roles in biosynthesis and cellular metabolism. Conversely, no significant differences were found among the group of cytoskeletal proteins.

Among the glycolytic enzymes, glyceraldehyde-3-phosphate dehydrogenase (G3P2) showed an average increase of 1.5-fold relative to the control map. However, the various isoforms increased to a different extent, with the highest level of 2.5-fold exhibited by isoform c (TABLE 3). Similarly, alpha-enolase displayed an average increase of 1.7-fold, with the greatest difference for isoform c. An increment was also observed for fructose bisphosphate aldolase (1.37-fold for ALFA a and 1.5-fold for isoform b) and for pyruvate kinase (1.74-fold for KPY1 and 1.9-fold for KPY2). By contrast, no essential differences were observed for triosephosphate isomerase (TPIS).

Among the group of chaperonins, one isoform of mitochondrial molecular chaperone heat-shock protein 60 (HSP60) was found almost differentially present in cancer cells, whereas disulfide isomerase ER-60 (ERP 60) and peptidil prolyl cis-trans isomerase (CYPH) showed increased levels of about twofold. A similar difference was found for elongation factor Tu (EFTU), thioredoxin (THIO), superoxide dismutase (SOD), oncosuppressor p53, and the MA32 glycoprotein, all proteins that play an active role in controlling cell proliferation and biosynthesis. Conversely, tumor rejection antigen 1 (TRA) and collagen binding protein (CBP2) were more expressed in HB2 cells.

Concerning proteins of unknown identity (marked U followed by the number assigned in the 2D maps in FIGS. 2 and 3), two were uniquely present in cancer cells, as already mentioned (U35 and U36), and 22 were highly overexpressed (FIG. 7). The proteins overexpressed, or uniquely present, in epithelial cells relative to cancer cells are shown in FIGURE 8.

DISCUSSION

The proteomic strategy, based on two-dimensional gel electrophoresis and related techniques for protein identification and quantification, is a growing field of research in a world-wide dimension. However, comprehensive protein profiling in cancer occurs at its beginning. This work has contributed to the knowledge of breast cancer

---

FIGURE 6. Histogram showing a pattern of differentially expressed proteins between neoplastic and normal epithelial cells. Values in the ordinate represent the percentage of volume (integration of outer diameter [OD] over the feature's area) of individual spots over the sum of total spot volumes in each map. *Bars* indicate the standard deviation of triplicate measurements, which were 5–10%. Correspondence between numbers (Nr) in the abscissa and protein identity (ID) is given in the table below the graph.

FIGURE 7. Relative abundances (Vol%) of a subset of protein spots with unknown identity, which are differentially expressed in normal and neoplastic cells. Graph highlights the protein spots more abundant in cancer cells relative to HB2 cells. The table below the graph lists the number of protein spots (corresponding to that assigned in the maps in FIGS. 5 and 6), with the pI and Mr coordinates. Standard deviation (not shown) of triplicate measurements was 5–10%.

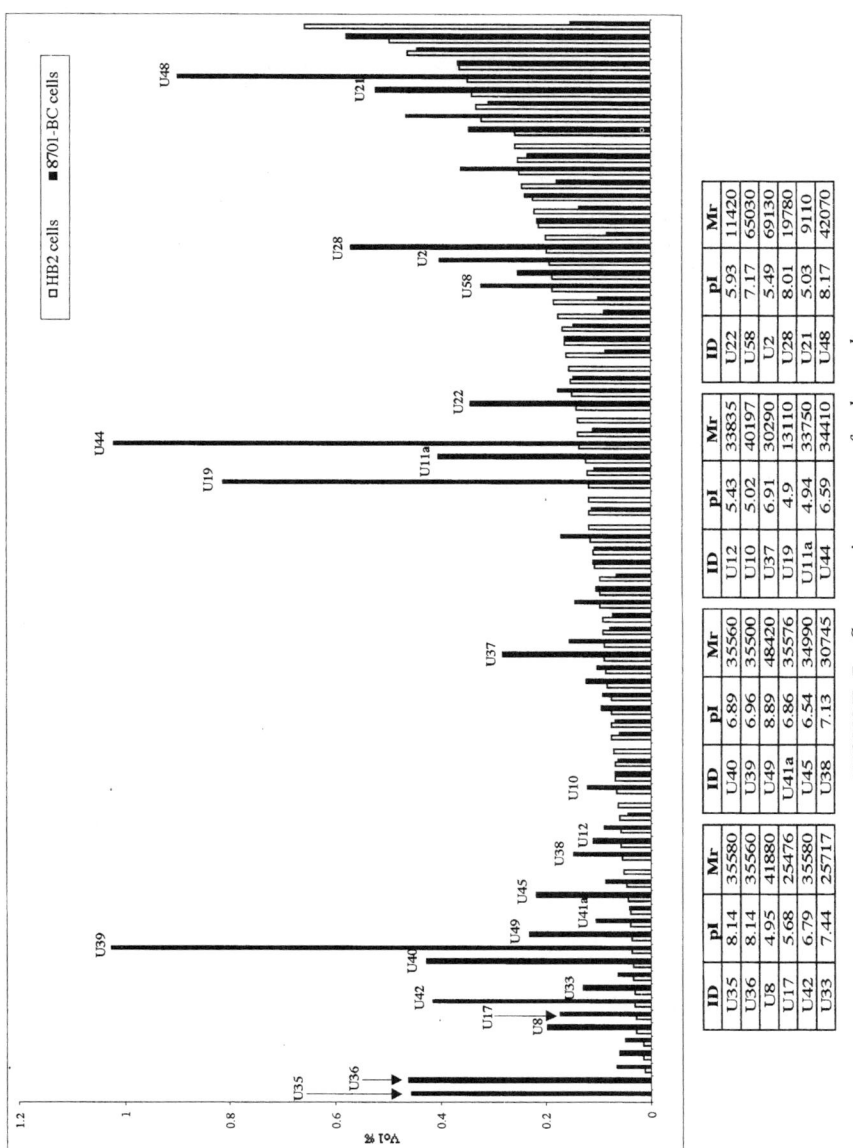

FIGURE 7. See previous page for legend.

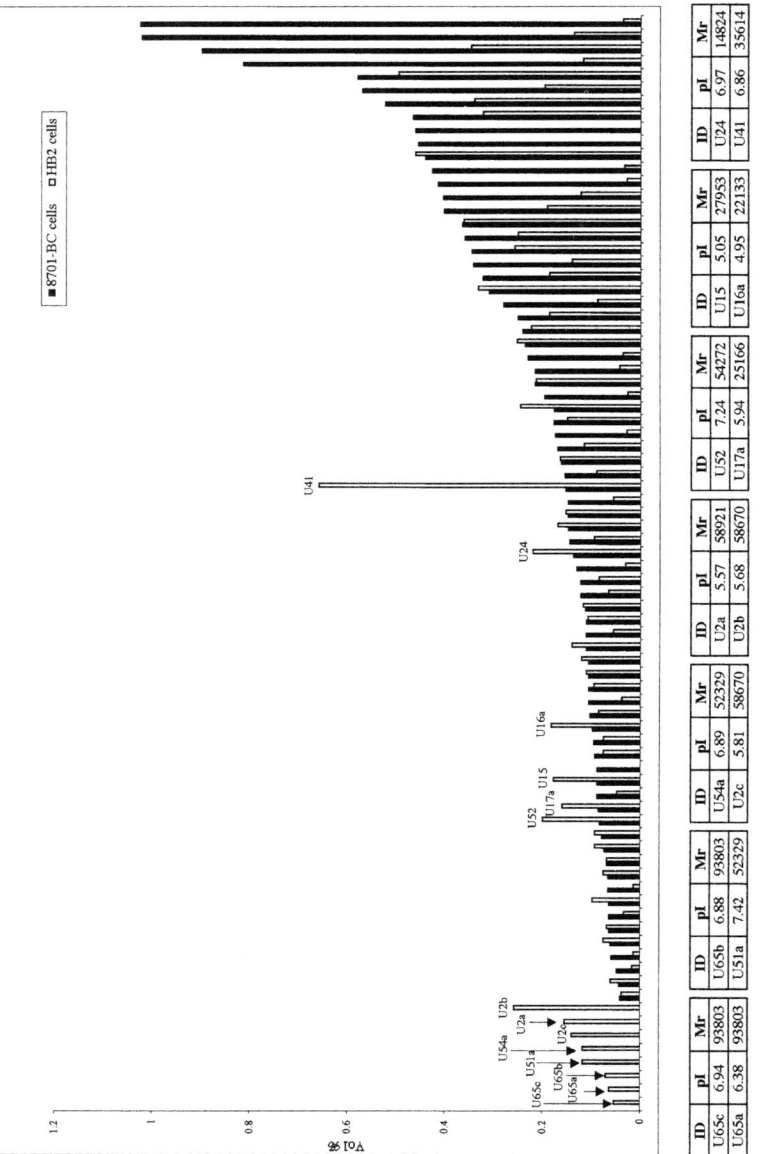

FIGURE 8. *See following page for legend.*

proteomics, using an *in vitro* model consisting of the well-characterized breast cancer cell line 8701-BC[5] and a human mammary epithelial cell line, HB2.[7]

Within the limitation of cultured cells, the two cell lines represent a suitable model, because each of them maintains in culture the specific features of their original *in vivo* status: HB2 cells display a polarized phenotype and are responsive to contact inhibition, whereas 8701-BC cells have pleomorphic morphology and overgrow, forming typical domes. Both of them express cytokeratin 8 and 18, which is typical of lumenal mammary cells. However, 8701-BC cells display isoelectric variants of the two cytokeratin forms, which are absent in normal cells (work in progress).

Within the experimental window of the 2D-IPG used, an average of 1,750 spots was detected by the Melanie system. To establish a significant area of overlapping between maps, we arbitrarily chose a subset of 140 representative spots, covering the 8% of the total protein complement in the maps. Fifty-eight proteins (including isoforms) were identified by gel matching with reference maps, immunodetection, or N-terminal microsequencing and were classified according to their major functions. Of these, 9 belong to the class of cytoskeletal proteins, 18 to chaperonins and affine proteins, 23 are proteins involved in metabolism and biosynthesis, and 8 are involved in regulatory functions.

Results of computer-assisted matching of the neoplastic cell protein profile versus the normal epithelial cell profile demonstrated that within our selected protein sample, 12 proteins, four of which were uniquely present in the cancer cells, were differentially expressed in the two cell lines. Among these were isoelectric variants of glutathione S-transferase (GSTP) and the ubiquitin carboxyl-terminal hydrolase isozyme (UBL 1). The latter is a thiol protease involved in the processing of both ubiquitin precursors and ubiquinated proteins. It is interesting that this enzyme was originally found in neurons and cells of the diffuse neuroendocrine system and their tumors; therefore, its presence and function in breast cancer cells deserve further study.

In measuring changes in relative intensity within the subset of 140 protein spots, we found differences in about 37% of them, that is, 44 proteins were more elevated in cancer cells and 9 in epithelial cells.

Interestingly, most proteins overexpressed in cancer cells belong to the group of glycolytic enzymes. Elevated levels of anaerobic metabolism, even in the presence of oxygen, known as the "Warburg effect" after the scientist's discovery seven decades ago, are a frequent clinical syndrome in oncologic patients.[13] However, the relative increment in glycolytic enzymes (or their isoforms) at the protein expression level was unexpected, because they are thought to be constitutively expressed by cells; in particular, G3P2 is used as one of the housekeeping genes to normalize transcriptional levels of other messengers in several experimental models.

Comparing our breast cancer cell map with that available on line (http://www.expasy.ch/ch2d/), we found that DIC tissues[17] consistently and reproducibly show in-

---

FIGURE 8. Relative abundance of the same group of protein spots shown in the previous figure. The graph highlights a subset of protein spots more abundant in HB2 cells than in neoplastic cells. The table below shows the numbers of protein spots (corresponding to the maps in FIGS. 5 and 6) with the pI and Mr coordinates. The standard deviation (not shown) of triplicate measurements was 5–10%.

creased levels of glycolytic enzymes in comparison with paired healthy tissues of the same patients. This observation allows us to conclude that the increased level of glycolytic enzymes *in vivo* is also maintained in cultured cancer cells and therefore may represent part of early oncogenic transformation in cancer rather than a mere adaptive response of tumor cells to the low oxygen supply in the host microenvironment.

This hypothesis is supported by recent molecular studies revealing that several of the multiple genetic alterations involved in tumor development directly affect glycolysis, which in turn increases the ability of tumor cells to recruit new blood vessel metabolism (Ref. 18 and references therein).

In conclusion, our current data have contributed to the knowledge of proteomic profiling of breast cancer cells. While indicating homologies with data already reported *in vivo*, they add new information on cancer-related proteomics, the knowledge of which will greatly enhance our understanding of molecular pathways involved in cancer development.

ACKNOWLEDGMENTS

This work was supported by AIRC and MURST (to I.P.M.). We thank Dr. Silvana Caricato (Centre of Experiemental OncoBiology, Palermo) for excellent technical assistance in cell culture preparation.

REFERENCES

1. DONEGAN, W.L. 1997. Tumor-related prognostic factors for breast cancer. Cancer J. Clin. **47:** 28–51.
2. LANDER, E.S., L.M. LINTON, B. BIRREN, *et al.* 2001. Initial sequencing and analysis of the human genome. Nature **409:** 860–921.
3. VENTER, J.C., M.D. ADAMS, E.W. MYERS, *et al.* 2001. The sequence of the human genome. Science **291:** 1304–1351.
4. EMMERT-BUCK, M., J.P. GILLESPIE, C.P. ORNSTEIN, *et al.* 2000. An approach to proteomic analysis of human tumors. Mol. Carcinog. **27:** 158–165.
5. MINAFRA, S., V. MORELLO, F. GLORIOSO, *et al.* 1989. A new cell line (8701-BC) from primary ductal infiltrating carcinoma of human breast. Br. J. Cancer **60:** 185–192.
6. MINAFRA, S., C. GIAMBELLUCA, M. ANDRIOLO & I. PUCCI-MINAFRA. 1995. Cell-cell and cell-collagen interactions influence gelatinase production by human breast carcinoma cell line 8701-BC. Int. J. Cancer **62:** 1–7.
7. BARTEK, J., J. BARTKOVA. N. KYPRIANOU, *et al.* 1991. Efficient immortalization of luminal epithelial cells from human mammary gland by introduction of simian virus 40 large tumor antigen with a recombinant retrovirus. Proc. Natl. Acad. Sci. USA **88:** 3520–3524.
8. BERDICHEVSKY, F., D. ALFORD, B. D'SOUZA & J. TAYLOR-PAPADIMITRIOU. 1994. Branching morphogenesis of human mammary epithelial cells in collagen gels. J. Cell Sci. **107:** 3557–3568.
9. PEROU, C.M., S.S. JEFFREY, M. VAN DE RIJN, *et al.* 1999. Distinctive gene expression patterns in human mammary epithelial cells and breast cancers. Proc. Natl. Acad. Sci. USA **96:** 9212–9217.
10. WILLIAMS, K., C. CHUBB, E. HUBERMAN & C.S. GIOMETTI. 1998. Analysis of differential protein expression in normal and neoplastic human breast epithelial cell lines. Electrophoresis **19:** 333–343.
11. GÖRG, A., W. POSTEL & S. GUNTHER. 1988. The current state of two dimensional electrophoresis with immobilized pH gradient. Electrophoresis **9:** 531–546.

12. BJELLQVIST, B., C. PASQUALI, F. RAVIER, *et al.* 1993. A nonlinear wide-range immobilized pH gradient for two dimensional electrophoresis and its definition in a relevant pH scale. Electrophoresis **14:** 1357–1365.
13. HOCHSTRASSER, D.F., M.G. HARRINGTON, A.C. HOCHSTRASSER, *et al.* 1988. Methods for increasing the resolution of two dimensional protein electrophoresis. Anal. Biochem. **173:** 424–435.
14. ALESSANDRO, R., S. MINAFRA, I. PUCCI MINAFRA, *et al.* 1993. Metalloproteinase and Timp expression by the human breast carcinoma cell line 8701-BC. Int. J. Cancer **55:** 250–255.
15. LUPARELLO, C., A. NOEL & I. PUCCI-MINAFRA. 1997. Intratumoral heterogeneity for hsp90beta mRNA levels in a breast cancer cell line. DNA Cell Biol. **16:** 1231–1236.
16. LUPARELLO, C., A.F. GINTY, J.A. GALLAGHER, *et al.* 1993. TGF-beta, urokinase and PTHrP expression in 8701-BC breast cancer cells and clones. Differentiation **55:** 73–80.
17. BINI, L., B. MAGI, B. MARZOCCHI, *et al.* 1997. Protein expression profiles in human breast ductal carcinoma and histologically normal tissue. Electrophoresis **18:** 2832–2841.
18. DANG, C.V. & G.L. SEMENZA. 1999. Oncogenic alterations of metabolism. Trends Biochem. Sci. **24:** 68–72.

Antiestrogenic Regulation of Transforming Growth Factor Beta Receptors I and II in Human Breast Cancer Cells

M. BUCK, J. VON DER FECHT, AND C. KNABBE

Dr. Margarete Fischer-Bosch-Institute of Clinical Pharmacology and Robert Bosch Hospital, Department of Clinical Chemistry, 70376 Stuttgart, Germany

ABSTRACT: To obtain more information about the interactions between antiestrogens and transforming growth factor beta (TGF-β) signaling, we analyzed the influence of different types of antiestrogens on the expression of TGF-β receptors I (TβRI) and II (TβRII). Our results show that antiestrogens selectively induce TβRII but not TβRI mRNA.

KEYWORDS: transforming growth factor-β; TGF-β; receptors; breast cancer; antiestrogens

INTRODUCTION

The antiestrogen tamoxifen is used in the treatment of breast cancer; however, its beneficial effect is often impaired by the development of antiestrogen resistance. The molecular mechanisms of antiestrogen action are still only partially understood. An important step seems to be the activation of transforming growth factor-β (TGF-β).[1] TGF-β is a strong inhibitor of proliferation of primary human mammary epithelial cells.[2] Its growth inhibitory effect on breast cancer cells varies considerably, and complete loss of the antiproliferative effect can be observed.[3] Antiestrogen resistance could therefore originate in defects in the TGF-β signal transduction pathway. To obtain more information about the interactions between antiestrogens and TGF-β signaling, we analyzed the influence of different types of antiestrogens on the expression of TGF-β receptors I (TβRI) and II (TβRII).

RESULTS

mRNA levels of the two TGF-β receptors were quantified using a one-tube Light-Cycler RT-PCR. Induction was calculated in comparison to untreated control cells. Treatment of MCF-7 cells with the nonsteroidal antiestrogen 4-hydroxytamoxifen, an

Address for correspondence: Dr. M. Buck, Dr. Margarete Fischer-Bosch-Institute of Clinical Pharmacology and Robert Bosch Hospital, Department of Clinical Chemistry, Auerbachstr. 110, 70376 Stuttgart, Germany. Voice: 0711/8101-3712; fax: 0711/859295.
miriam.buck@ikp-stuttgart.de

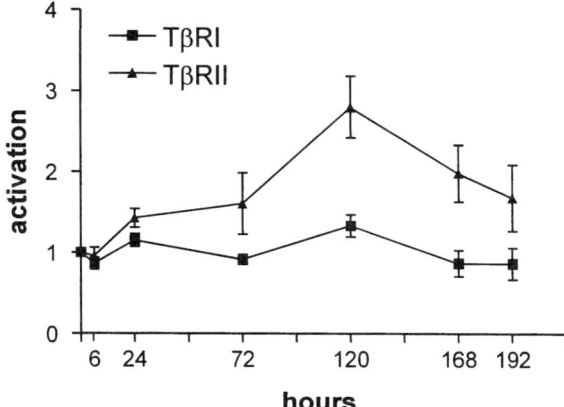

FIGURE 1. 4-Hydroxytamoxifen differentially regulates mRNA expression of TβRI and TβRII. Cells were treated for the indicated time periods with the nonsteroidal antiestrogen 4-hydroxytamoxifen (10^{-7} M). mRNA levels were quantified using a one-tube RT-PCR on the LightCycler. mRNA induction was calculated in comparison with untreated control cells. Data are given as mean ± SEM of five independent experiments.

active metabolite of tamoxifen, leads to slow induction of TβRII mRNA, which begins 24 hours after treatment. After 120 hours, a nearly threefold induction is reached, which immediately starts to decrease again (FIG. 1). TβRI mRNA levels are not influenced by treatment with 4-hydroxytamoxifen (FIG. 1). Treatment of MCF-7 cells with the steroidal antiestrogen ICI 182 780 leads to a steady rise in TβRII mRNA levels over the observed time period. A nearly ninefold induction is reached after 168 hours of treatment (FIG. 2). The mRNA levels of TβRI remain unchanged (FIG. 2).

To gain insight into the molecular mechanisms leading to the induction of TβRII, we started to analyze the TβRII promoter. MCF-7 cells were transiently transfected with a vector construct containing the TβRII promoter in front of a luciferase gene. Directly after transfection the cells were treated with 4-hydroxytamoxifen or ICI 182 780 for 120 hours. 4-Hydroxytamoxifen causes slight activation of the construct. Treatment with ICI 182 780 leads to a nearly fourfold induction (FIG 3).

DISCUSSION

Previous data from our group showed that activation of TGF-β represents an important step in the mechanism of antiestrogen action.[1,4] We have now characterized the influence of antiestrogens on another component of the TGF-β signal transduction pathway, the TGF-β receptor complex composed of TβRI and TβRII.

Our results show that antiestrogens selectively induce TβRII but not TβRI mRNA. The induction of TβRII mRNA is not an immediate transcriptional event, as short-term treatment of 6 hours has no effect, and the highest level of induction is reached not earlier than 120 (4-hydroxytamoxifen) to 168 (ICI 182 780) hours after treatment.

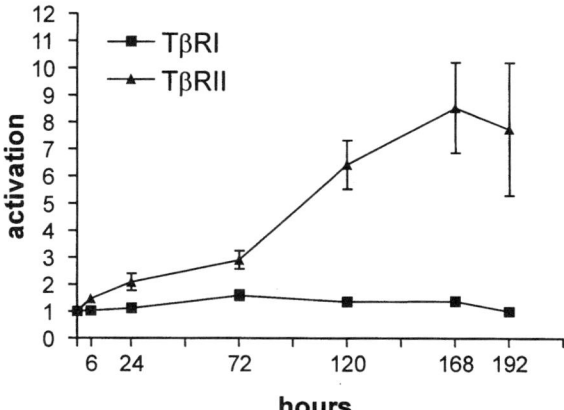

FIGURE 2. ICI 182 780 differentially regulates the mRNA expression of TβRI and TβRII. Cells were treated for the indicated time periods with the steroidal antiestrogen ICI 182 780 (10^{-7} M). mRNA levels were quantified using a one-tube RT-PCR on the Light-Cycler. mRNA induction was calculated in comparison with untreated control cells. Data are given as mean ± SEM of five independent experiments.

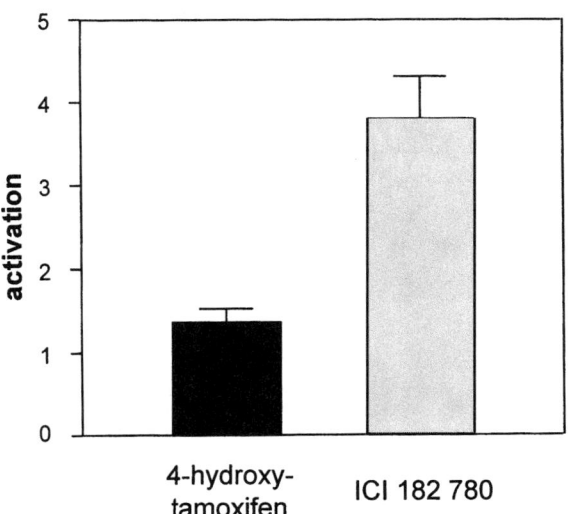

FIGURE 3. Antiestrogen induced activation of the TβRII promoter. MCF-7 cells were transfected with the TβRII promoter construct (nucleotids −2140 to 2). After transfection, the cells were treated for 5 days with 4-hydroxytamoxifen (10^{-7} M) or ICI 182 780 (10^{-7} M). Activation of the promoter construct was calculated in comparison with untreated control cells.

The two different types of antiestrogens used in this study show different effects on the extent of TβRII mRNA induction. The steroidal antiestrogen ICI 182 780 has a much stronger inductive effect on TβRII mRNA levels than does the nonsteroidal antiestrogen 4-hydroxytamoxifen. The level of mRNA induction seems to reflect the growth inhibitory potential of the antiestrogens. In MCF-7 cells 4-hydroxytamoxifen usually leads to 40% growth inhibition after 7 days of treatment, ICI 182 780 to over 80% growth inhibition. As TβRII is responsible for ligand binding, upregulation of the receptor represents a mechanism to render cells more sensitive to the effects of TGF-β^5 and as our results suggest at the same time to the effects of antiestrogens.

The kinetics of TβRII induction suggest an indirect transcriptional event. In order to characterize the mechanisms leading to this effect and to the differential activation of the receptor by the two antiestrogens we started to analyze the TβRII promoter. The first experiments confirm that at least for ICI 182 780 the induction of TβRII mRNA is regulated on the promoter level.

ACKNOWLEDGMENTS

This work was supported by the Deutsche Forschungsgemeinschaft (DFG KN 228/2-1) and the Robert-Bosch Stiftung.

REFERENCES

1. KNABBE, C., M.E. LIPPMAN, L.M. WAKEFIELD, *et al.* 1987. Evidence that transforming growth factor-beta is a hormonally regulated negative growth factor in human breast cancer cells. Cell **48:** 417–428.
2. BASOLO, F., L. FIORE, F. CIARDIELLO, *et al.* 1994. Response of normal and oncogene-transformed human mammary epithelial cells to transforming growth factor beta 1 (TGF-beta 1): lack of growth-inhibitory effect on cells expressing the simian virus 40 large-T antigen. Int. J. Cancer **56:** 736–742.
3. ZUGMAIER, G., B.W. ENNIS, B. DESCHAUER, *et al.* 1989. Transforming growth factors type beta 1 and beta 2 are equipotent growth inhibitors of human breast cancer cell lines. J. Cell Physiol. **141:** 353–361.
4. KNABBE, C., A. KOPP, W. HILGERS, *et al.* 1996. Regulation and role of TGF beta production in breast cancer. Ann. N.Y. Acad. Sci. **784:** 263–276.
5. SUN, L., G. WU, J.K. WILLSON, *et al.* 1994. Expression of transforming growth factor beta type II receptor leads to reduced malignancy in human breast cancer MCF-7 cells. J. Biol. Chem. **269:** 26449–26455.

Objective Response to Treatment as a Potential Surrogate Marker of Survival in Breast Cancer

PAOLO BRUZZI

Unit of Clinical Epidemiology and Trials, National Cancer Research Institute, 16132 Genoa, Italy

ABSTRACT: Until recently, objective tumor response to chemotherapy was used as the primary endpoint in phase II trials aimed at assessing the anti-tumor activity of new drugs. However, it was not accepted as a surrogate endpoint of survival for efficacy trials in solid tumors, and it was not believed to be associated with survival benefit. The recent demonstration that objective response is indeed a valid surrogate endpoint of survival in colorectal cancer, together with strong indirect evidence supporting a similar role of response in breast cancer, opens new possibilities for both the design of trials in metastatic breast cancer and the clinical decision in individual patients with the disease.

KEYWORDS: surrogate endpoints; objective response; breast cancer

INTRODUCTION

Twenty years ago, oncologists still used to compute survival curves of advanced cancer patients, where the outcome of those who responded to a particular chemotherapeutic regimen was contrasted with that of patients who did not. The longer survival of responders was interpreted as a demonstration of the beneficial effect of chemotherapy. Eventually, biostatisticians were able to convince clinicians that these comparisons were meaningless for two main reasons[1]: (1) only patients who survived long enough could respond to treatment, and (2) both response and survival could be related to a third, unknown prognostic factor, and the longer survival of responders could be due to this third factor. Chemotherapy, under this hypothesis, was assumed simply to unmask those patients who were going to live longer in the absence of treatment.

The first bias could easily be overcome[2] with the use of techniques such as landmark or multivariate regression methods (e.g., treating response as a time-dependent covariate), but the second hypothesis could neither be confirmed nor discarded. Strong, although indirect, confirmation of its validity apparently came from the initial randomized trials in metastatic solid tumors, which consistently showed that the substantial increases in response rates obtained with newer, more aggressive chemotherapeutic regimens did not translate into detectable improvements in survival.[3–5]

Address for correspondence: Dr. Paolo Bruzzi, Unit of Clinical Epidemiology and Trials, National Cancer Research Institute, L.go R. Benzi n.10, 16132 Genoa, Italy. Voice: +39 0105737477; fax: +39 010354103.
paolo.bruzzi@istge.it

Consequently, it was assumed that attainment of a clinical response in a patient with a metastatic solid cancer was not associated with longer survival. In the following years, comparisons of survival in responders and nonresponders were no longer accepted at scientific meetings or in papers published in referenced medical journals. Objective response to treatment was accepted as the standard endpoint for assessing the activity of a chemotherapeutic regimen, but it was useless as far as efficacy was concerned. Meanwhile, oncologists continued to use the most active regimens in the hope of obtaining a clinical response, but neither scientific journals nor regulatory agencies would accept a treatment as standard solely on the basis of an increased response rate.

RESPONSE TO TREATMENT AND PROLONGED SURVIVAL

In sharp contrast to this official position of oncologists and statisticians, it is becoming increasingly clear that in solid tumors, response to treatment does indeed prolong survival. Evidence is almost definitive in colorectal cancer and is probably true for most other solid tumors. There were many signs of this impending dramatic change of perspective. Meta-analyses of randomized trials began to show a survival benefit in patients assigned to more active treatment for colorectal cancer, breast cancer, and even lung cancer.[6–9] This benefit was too short in duration (a few months) to be detected in individual trials and also to warrant the use of chemotherapy in all patients with advanced disease. Yet, the obvious question was: is this small increase in survival shared by all patients exposed to chemotherapy? The opposite explanation was much more plausible: little or no benefit (or even some harm, because of toxicity) is expected in those who do not respond to the treatment, whereas only patients who respond may derive a survival benefit from treatment. According to this hypothesis, any effect of a chemotherapeutic regimen on survival is equal to the survival gain in responders times the proportion of responders. Consequently, if in a trial comparing active treatment with no treatment we observed a response rate of 25% and an overall survival gain of 3 months, this implies that on average, response prolongs survival of responders by at least 1 year. Furthermore, in randomized trials comparing different anticancer treatments, each with some degree of activity, the expected difference in survival would depend on the difference in the proportion of responders. In most of these trials the difference in the proportion of responders was below 15–20%. As a consequence, even if the response was associated with a survival benefit of clinical relevance for the individual patient who responds, the expected overall survival benefit for the whole treated population could not be more than a few weeks or months, well below the level of detectability (= power) of most trials. These considerations provided a possible explanation for the lack of a consistent effect on survival in randomized trials in advanced patients. However, this was a hypothesis and not proven. The possibility of strong support for this hypothesis came from the theory of surrogate endpoints[10]: an endpoint (in this instance a response) is a valid surrogate endpoint of the true endpoint (i.e., survival) if, and only if: (a) it is correlated with both treatment and the true endpoint, and (b) its correlation with the true endpoint is independent of treatment. In simple terms, for a response to be a valid surrogate endpoint for survival, (a) effective treatment should be associated with increased response rates and longer survival in responders than in nonresponders, and (b) survival among responders to treatment with different response rates should be the same, and survival among nonresponders to these treatments should be the same. Demonstration of the latter is impossible, because in statistics it is notoriously impossible to prove equivalence. However, if the results of a very large study show, with sufficient precision, that after stratification by response status, survival is similar in groups of patients treated with regimens of different activity, this could be considered a strong argument in favor of the hypothesis that anticancer treatments work in metastatic patients by inducing a detectable response.

RESPONSE AS A SURROGATE ENDPOINT

This argument is now available. The results of meta-analysis presented in the July 2000 issue of *The Lancet*[11] indicate that in advanced colorectal cancer, response to 5-fluorouracil–based chemotherapy is a valid surrogate endpoint for the effect of chemotherapy on survival. This demonstration has two implications: in the future, it will be possible to assume that cytotoxic regimens associated with an increased response rate in colorectal cancer cause an improvement in survival. As a consequence, it will be possible to use objective response as a surrogate endpoint for survival in chemotherapy trials in colorectal cancer, with obvious advantages in both trial size and duration.

The decision to use chemotherapy in patients with metastatic colorectal cancer will no longer be based on the overall survival advantage of, for example, 4 months, but on a possible survival advantage of more than 1 year, conditional on the achievement of a response, with a probability of response of about 30%.

Many cancer patients who refuse a toxic treatment warranting but a few more months of life would possibly be much more interested if the same treatment could prolong life for much longer, even though the probability of obtaining this benefit is small (e.g., 20%).

Indirect evidence supporting a similar role for objective response in breast cancer is overwhelming[7,12–15]: a survival advantage has been seen in several trials in which the difference in response rate between the two treatment arms was above 10–15%, and several meta-analyses of chemotherapeutic trials in advanced breast cancer indicated a survival advantage of more active treatments. Finally, long-term survivors of advanced breast cancer are almost exclusively patients who had a complete response to first-line treatment for metastatic disease.

Thus far, however, no formal validation of an objective response as a surrogate endpoint in breast cancer has been attempted. As previously stated, validation of a surrogate endpoint requires the demonstration that the effect of a treatment on survival is adsorbed by the surrogate endpoint. In the present context, it is necessary to confirm that responders live longer than nonresponders, independently of treatment, and to show that the survival of patients who responded (and who did not respond) to treatment is independent of the activity of the treatment that induced the response. This implies the availability of the results of a large randomized trial (or better, of a series of trials) comparing regimens with different activity. It is to be expected that the results of validation studies of this kind, based on the large databases of clinical trials in advanced breast cancer, will soon be published, with remarkable implications for both research strategies and clinical management of individual breast cancer patients.

REFERENCES

1. OYEM, R.K. & M.F. SHAPIRO. 1984. Reporting results from chemotherapy trials. Does response make a difference in patient survival? JAMA **252:** 2722–2725.
2. BUYSEM, M. & P. PIEDBOIS. 1996. On the relationship between response to treatment and survival time. Stat. Med. **15:** 2797–2812.
3. SORENSENM, J.B., J.H. BADSBERG & H.H. HANSEN. 1989. Response to cytostatic treatment in inoperable adenocarcinoma of the lung: critical implications. Br. J. Cancer **60:** 389–393.
4. KEMENY, N., J.J. LOKICH, N. ANDERSON & J.D. AHLGREN. 1993. Recent advances in the treatment of advanced colorectal cancer. Cancer **71:** 9–18.
5. BAILAR, J.C., 3RD, & E.M. SMITH. 1986. Progress against cancer? N. Engl. J. Med. **314:** 1226–1232.
6. SIMMONDS, P.C. 2000. Palliative chemotherapy for advanced colorectal cancer: systematic review and meta-analysis. Colorectal Cancer Collaborative Group. Br. Med. J. **321:** 531–535.
7. FOSSATI, R., C. CONFALONIERI, V. TORRI, et al. 1998. Cytotoxic and hormonal treatment of metastatic breast cancer: a systematic review of published randomized trials involving 31,510 women. J. Clin. Oncol. **16:** 3439–3460.
8. NON-SMALL CELL LUNG CANCER COLLABORATIVE GROUP. 1995. Chemotherapy in nonsmall cell lung cancer: a meta-analysis using updated data on individual patients from 52 randomised clinical trials. Br. Med. J. **311:** 899–909.
9. LILENBAUM, R.C., P. LANGENBERG & K. DICKERSIN. 1998. Single agent versus combination chemotherapy in patients with advanced nonsmall cell lung carcinoma: a meta-analysis of response, toxicity, and survival. Cancer **82:** 116–126.
10. BUYSE, M. & G. MOLENBERGHS. 1998. Criteria for the validation of surrogate endpoints in randomized experiments. Biometrics **54:** 1014–1029.
11. BUYSE, M., P. THIRION, R.W. CARLSON, et al. 2000. Relation between tumour response to first-line chemotherapy and survival in advanced colorectal cancer: a meta-analysis. Meta-Analysis Group in Cancer. Lancet **356:** 373–378.
12. A'HERN, R.P., S.R. EBBS & M.B. BAUM. 1988. Does chemotherapy improve survival in advanced breast cancer? A statistical overview. Br. J. Cancer **57:** 615–618.
13. GREENBERG, A.C., G.N. HORTOBAGYI, T.L. SMITH, et al. 1996. Long-term follow-up of patients with complete remission following combination chemotherapy for metastatic breast cancer. J. Clin. Oncol. **14:** 2197–2205.
14. PIERGA, J.Y., M. ROBAIN, M. JOUVE, et al. 2000. Response to chemotherapy is a major parameter-influencing long-term survival of metastatic breast cancer patients. Ann. Oncol. **12:** 231–237.
15. BERGH, J., P.E. JONSSON, B. GLIMELIUS & P. NYGREN. 2001. A systematic overview of chemotherapy effects in breast cancer. Acta Oncol. **40:** 253–281.

Nutrition and Prostate Cancer
A Review

LEONARD A. COHEN

American Health Foundation, Valhalla, New York 10595, USA

ABSTRACT: Despite intense efforts, little is known about the etiology of prostate cancer, and treatment of advanced forms of the disease has had limited success. Nonetheless, epidemiologic studies combined with animal model and *in vitro* experiments indicate that natural components of the diet, including n-3 PUFA, the carotenoid lycopene, and the trace element selenium, may serve as chemopreventive agents that suppress the growth and dissemination of neoplastic prostate cells. Until further study, however, soy isoflavones should be viewed with some caution, especially as adjuvant's to chemotherapy, in patients with hormone-refractory prostate cancer. Future studies, using different forms and doses of selenium and tomato carotenoids, may shed new light on the etiology and prevention of prostate cancer.

KEYWORDS: nutrition; prostate cancer; soy isoflavones; selenium; lycopene

INTRODUCTION

Prostate cancer is the third most frequently diagnosed cancer in males in Western industrialized countries.[1] In the United States, it is the most common cancer in males and, except for lung cancer, is the leading cause of death from cancer.[2] Although the etiology of prostate cancer is unknown, several risk factors including age, race, and diet have been identified.[3] Other risk factors include polymorphic repeats in the androgen receptor gene[4] and high circulating concentrations of androgens[3] and IGF-1.[5] In addition, mutations in a number of tumor suppressor genes, such as p53, BRCA1, and WAF-1/CIP1, have been implicated in prostate cancer.[6] However, none of the known risk factors alone or in combination can explain the high incidence of prostate cancer in Western industrialized countries, and success in the treatment of advanced hormone-refractory prostate cancer has been limited.[3]

DIETARY FACTORS AND PROSTATE CANCER

Currently, over 100 clinical trials are underway in the United States, focusing largely on agents that interact with androgen metabolism and receptor function.[7,8] Regarding diet, several epidemiologic studies have demonstrated a positive associa-

Address for correspondence: Dr. Leonard A. Cohen, American Health Foundation, 1 Dana Road, Valhalla, New York 10595, USA. Voice: 914-789-7154; fax: 914-592-6317.
Lcohen@AHF.org

tion between prostate cancer risk and fat intake.[9–14] Both the quantity and quality of fat ingested appear to play a role. For example, there are indications that increased risk of prostate cancer is associated with intake of animal and saturated fat and that n-6 polyunsaturated fatty acids (PUFA) promote prostate cancer,[9–12] while n-3 PUFA and n-9 monounsaturates are either neutral or protective.[13,14] Mechanistic studies using animal models and cultured cells suggest that lipoxygenase products of the n-6 PUFA arachidonic acid play a regulatory role in prostate cancer tumor growth, apoptosis, and angiogenesis.[15–24] N-3 fats such as EPA (C 20:5, n-3) and DHA (C 22:6, n-3) appear to inhibit prostate cancer growth by inhibiting the n-6 lipoxygenase pathway.[16–20] The precise role of dietary fat in cancer, however, remains a matter of controversy.[25,26]

Evidence that dietary antioxidants may confer protection has also been reported. The ATBC trial, for example, reported that prostate cancer was reduced by 32% in men receiving an α-tocopherol supplement compared to a placebo.[27] The Clark Study,[28,29] which involved ingestion of 200 µg Se as a selenized yeast preparation, although designed to test for squamous cell carcinoma prevention, resulted in an unexpected 60% reduction in prostate cancer. Also, Kristal et al.[30] reported a significant reduction in prostate cancer in men receiving a combination of Zn, vitamin C, and vitamin E in a cohort of men in Washington State. Interest in the possible protective effects of tomatoes and the major carotenoid in tomatoes, namely, the acyclic, non-vitamin A precursor lycopene, is based largely on epidemiologic studies linking tomato consumption and high serum lycopene levels with decreased risk of gastrointestinal tract,[31] lung,[32] and prostate cancer.[33–35]

The focus of this discussion is on the two aforementioned areas, namely, the role of the trace element selenium and of lycopene, the major carotenoid in tomatoes, and on soy isoflavones in prostate cancer prevention.

SOY ISOFLAVONES

Epidemiologic studies indicate that Asian men have a significantly lower incidence of prostate cancer than Western men.[3] One explanation for this difference is that Asian men consume high levels of soy products, which are rich in isflavones such as genistein and daidzein.[36,37] In model studies, genistein has been shown to act as a protein kinase inhibitor,[36–38] an inducer of apoptosis[39] and cell differentiation, and an antiangiogenic agent and topoisomerase inhibitor.[37] In addition, it functions as a phytoestrogen, serving as a weak antiestrogen and an estrogen agonist.[37,40] Animal model[41] and cell culture studies[38] have shown that soy isoflavones inhibit prostate cancer growth, and based on available evidence, we have suggested that soy supplements be used as a chemopreventive agent in patients with prostate cancer.[42] Current evidence suggests that soy may act on the development of autochthonous rat tumors[41] and androgen-dependent human prostate cancer xenografts,[43] but there are no published reports on the effects of soy isoflavones on androgen-independent rat prostate cancer tumor growth. We addressed this question by the use of the AT-1 androgen-independent prostate tumor model developed by Isaacs et al.[44] Using AT-1 cells inoculated subcutaneously into male Copenhagen rats, it was found that a soy protein concentrate containing genistein 1.07 mg/g and daidzein 0.52 mg/g fed in the AIN-93M diet at 20% and 10% by weight significantly enhanced tumor growth

TABLE 1. Effects of soy protein isolate on prostate tumor growth[a]

Group (n)	Teatment	Percent increase from baseline		
		Mean	SD	Median
1	Soy 20%	1360	(684)	1250
2	Soy 10%	1350	(624)	994
3	Soy 5%	724	(289)	642
4	Soy 0%	633	(283)	602

[a]The SPI (Protein Technologies Inc., St. Louis, MO) contained 2.89 mg/g total isoflavones, (1.67 mg/g genistein and 0.52 mg/g daidzein) approximately 50% in conjugated and 50% in unconjugated form. When added to the diet at 20%, 10%, and 5% this amounted to an intake of 9.2, 4.6, and 2.3 mg total isoflavones/day/rat. AT-1 cells were inoculated sc at 0.8×10^6 cells/rat.
[b]Statistical analysis:
  I Group 4 (Control) <Group 1, $p < 0.01$; Group 2, $p < 0.05$; Group 3, NS by ANOVA followed by Dunnett's test.
  II Group 4 (Control) <Group 1, $p < 0.01$; Group 2, $p < 0.0005$; Group 3, NS by median test.

(TABLE 1) compared to the findings in untreated controls. No effect was observed when the concentrate was fed at 5%. Levels of genistein and daidzein in urine reflected dietary intake, and body weight gains were similar in each group, indicating that the presence of isoflavones did not influence food intake.

Explanations for these results are currently speculative. Because the AT-1 tumor is not androgen responsive, there is no reason to believe that the enhancing effect of genistein or daidzein is due to the effects of the level of the androgen receptor.[45] However, because genistein, daidzein, and its metabolite equol may act as estrogen agonists,[37,40] the presence of high levels of isoflavones may exert effects associated with estrogen-response elements in prostate tumors. Until further animal model studies are completed, these results in the rat model suggest that clinical intervention with isoflavones in patients with prostate cancer should proceed with caution, particularly in men with advanced androgen-independent prostate cancer.

SELENIUM

The connection between selenium and cancer was originally demonstrated by correlational studies relating Se levels in crops with cancer mortality rates[46] and epidemiologic studies linking increased cancer risk with low blood Se levels.[47] Moreover, a variety of animal model studies, primarily in breast cancer models, have shown that dietary supplementation with 3-5 PPM Se resulted in significant inhibition of tumor development.[46] Current interest in Se and prostate cancer, however, is based largely on the landmark clinical intervention study by Clark et al.[28,29] in 1996 which demonstrated that supplementation with 200 µg Se/day in the form of selenized yeast resulted in a 60% decrease in prostate cancer over a mean period of 4.5 years.

It is well known that Se acts as a cofactor for the antioxidant enzyme glutathione peroxidase.[48] However, recent evidence suggests that Se serves key functions other than as a cofactor to antioxidant enzymes.[48] For example, Se is metabolized to bioactive metabolites, mainly methylated forms such as methylselenium and S-methylselenocysteine,[49–51] which appear to act at the level of transcription factor NFκB,[52] signal transduction,[53,54] cell cycle checkpoints,[55] and apoptosis,[56] and evidence indicates that Se may substitute for sulfur in key signaling enzymes such as tyrosine kinase.[57] Hence, selenium's role in antioxidant function may not be its major function in cancer chemoprevention. Supporting this view is the work of Jiang et al.[58] who reported that administration of Se-methylselenocysteine significantly reduced mammary tumor angiogenesis, as evidenced by decreased intratumoral microvessel density and tumor vascular endothelial growth factor (VEGF) production. In addition, methylseleninic acid, a precursor of methylselenenol, was shown by the same investigators[59] to decrease the gelatinolytic activity of matrix metalloproteinase using human endothelial cell assay, providing further evidence that Se metabolites play a role in regulating neoangiogenesis.[59]

Clinical intervention studies currently underway, on the protective role of Se in prostate cancer, involve a follow-up of the original Clark cohort and new trials among men with negative biopsies, those with high-grade prostatic intraepithelial neoplasia (PIN), and men with prostate cancer who have chosen watchful waiting rather than active intervention.[60] The outcome of these studies are awaited with great interest.

LYCOPENE

Lycopene is the most prominent carotenoid in tomatoes and is among the major carotenoids present in human milk and serum.[61] A prospective cohort study by Giovannucci et al.[33] indicated that the intake of tomatoes and tomato products was inversely related to the risk of prostate cancer particularly in men with extraprostatic cancer. Interestingly, in the same study, no association was found between overall fruit and vegetable intake and risk of prostate cancer. Also of interest was the finding that the strongest association was with cooked or processed rather than raw tomatoes, indicating that carotenoids must be released from their intracellular compartment in order to facilitate their absorption.

Interest in lycopene, which is one of six carotenoids in tomatoes,[61] is based largely on the fact that lycopene is an efficient single oxygen quencher[62] and was shown to reduce mutagenesis in the Ames test.[63] Using multilamellar liposomes, the antioxidant activity of lycopene was shown to be even greater than that of α-tocopherol,[64] and mixtures of lycopene and lutein were more effective than lycopene alone. Because reactive oxygen species have been implicated in the carcinogenic process, lycopene's potent antioxidant activity focused interest in its possible role as a cancer preventive agent.

Lycopene in association with vitamin E was shown to inhibit proliferation of cultured neoplastic prostate cells,[65] and in vitro studies suggest that lycopene inhibits gap junction communication,[66,67] activates phase II enzymes,[68] and suppresses eicosanoid metabolism by blocking COX-2 synthesis.[69] Until now, most reported studies in both animal models and cell cultures have focused on cancers other than that of the prostate. Lycopene is readily taken up by the prostate gland in man and rats in ng/g amounts.[70,71] Studies by Clinton et al.[71] and Stahl et al.[72] indicate that lycopene is found in the human prostate gland primarily in the cis form despite the fact that in the diet lycopene is largely in the trans form. The significance of this transformation remains to be determined.

In summary, until now, studies have examined tomato products and lycopene intake or circulating lycopene levels in relation to prostate cancer risk.[33,34,47] Data suggest that high tomato consumption or high circulating lycopene levels are associated with a 30–40% reduction in risk, especially of extraprostatic prostate cancer. However, not all studies are supportive,[73–75] and one by Gann *et al.*[35] suggested that a significant inverse association with prostate cancer could only be observed in those men with the highest plasma levels of lycopene. It remains to be determined whether the benefits derived from tomato product consumption are due to lycopene *per se* or to the entire complement of carotenoids present in tomatoes.[34] Moreover, earlier studies have shown that the best effects of tomato consumption occurred in prostate cancer patients exhibiting the more lethal, advanced forms of the disease. It remains to be seen if men with early stage prostate cancer also can benefit from increased tomato lycopene consumption.

REFERENCES

1. PARKIN, D. 1999. Estimate of the worldwide incidence of 25 major cancers in 1990. Int. J. Cancer **80:** 827–841.
2. GREENLEE, R.T., T. MURRAY, S. BOLDEN, *et al.* 2000. Cancer statistics, 2000. CA Cancer J. Clin. **50:** 7–323.
3. SPITZ, M., S. STROM, Y. YAMURA, *et al.* 2000. Epidemiologic determinants of clinically relevant prostate cancer. Int. J. Cancer **89:** 259–264.
4. STANFORD, J., J. JUST, M. GIBBS, *et al.* 1997. Polymorphic repeats in the androgen receptor gene: molecular markers of prostate cancer risk. Cancer Res. **57:** 1194–1198.
5. SIGNORELLO, L., K. BRISMAR, R. BERGSTROM, *et al.* 1999. Insulin-like growth factor-binding protein-1 and prostate cancer. J. Natl. Cancer Inst. **91:** 1965–1967.
6. GAO, X., A.T. PORTER & K.V. HONN. 1997. Involvement of multiple tumor suppressor genes and 12-lipoxygenase in human prostate cancer. Therapeutic implications. Adv. Exp. Med. Biol. **407:** 41–53.
7. TINDALL, D. & P. SCARDINO. 1999. Defeating prostate cancer: crucial directions for research: excerpt from the report of the Prostate Cancer Progress Research Group. Prostate **38:** 166–171.
8. BRAWLEY O.W. & H. PARNES. 2000. Prostate cancer prevention trials in the USA. Eur. J. Cancer **36:** 1312–1315.
9. KOLONEL, L., A. NOMURA & R. COONEY. 1999. Dietary fat and prostate cancer: current review. J. Natl. Cancer Inst. **91:** 414–428.
10. KOLONEL, L.N., C.N. YOSHIZAWA & J. H. HANKIN. 1988. Diet and prostatic cancer: a case-control study in Hawaii. Am. J. Epidemiol. **127:** 999–1012.
11. GIOVANNUCCI, E., E.B. RIMM, G.A. COLDITZ, *et al.* 1993. A prospective study of dietary fat and risk of prostate cancer. J. Natl. Cancer Inst. **85:** 1571–1579.
12. GODLEY, P.A., M.K. CAMPBELL, P. GALLAGHER, *et al.* 1996. Biomarkers of essential fatty acid consumption and risk of prostatic carcinoma. Cancer Epidemiol. Biomarkers Prev. **5:** 889–895.
13. NORRISH, A.E., C.M. SKEAFF, G.L. ARRIBAS, *et al.* 1999. Prostate cancer risk and consumption of fish oils: a dietary biomarker-based case-control study. Br. J. Cancer **81:** 1238–1242.
14. NORRISH, A.E., R.T. JACKSON, S.J. SHARPE & C.M. SKEAFF. 2000. Men who consume vegetable oils rich in monounsaturated fat: their dietary patterns and risk of prostate cancer. Cancer Causes Control **11:** 609–615.

15. ROSE, D.P. & J.M. CONNOLLY. 1999. Omega-3 fatty acids as cancer chemopreventive agents. Pharmacol. & Therapeutics **83:** 217–244.
16. ROSE, D.P. & J.M. CONNOLLY. 1991. Effects of fatty acids and eicosanoid synthesis inhibitors on the growth of two human prostate cancer cell lines. Prostate **18:** 243–254.
17. GAO, X., D.J. GRIGNON, T. CHBIHI, et al. 1995. Elevated 12-lipoxygenase in mRNA expression correlates with advanced stage and poor differentiation of human prostate cancer. Urology **46:** 227–237.
18. ANDERSON, K.M., T. SEED, M. VOS, et al. 1998. 5-Lipoxygenase inhibitors reduce PC-3 cell proliferation and initiate nonnecrotic cell death. Prostate **37:** 161–173.
19. GOSH, J. & C.E. MEYERS. 1998. Inhibition of arachidonate 5-lipoxygenase triggers massive apoptosis in human prostate cancer cells. Proc. Natl. Acad. Sci. USA. **95:** 13182–13187.
20. HONN, K.V., D.G. TANG, X. GAO, et al. 1994. 12-lipoxygenases and 12(S)-HETE; role in cancer metastasis. Cancer Metastasis Rev. **13:** 365–396.
21. HERRMANN, J.L., D.G. MENTER, A. BEHAM, et al. 1997. Regulation of lipid signaling pathway for cell survival and apoptosis by bcl-2 in prostate carcinoma cells. Exp. Cell Res. **234:** 442–451.
22. HAU, L.-X., Y.U. SHEN, A. KIRSCHENBAUM & A.C. LEVINE. 1998. NS398, a selective cyclooxygenase-2 inhibitor, induces apoptosis and down-regulates bcl-2 expression in LNCaP cells. Cancer Res. **58:** 4245-4249.
23. HUGHES-FULFORD, M., Y. CHEN & R.R. TJANDRAWINATA. 2001. Fatty acid regulates gene expression and growth of human prostate cancer PC-3 cells. Carcinogenesis **22:** 701–707.
24. ATTIGA, F.A., P.M. FERNANDEZ, A.T. WEERARATNA, et al. 2000. Inhibitors of prostaglandin synthesis inhibit human prostate tumor cell invasiveness and reduce the release of matrix metalloproteinases. Cancer Res. **60:** 4629–4637.
25. ZHOU, J.R. & G.L. BLACKBURN. 1997. Bridging animal and human studies: what are the missing segments in dietary fat and prostate cancer? Am. J. Clin. Nutr. **66:** 1572–1580.
26. TAUBES, G. 2001. The soft science of dietary fat. Science **291:** 2536–2545.
27. HEINONEN, O.P., D. ALBANES, J. VIRTAMO, et al. 1998. Prostate cancer and supplementation with α-tocopherol and β-carotene: incidence and mortality in a controlled trial. J. Natl. Cancer Inst. **90:** 440–446.
28. CLARK, L.C., G.F. COMBS, JR., B.W. TURNBULL, et al. 1996. Effects of selenium supplementation for cancer prevention in patients with carcinoma of the skin. A randomized controlled trial. Nutritional Prevention of Cancer Study Group. J. Am. Med. Assoc. **276:** 1957–1963.
29. CLARK, L.C., B. DALKIN, A. KRONGRAD, et al. 1998. Decreased incidence of prostate cancer with selenium supplementation: results of a double-blind cancer prevention trial. Br. J. Urol. **81:** 730–734.
30. KRISTAL, A.R., J.L. STANFORD, J.H. COHEN, et al. 1999. Vitamin and mineral supplement use is associated with reduced risk of prostate cancer. Cancer Epidemiol. Biol. & Prev. **8:** 887–892.
31. LA VECCHIA, C. 1998. Mediterranean epidemiological evidence on tomatoes and the prevention of digestive tract cancers. Proc. Soc. Exp. Biol. Med. **218:** 125–128.
32. MICHAUD, D.S., D. FESKANICHI, E.B. RIMM, et al. 2000. Intake of specific carotenoids and risk of lung cancer in 2 prospective US cohorts. Am. J. Clin. Nutr. **72:** 990–997.
33. GIOVANNUCCI, E., A. ASCHERIO, E.B. RIMM, et al. 1995. Intake of carotenoids and retinol in relation to risk of prostate cancer. J. Natl. Cancer Inst. **87:** 1767–1776.
34. GIOVANNUCCI, E. 1999. Tomatoes, tomato-based products, lycopene and cancer. Review of the epidemiologic literature. J. Natl. Cancer Inst. **91:** 317–331.
35. GANN, P.H., J. MA, E. GIOVANNUCCI, et al. 1999. Lower prostate cancer risk in men with elevated plasma lycopene levels: results of a prospective analysis. Cancer Res. **59:** 1225–1230.
36. FOURNIER, D.B., J.W. ERDMAN & G.B. GORDON. 1998. Soy, its components and cancer prevention: a review of the *in vitro*, animal and human data. Cancer Epidemiol. Biomarkers Prev. **7:** 1055–1065.

37. BARNES, S., G. PETERSON, C. GRUBBS & K. SETCHELL. 1998. Potential role of dietary isoflavones in the prevention of cancer. Adv. Exp. Med. Biol. **354:** 135–147.
38. PETERSON, G. & S. BARNES. 1993. Genistein and biochanin A inhibit the growth of human prostate cancer cells but not epidermal growth factor receptor tyrosine autophosphorylation. Prostate **22:** 335–345.
39. DAVIS, J.N., B. SINGH, M. BHUIYAN & F.H. SARKAR. 1998. Genistein up-regulation of p21^{WAF1}, down-regulation of cyclin B, and induction of apoptosis in prostate cancer cells. Nutr. & Cancer **32:** 123–131.
40. ROSENBERG ZAND, R.S., D.J.A. JENKINS & E.P. DIAMANDIS. 2000. Agonistic activity of flavonoids and related compounds on steroid hormone receptors. Breast Cancer Res. Treat. **62:** 35–49.
41. WANG, J., I.-E. ELTOUM & C. LAMARTINIERE. 2001. Dietary genistein suppresses chemically induced prostate cancer development in Lobund-Wistar rats (Abstr. 2484). Cancer Res. **42:** 461.
42. WYNDER, E.L., D.P. ROSE & L.A. COHEN. 1994. Nutrition and prostate cancer: a proposal for dietary intervention. Nutr. & Cancer **22:** 1–10.
43. ZHOU, J.R., E.T. GUGGER. T. TANKA, *et al.* 1999. Soybean phytochemicals inhibit the growth of transplantable human prostate carcinoma and tumor angiogenesis in mice. J. Nutr. **129:** 1628–1635.
44. ISAACS, J.T., W.D.W. HESTON, R.M. WEISSMAN & D.S. COFFEY. 1978. Animal models of the hormone-sensitive and in-sensitive prostatic adenocarcinomas. Dunning 3327-H, R-3327-111, and R3327-AT. Cancer Res. **38:** 4353–4359.
45. ROSENBERG ZAND, R.S., D.J. JENKINS & E.P. DIAMANDIS. 2000. Genistein: a potential natural anti-androgen. Clin. Chem. **46:** 887–888.
46. EL-BAYOUMY, K., O.-S. SOHN, C.V. RAO, *et al.* 1995. Chemoprevention of cancer by organoselenium compounds. J. Cell Biochem. (Suppl) **22:** 92–100.
47. NOMURA, A.M.Y., J. LEE, G. STEMMERMANN & J.F. COOMBS, JR. 2000. Serum selenium and subsequent risk of prostate cancer. Cancer Epidemiol. Biomarkers & Prev. **9:** 883–887.
48. ALLAN, C.B., G.M. LACOURCIERE & T.C. STADTMAN. 1999. Responsiveness of selenoproteins to dietary selenium. Annu. Rev. Nutr. **19:** 1–16.
49. GANTHER, H.E. 1986. Pathways of selenium metabolism including respiratory excretory products. J. Am. Coll. Toxocol. **5:** 1–5.
50. IP, C. & H.E. GANTHER. 1990. Activity of methylated forms of selenium in cancer prevention. Cancer Res. **50:** 1206–1211.
51. IP, C., H.J. THOMPSON, Z. ZHU & H.E. GANTHER. 2000. *In vitro* and *in vivo* studies of methylseleninic acid: evidence that a monomethylated selenium metabolite is critical for cancer chemoprevention. Cancer Res. **60:** 2882–2886.
52. MAKROPOULOS, V., T. BRÜNING & K. SCHULZE-OSTHOFF. 1996. Selenium-mediated inhibition of transcription factor NF-κB and HIV-1 LTR promoter activity. Arch. Toxicol. **70:** 227–283.
53. STAPLETON, S.R., G.L. GARLOCK, L. FOELLMI-ADAMS & R.F. KLETZIEN. 1997. Selenium: potent stimulator of tyrosyl phosphorylation and activator of MAP kinase. Biochim. Biophys. Acta **1355:** 259–269.
54. ADLER, V., M.R. PINCUS, S. POSNER, *et al.* 1996. Effects of chemopreventive selenium compounds on Jun N-kinase activities. Carcinogenesis **17:** 1849–1854.
55. KAECK, M., L. JUNXUAN, R. STRANGE, *et al.* 1997. Differential induction of growth arrest inducible genes by selenium compounds. Biochem. Pharmacol. **53:** 921–926.
56. LU, J., M. KAECK, C. JIANG, *et al.* 1994. Selenite induction of DNA strand breaks and apoptosis in mouse leukemic L 12110 cells. Biochem. Pharmacol. **47:** 1531–1535.
57. GOPALAKRISHNA, R., U. GUNDIMEDA & Z.-H. CHEN. 1997. Cancer-preventive selenocompounds induce a specific redox modification of cysteine-rich regions in Ca^{2+}-dependent isoenzymes of protein kinase C. Arch. Biochem. Biophys. **348:** 25–36.
58. JIANG, C., W. JIANG, C. IP, *et al.* 1999. Selenium–induced inhibition of angiogenesis in mammary cancer at chemopreventive levels of intake. Mol. Carcinogenesis **26:** 213–225.
59. JIANG, C., H. GANTHER & J. LU. 2000. Monomethylselenium-specific inhibition of MMP-2 and VEGF expression: implications for angiogenic switch regulation. Mol. Carcinogenesis **29:** 236–250.

60. DALKIN, B.W., A.J. LILLICO, M.E. REID, et al. 2001. Selenium and chemoprevention against prostate cancer: an update on the Clark results (abstr. 2478). Cancer Res. **42:** 460.
61. KHACHIK, F., C.J. SPANGLER, J.C. SMITH, JR., et al. 1997. Identification, quantification, and relative concentrations of carotenoids, and their metabolites in human milk and serum. Anal. Chem. **69:** 1873–1881.
62. DIMASCIO, P., S. KAISER & H. SIES. 1989. Lycopene as the most efficient biological carotenoid singlet oxygen quencher. Arch. Biochem. Biophys. **274:** 532–538.
63. WEISBURGER, J.H., L. DOLAN & B. PITTMAN. 1998. Inhibition of PhIP mutagenicity by caffeine, lycopene, daidzein, and genistein. Mut. Res. **416:** 125–128.
64. STAHL, W., A. JUNGHAMS, B. DE BOER, et al. 1998. Carotenoid mixtures protect multilamellar liposomes against oxidative damage: synergistic effects of lycopene and lutein. FEBS Lett. **427:** 305–308.
65. PASTERI, M., H. PFANDER, D. BOSCOBOINITE & A. AZZI. 1998. Lycopene in association with alpha-tocopherol inhibits at physiological concentrations proliferation of prostate carcinoma cells. Biochem. Biophys. Res. Commun. **250:** 582–585.
66. BERTRAM, J.S. 1999. Carotenoids and gene regulation. Nutr. Rev. **57:** 182–191.
67. STAHL, W., J. VON LAAR, H.D. MARTIN, et al. 2000. Stimulation of gap junctional communication: comparison of acyclo-retinoic acid and lycopene. Arch. Biochem. Biophys. **323:** 271–274.
68. BREINHOLT, V., S.T. LAURIDSEN, B. DAVESHVAR & J. JAKOBSEN. 2000. Dose-response effects of lycopene on selected drug-metabolizing enzymes in the rat. Cancer Letts. **154:** 201–210.
69. CACCIOLA, S.A., L.A. COHEN & K. KASHFI. 1999. Lycopene inhibits proliferation and regulates cyclooxygenase-2 gene expression in neoplastic rat mammary epithelial cells. FASEB J. **13:** Abstr. 441.2.
70. ZHAO, Z., F. KHACHIK, J.P. RICHIE & L.A. COHEN. 1998. Lycopene uptake and tissue disposition in male and female rats. Proc. Soc. Exp. Biol. Med. **218:** 109–114.
71. CLINTON, S.K., C. EMENHISER, S.J. SCHWARTZ, et al. 1996. cis-trans Lycopene isomers, carotenoids, and retinol in the human prostate. Cancer Epidemiol. Biomarkers & Prev. **5:** 823–833.
72. STAHL, W., W. SCHWART, A.R. SUNDQUIST & H. SIES. 1992. Cis-trans isomers of lycopene and β-carotene in human serum and tissues. Arch. Biochem. Biophys. **294:** 173–177.
73. NORRISH, A.E., R.T. JACKSON, S.J. SHARPE & C.M. SKEAFF. 2000. Prostate cancer and dietary carotenoids. Am. J. Epidemiol. **151:** 119–123.
74. KRISTAL, A.R. & J.H. COHEN. 2000. Invited Commentary: tomatoes, lycopene, and prostate cancer. How strong is the evidence? Am. J. Epidemiol. **151:** 124–127.
75. COHEN, J.H., A.R. KRISTAL & J. STANFORD. 2000. Fruit and vegetable intakes and prostate cancer risk. J. Natl. Cancer Inst. **92:** 61–68.

Intercellular Communication and Human Prostate Carcinogenesis

GIUSEPPE CARRUBA,[a] ROSALBA STEFANO,[a] LETIZIA COCCIADIFERRO,[b] FRANCESCA SALADINO,[a] ANTONIETTA DI CRISTINA,[b] ERIK TOKAR,[c] SALMAAN T.A. QUADER,[c] MUKTA M. WEBBER,[c] AND LUIGI CASTAGNETTA[a,b]

[a]*Department of Experimental Oncology and Clinical Application, University Medical School, Palermo, Italy*

[b]*Unit of Experimental Oncology & Palermo Branch of IST-GE and Department of Clinical Oncology, A.R.N.A.S., "M. Ascoli" Cancer Hospital Center, Palermo, Italy*

[c]*Departments of Zoology and Medicine, Michigan State University, East Lansing, Michigan 48824, USA*

ABSTRACT: Gap-junction–mediated intercellular communication (GJIC) is required for completion of embryonic development, tissue homeostasis, and regulation of cell proliferation and death. Although, as emphasized in several reports, defects or disruption of GJIC may be important in carcinogenesis, the potential role of GJIC in the onset and progression of human prostate cancer remains ill-defined. The gap junction channel-forming connexins (Cx) comprise a multigene family of highly conserved proteins that are differentially expressed in a tissue- and development-specific manner; changes in connexin expression are also commonly seen during cellular differentiation. However, when multiple connexins are concurrently expressed, gap junction channels may consist of more than one connexin species. This is important, because only certain pairings give rise to functional channels. In our studies, we investigated GJIC in a panel of both nontumorigenic (RWPE-1) and malignant (RWPE-2, LNCaP, DU-145) human prostate epithelial cells, compared to a normal rat liver epithelial F344 (WB-1) cell line, as it was found to be junctionally proficient. In addition, expression and regulation of Cx43 and Cx32 were also inspected using western blot analysis. The ability of hormones, antihormones, and the antihypertensive drug forskolin to restore GJIC in nontumorigenic and malignant human prostate epithelial cells was examined by the scrape-loading/dye transfer (SL/DT) or fluorescence recovery after photobleaching (FRAP) methods using an Ultima laser cytometer. Results from both assays showed that neither nontumorigenic nor malignant prostate cells have functional GJIC. However, both estrone (E1) and forskolin (FK) induced a significant increase (4.4- and 2.8-fold, respectively) in cell-cell communication only in the RWPE-1 cells. Interestingly, the use of Matrigel, a solubilized basement membrane, as substrate for cell attachment and growth resulted in the rescue of GJIC activity in RWPE-1 cells, as revealed by the SL/DT method. Furthermore, E1 induced a twofold increase in connexin 43 (Cx43), whereas forskolin caused a 50% reduction in Cx32 expression in RWPE-1 cells. These data suggest that agents

Address for correspondence: Giuseppe Carruba, M.D., Ph.D., Unit of Experimental Oncology, "M. Ascoli" Cancer Hospital Center, Via Parlavecchio 139, 90127 Palermo, Italy. Voice: +39 091 666-4346; fax: +39 091 666-4352.
lucashbl@unipa.it

that increase Cx43:Cx32 ratio may restore GJIC in junctionally deficient cells, providing a basis for the development of new strategies for the prevention and treatment of human prostate cancer.

KEYWORDS: prostate cancer; connexin; gap junction; intercellular communication; carcinogenesis

BACKGROUND

Prostate cancer has become the most common neoplasm in men in the United States. An estimated 198,100 new cases and 31,500 deaths from this disease were expected in the year 2001.[1] In Italy, the incidence of prostate cancer has continuously been increasing in the last decade, with an estimate of nearly 13,000 new cases (corresponding to 10% of all male cancers) and 6,800 deaths in 1994.[2] Despite these alarming figures, the causes of prostate cancer in humans remain largely unknown. Studies of prostatic carcinoma have been limited in the past because of the lack of suitable animal and cell culture models. In this respect, the availability of malignant and, especially, nonneoplastic human prostate epithelial cell lines may allow important advances and provide a consistent and reproducible source for prostate studies.

The multistep carcinogenesis of human solid tumors, including prostate cancer, is a complex, lengthy process, leading to conversion of a normal cell to a metastasizing, invasive cancer cell. According to the operational concepts of initiation→ promotion→progression, this process involves dramatic alteration in cell phenotypes, including the inability to terminally differentiate, the loss of growth control or contact inhibition, and the acquired invasive/metastatic potential. Concurrent evidence in the literature supports the theory that cancer is a stem cell disease or a disease of differentiation. In this concept, the initiation phase, where mutagens are assumed to induce ostensibly irreversible genetic changes in the cell, would prevent or partially block the ability of a stem cell to terminally differentiate. Conversely, the promotion phase is a potentially interruptible or reversible process whereby promoters, which act operationally as mitogens rather than mutagens, induce clonal amplification of the single initiated stem cell that is unable to terminally differentiate but can still self-renew. The progression phase converts a promoter-dependent, premalignant initiated cell to a malignant and tumor promoter-independent cell through additional genetic/epigenetic alteration. Because the terminal differentiation pathway is associated with the appearance of the gap-junctional intercellular communication (GJIC), it has been speculated that any agent capable of disrupting GJIC or preventing its formation may play a role in carcinogenesis. Several tumor promoters, a wide spectrum of chemicals, drugs, environmental pollutants, a variety of toxicants, as well as hormones and growth factors, have all been shown to inhibit GJIC.[3–5]

The identification of agents capable of preventing GJIC disruption in junctionally proficient cells, restoring GJIC in gap junctionally deficient cells, and reducing proliferative activity of cells or increasing their apoptotic rates, or both may provide significant insights into our understanding of the carcinogenetic process. Furthermore, this may eventually lead to the development of novel chemopreventive measures and to the improvement of current therapeutic strategies in human prostate cancer. The availability of a wide panel of nontumoral (immortalized), chemically transformed, and cancer-derived prostate epithelial cell lines represents an invaluable tool for accurately investigating various steps in multistage carcinogenesis of the human prostate.

INTERCELLULAR COMMUNICATION: THE CELLULAR WEB

From an evolutionary standpoint, single cell organisms survived changes in the environment by adaptively responding to physical (temperature and radiation) and chemical (nutrients, toxins, and toxicants) agents through intracellular signals leading to modification of cell proliferation. In multicellular organisms, the fine tuning of growth and differentiation processes had to occur after fertilization of the egg cell to organize and orchestrate the collection of pluripotent stem, progenitor, and differentiated cells during embryonic/fetal development, sexual maturation, and adulthood/aging of the individual organism. That tuning of specific cell/tissue and organ system functions is referred to as homeostasis.

In multicellular organisms, three distinct forms of communication have homeostatic control of major cell functions, namely, cell growth and differentiation, apoptosis, and adaptive responses of differentiated cells. Extracellular communication is involved in the secretion of hormones, growth factors, cytokines, and neurotransmitters from one cell to another, over distance and space. The intracellular communication triggered in the cell by these extracellular effectors involves a modification of a variety of second messengers (including cAMP, Ca^{2+}, reactive oxygen species, nitric oxide, etc.) that set off different signal transduction systems, such as protein kinase C and mitogen-activated protein kinases. This intracellular network may either increase or diminish the third form of cell communication, gap-junctional intercellular communication (GJIC).[6] The GJIC, which functions through direct cytoplasmic continuity between adjacent cells, is required for completion of embryonic development, maintenance of tissue homeostasis, and regulation of normal cell growth.[7–9] A family of highly evolutionarily conserved genes, termed gap junction genes, code for peptides, the connexins, which self-assemble into hexamers forming a hemichannel unit, called connexon. Two adjacent connexons from contiguous cells attach end to end to give rise to a hydrophilic membrane channel through which ions and small molecules (below 1,000 daltons) may equilibrate the cytoplasms and synchronize the metabolic activities of coupled cells.

Several reports have emphasized that disruption of GJIC may be important in carcinogenesis. Evidence is consistent that various oncogenes (e.g., *ras*, *raf*, *neu*, and *src*),[10,11] some tumor suppressor genes (such as *p53* and *pRb*),[12] different tumor-promoting chemicals (e.g., phenobarbital and phorbol esters),[13] and several antitumor-promoting agents (including retinoids and dexamethasone),[14] which are all known to inhibit or enhance apoptosis, can also respectively inhibit or enhance GJIC at the transcriptional, translational, or posttranslational level. In this respect, GJIC may have a permissive role in apoptosis by facilitating the information trafficking needed to trigger cell death. On the other hand, transfection of different gap junction genes into a variety of noncommunicating tumor cells increases genetic stability, restores some or most growth control, and suppresses tumorigenicity of cells.[15,16] All of the foregoing evidence would imply that gap junction genes could be considered a novel family of tumor suppressor genes. It could be speculated that alteration of

GJIC may represent a nongenotoxic mechanism that plays a role in tumor promotion, also by inhibiting apoptosis.[17]

HUMAN PROSTATE EPITHELIAL CELL SYSTEMS

In our studies, we have used a panel of both nontumorigenic and malignant human prostate epithelial cells. The RWPE-1 and RWPE-2 cell lines were originally established from nontumoral human prostate tissue samples obtained from patients who underwent cystoprostatectomy for bladder cancer, and then immortalized by: (1) transfection with human papilloma virus 18 (HPV18) for RWPE-1 cells;[18] and (2) a combination of HPV18 and Kirsten murine sarcoma virus containing the activated Ki-*ras* oncogene for RWPE-2 cells.[18] The LNCaP.FGC and DU-145 human prostate cancer cells were obtained from the American Type Culture Collection (Rockville, MD). For the GJIC studies, all of the aforementioned cells were compared to a normal rat liver epithelial F344 (WB-1) cell line, as it has been found to be junctionally proficient.[19]

The nontumorigenic cell lines represent a unique model for studies on the regulation of prostate cell growth and differentiation, because they retain the ability to grow in response to both androgens and peptide growth factors (including EGF and TGF-β) and express both PSA and androgen receptor.[19] More importantly, RWPE-1 cells undergo acinar morphogenesis in three-dimensional matrix cultures, similar to normal human prostatic epithelium *in vivo*.[20,21] This cell model has a twofold value. Firstly, immortalization is a necessary event in the multistep process of carcinogenesis; therefore, studies using immortalized cells may provide important clues for a deeper understanding of neoplastic transformation. Secondly, there is multiple, although controversial, evidence that sexually transmitted human papilloma viruses may play a role in the etiology of prostate cancer in humans.[22,23]

GAP-JUNCTION–MEDIATED INTERCELLULAR COMMUNICATION STUDIES

For GJIC, cells were examined either under standard conditions or following a 48-hour exposure to test agents including: (a) estradiol (E_2, 1 μM); (b) estrone (E_1, 1 μM); (c) the antiestrogen tamoxifen (1 μM); (d) the synthetic estrogen diethylstilbestrol (DES, 15 μM); (e) the synthetic androgen R1881 (1 μM); (f) the pure antiandrogen casodex (1 μM); and (g) the antihypertensive drug forskolin (FK, 30 μM). Control cell cultures received relevant vehicle (DMSO for FK; ethanol for all other treatments) alone (0.01% v/v).

GJIC activity was assessed using two different approaches: the scrape-loading/dye transfer (SL/DT)[24] and the fluorescence recovery after photobleaching (FRAP)[25] assays. In the SL/DT assay, junctional communication was measured as the extent of diffusion of fluorescent, membrane-impermeable, lucifer yellow dye, after cell monolayers were scraped using a surgical blade and exposed to dye for a few minutes at room temperature. In the FRAP assay, cells were incubated with 5,6-carboxyfluorescein diacetate for 15 minutes at 37°C, the dye transfer visualized us-

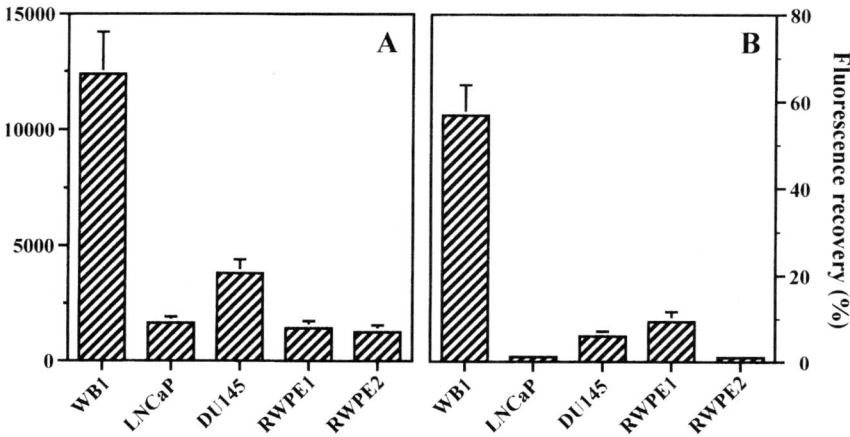

FIGURE 1. SL/DT (**A**) and FRAP (**B**) analysis of GJIC activity in nontumorigenic and malignant human prostate epithelial cells. Values represent average positive areas (μm^2) for SL/DT and percentage of recoveries of fluorescence after photobleaching for FRAP. For methodologic details see text.

ing a 488-nm laser beam to bleach selected cells, and recovery of fluorescence monitored over time using an Ultima laser cytometer.

Using both SL/DT and FRAP assays, we observed that neither nontumorigenic nor malignant prostate cells exhibited efficient cell-cell communication under basic conditions, whereas, as expected, WB-1 cells showed GJIC activity (FIG. 1). However, RWPE-1 cells showed 10% recovery of fluorescence after photobleaching, provided the observation time was extended to 1 hour. This evidence implies that RWPE-1 cells may at least partly retain functional GJIC.

In separate experiments, we investigated the potential induction of GJIC by various test agents. A 48-hour exposure of cells to both forskolin and estrone resulted in a significant ($p < 0.0001$) rise in junctional transfer in RWPE-1 cells compared to untreated cells. This was confirmed using either the SL/DT (FIG. 2) or the FRAP method (FIG. 3). In the former, a three- and fourfold increase in dye transfer was respectively observed for FK and E1; in the latter, fluorescence recovery values with FK (27%) and E1 (35%) were significantly greater than those in controls (around 3%). Treatment of cells with all remaining test agents (E_2, DES, TAM, and R1881) did not induce any significant change in GJIC activity in any of the cell lines studied (not shown).

THE CONNEXINS: PROTEINS "ON-LINE"

The gap-junction channel-forming connexins comprise a multigene family with at least 13 members in mammals.[26,27] Connexins (Cx) are differentially expressed in a cell-, tissue-, and development-specific manner; changes in connexin expression are also commonly seen during cellular differentiation. Despite the presence of high-

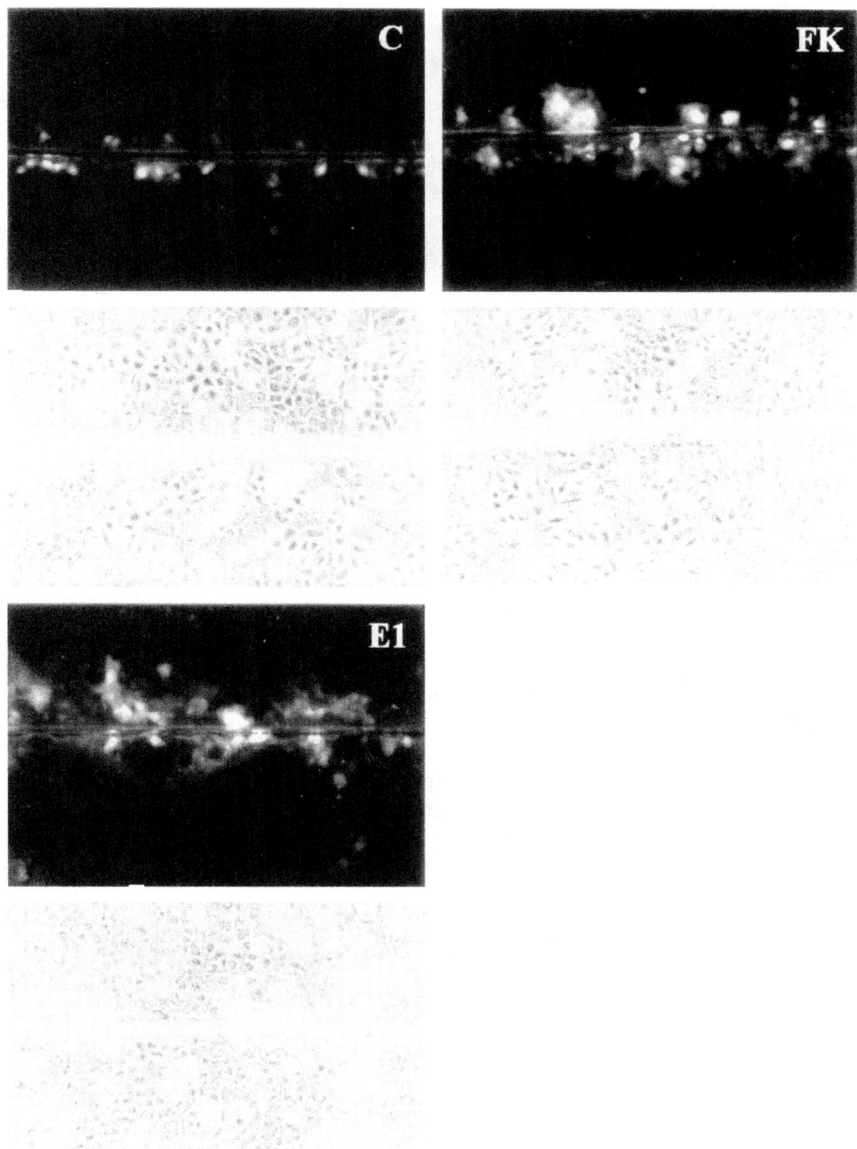

FIGURE 2. Effects of forskolin (FK) and estrone (E1) on GJIC activity in RWPE-1 cells. Cells were incubated for 24 hours in the presence of relevant treatment, and then junctional transfer was assessed by the SL/DT method, as described in Material and Methods. Control cell cultures (C) received vehicle (DMSO for FK, ethanol for E1) alone. For each condition, fluorescence is shown in the upper figure, phase contrast in the lower.

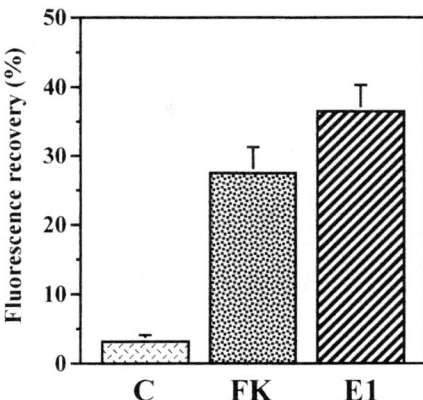

FIGURE 3. FRAP analysis of GJIC activity in RWPE-1 cells. Cells were incubated for 48 hours in the presence of 30 µM forskolin (FK) or 1 µM estrone (E1), and then junctional transfer was assessed by the FRAP method. Control cell cultures (C) received vehicle alone. Values represent average percentage of recoveries of fluorescence after photobleaching.

ly conserved sequences within different connexins, the diversity of these proteins is not due to alternative splicing of their mRNAs; instead, there appears to be one gene for each connexin. In those cells in which multiple connexins are expressed, gap-junction hemichannels may consist of more than one connexin species (heteromeric connexons) or they may be composed of a single connexin (homomeric connexons). Heteromeric channels, unlike homomeric ones, may have distinct permeability and regulatory properties, thus providing various additional options for regulating the type of signals that pass throughout. Heterotypic channels, consisting of two different connexons (both homomeric and heteromeric), have also been described.[28] This is worth mentioning, because only certain heterotypic pairings give rise to functional channels (e.g., Cx43/Cx26 or Cx32/Cx26, but not Cx43/Cx32).[27]

In our studies, we used western blot analysis to determine if either FK or E1 increases GJIC activity in RWPE-1 cells by regulating connexin expression, including Cx43, Cx32, and Cx26. Greater amounts of Cx43 were found in RWPE-1 cells with respect to their malignant, *Ki-ras*–transformed derivative, RWPE-2 cells. Conversely, higher expression levels of Cx32 were found in RWPE-2 than in RWPE-1 cells, whereas no expression of Cx26 could be detected in the two cell lines (FIG. 4). The presence of differentially phosphorylated species of Cx43 was observed in RWPE-1 cells only. It has repeatedly been reported that the phosphorylation status of gap junction proteins plays a crucial role in the regulation of a variety of connexin processes, including trafficking, assembly/disassembly, degradation, and the gating of gap junction channels.[29,30] In particular, Cx43 is translated as a 42-kDa protein that is efficiently phosphorylated to a 46-kDa species in junctionally competent, but not junctionally deficient cells.[31] On the other hand, tyrosine phosphorylarion of connexin proteins induced by the v-*src* oncogene results in complete inhibition of Cx43 channels, whereas Cx32 channels are unaffected.[32]

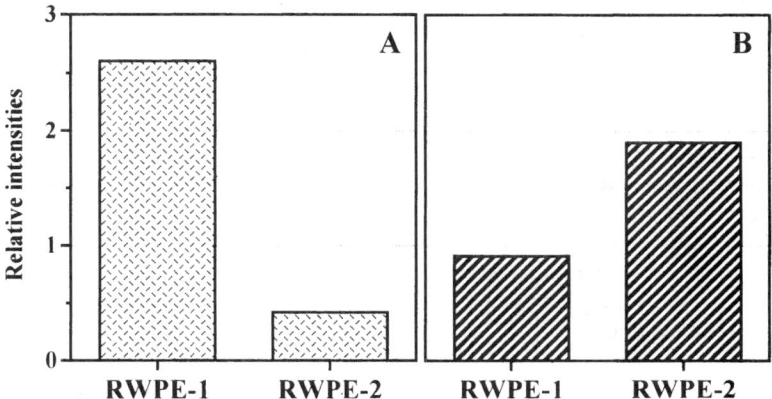

FIGURE 4. Western blot analysis of Cx43 (**A**) and Cx32 (**B**) expression in RWPE-1 and RWPE-2 cells. Values represent densitometric quantification of relative intensities for Cx32 and Cx43 in RWPE-1 and RWPE-2 cells after normalization for α-tubulin.

As illustrated in FIGURE 5, in RWPE-1 cells, E1 induced a significant increase in the expression of Cx43 and its differentially phosphorylated species, whereas FK did not change the expression levels of Cx43. Conversely, both E1 and FK reduced Cx32 expression in RWPE-1 cells. In the RWPE-2 cell line, FK induced a consistent increase in Cx43 with no changes in Cx32 expression, whereas E1 did not modify either Cx43 or Cx32 expression in this cell line (not shown). This evidence indicates that E1 may rescue GJIC activity in RWPE-1 cells through upregulation of Cx43 and reduction of Cx32 expression. In particular, it could be speculated that agents capable of increasing Cx43 (E1) or decreasing Cx32 (E1 and FK), or both, thus eventually leading to a rise of Cx43 to Cx32 ratio, may restore intercellular communication

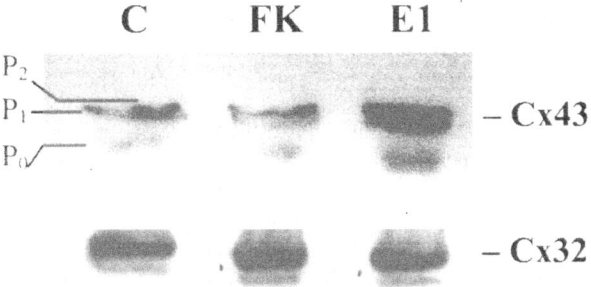

FIGURE 5. Western blot analysis of Cx43 and Cx32 regulation in RWPE-1 cells. Immunoblots show expression of Cx32 and Cx43 in control (C) cell cultures and after treatment with 30 μM FK or 1 μM E1. P_0-P_2 indicate the differentially phosphorylated species of Cx43.

in junctionally deficient cells. The relevance of Cx43 and Cx32 balance has been emphasized by recent evidence that adult prostates of neonatally estrogenized rats exhibit a marked decrease in Cx32 and a sustained increase in Cx43 expression, leading to significant changes in GJIC.[33] It is worth noting that both FK and E1 have been reported to increase intracellular levels of cAMP in human prostate cells,[34,35] suggesting that cAMP-dependent signal transduction pathways could also be involved in the regulation of connexin expression and junctional communication.

We have observed that FK did not induce any change in GJIC activity in RWPE-2 cells despite an over threefold increase in the expression of Cx43 in this cell line. The presence of differentially phosphorylated Cx43 species solely in RWPE-1 but not RWPE-2 cells may represent an essential prerequisite for restoration of intercellular communication.

SUBSTRATE FOR ANCHORAGE-DEPENDENT CELL GROWTH AND DIFFERENTIATION: THE MATRIGEL BASEMENT MEMBRANE MATRIX

It is self-evident that cell cultures, mostly heterogeneous by nature, are invariably exposed to the selective pressures of an otherwise artificial environment and usually grow attached to an unnatural substrate. Therefore, care should be taken when extrapolating experimental data from the *in vitro* to the *in vivo* condition. The use of Matrigel, a solubilized basement membrane containing laminin, collagen IV, and heparan sulfate proteoglycans, instead of plastic, may help mimic the interaction of cultured cells with the extracellular matrix.[21] In particular, Matrigel allows attachment and differentiation of both normal and transformed epithelial cells, influences their gene expression, and provides a useful model system for cell invasion and angiogenesis assays.[36–38] Our recent studies indicated that the noninvasive RWPE-1 human prostate epithelial cell line undergoes acinar morphogenesis in three-dimensional matrix cell cultures, laminin-1 and a functional $\alpha 6\beta 1$ integrin receptor being required for cell polarization and acinar formation.[21,39]

Based on the assumption that terminal differentiation of stem or progenitor cells is associated with the appearance of GJIC and that Matrigel facilitates cell differentiation, we examined the potential of this basement membrane matrix to restore intercellular communication in nontumorigenic, immortalized RWPE-1 human prostate epithelial cells. As illustrated in FIGURE 6, RWPE-1 cells show dramatic morphologic changes when cultured on Matrigel rather than plastic, giving rise to acinar-like structures (FIG. 6B) instead of the customary cell monolayer (FIG. 6A). More importantly, the assessment of GJIC activity using the SL/DT method reveals that the use of Matrigel as a substrate for cell attachment and growth results in the rescue of GJIC activity in RWPE-1 cells (FIG. 6C), whereas the same cells grown on plastic do not show, as expected, any detectable junctional transfer of dye (FIG. 6D). This evidence demonstrates the concept that intercellular communication may have a role in the terminal differentiation pathway and, at same time, may support the use of Matrigel as a helpful tool in studying the ability of various agents to prevent GJIC disruption in junctionally proficient cells.

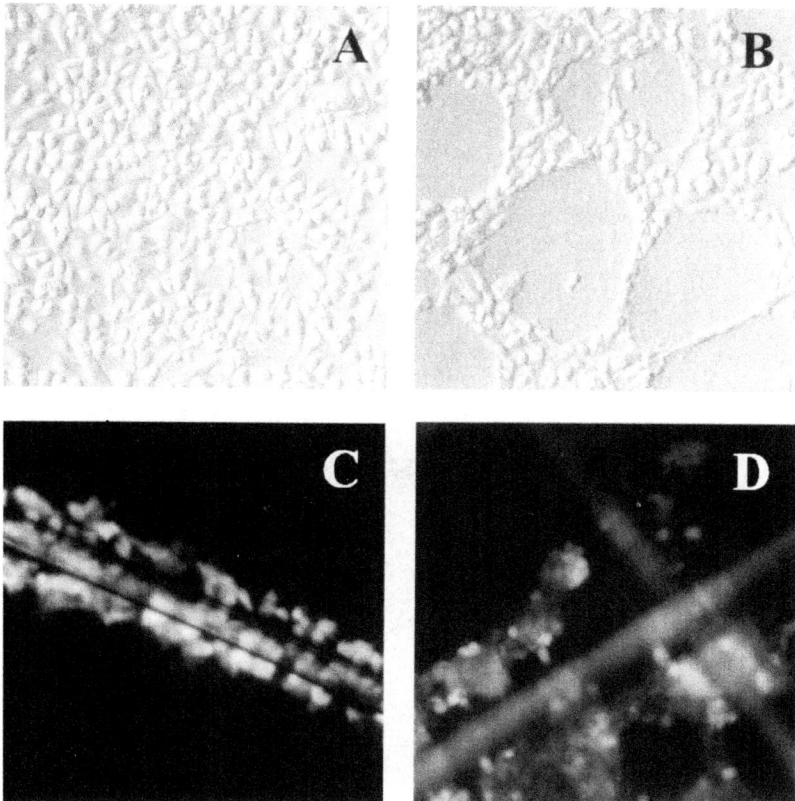

FIGURE 6. Effects of Matrigel on RWPE-1 cell differentiation and junctional activity. Cells were grown either on plastic (**A** and **C**) or Matrigel (**B** and **D**). Morphologic changes are shown in **A** and **B**; variations of GJIC activity, as assessed by the SL/DT method, are illustrated in **C** and **D**.

HUMAN PROSTATE CARCINOGENESIS AND INTERCELLULAR COMMUNICATION: FACTS AND PERSPECTIVES

It is well established that carcinogenesis for any human cancer, including human prostate cancer, is a multistep, multimechanism process involving the interaction of genetic (e.g., protooncogenes and tumor suppressor genes), endogenous (i.e., hormones and growth factors), and environmental (e.g., diet, radiation, and chemical pollutants) factors. Several well documented theories of carcinogenesis have been used to explain the multistage, multimechanism process of carcinogenesis, namely, the stem cell theory,[40,41] the theory of cancer as a disease of differentiation or oncogeny as partially blocked ontogen,[42] and the initiation/promotion/progression theory.[43] The age-old nature versus nurture concept has now been resolved, showing that nature and nurture, that is, genes and environmental factors, must interact to bring about cancer.[44] Lastly, the mutation versus epigenetic theories of carcinogenesis highlight the possible mechanisms that could convert a normal cell into a malignant one.

One critical assumption in the assessment of cancer risk involves the identification of the target cells for the carcinogenic process. Is any cell in all tissues potentially capable of being converted to a cancer cell? Or, are there only a few special types of cells that can undergo tumorigenic transformation? According to the theory of oncogeny as partially blocked ontogeny, also supported by that of cancer as a disease of differentiation, stem cells and/or their progenitor cell derivatives may represent the target cells. Stem cells represent a distinctive cell compartment that has the peculiar feature of dividing asymmetrically: one daughter cell goes down a terminal differentiation pathway, the other one retains stem cell properties, thus maintaining the stem cell pool.

Within this framework, the concept of carcinogenesis is viewed as a stem or a progenitor cell being exposed to an initiating agent that induces a stable alteration (a mutation or an epigenetic repression at the transcriptional level) of a protooncogene or a tumor suppressor gene (initiation phase) that controls terminal differentiation of the cell but does not disturb the regulation of its proliferative ability. This initiation or mutation of a critical gene controlling the terminal differentiation pathway would confer the status of immortalization, but not neoplastic transformation, on this cell. As long as this initiated stem-like cell is communicating with neighbor normal cells (heterologous GJIC) or with other initiated cells (homologous GJIC), there will be no cell proliferation. Exposing this initiated cell to agents that could cause this cell to proliferate but not terminally differentiate or undergo apoptosis would inhibit GJIC in a sustained but reversible fashion, leading to an accumulation of partially differentiated cells (oncogeny as partially blocked ontogeny). During this clonal expansion, or the promotion phase of carcinogenesis, additional genetic/epigenetic events could cause more activation of oncogenes or inactivation of tumor suppressor genes, which brings about genetic and stable inhibition of GJIC and results in the appearance of a malignant phenotype (the progression phase of carcinogenesis).

A variety of agents, including hormones and growth factors, may affect connexin gene expression and both formation and activity of gap junction channels in various cell systems. Unfortunately, little information is available on the potential role of GJIC disturbances in the development of human prostate cancer and its progression from an androgen-responsive towards an androgen-refractory state. In this framework, the availability of a wide panel of prostate epithelial cell lines (from normal pluripotent stem cells to the transformed, highly tumorigenic cells) may provide a unique model system to obtain significant insights into the carcinogenetic process of the human prostate. Particularly agents that prevent GJIC disruption in junctionally proficient cells or retrieve GJIC in junctionally deficient cells, such as retinoids,[45,46] may be considered for the development of new strategies in both prevention and treatment of prostate cancer.

ACKNOWLEDGMENTS

These studies were partly supported by the Italian Association for Cancer Research (AIRC) and the National Research Council (CNR).

REFERENCES

1. GREENLEE, R., M. HILL-HARMON, T. MURRAY, et al. 2001. Cancer statistics, 2001. CA Cancer J. **51:** 15–36.
2. VANNONI, F., A. BURGIO, L. QUATTROCIOCCHI, et al. 1999. Social differences and indicators of perceived health, chronic diseases, disability and life style in the 1994. ISTAT National Health Interview Survey. Epidemiol. Prev. **23:** 215–229.
3. TROSKO, J., C. CHANG, B. UPHAM, et al. 1998. Epigenetic toxicology as toxicant-induced changes in intracellular signalling leading to altered gap junctional intercellular communication. Toxicol. Lett. **102-103:** 71–78.
4. WILSON, M., T. CLOSE & J. TROSKO. 2000. Cell population dynamics (apoptosis, mitosis, and cell-cell communication) during disruption of homeostasis. Exp. Cell Res. **254:** 257–268.
5. RUCH, R. & J. TROSKO. 2001. Gap-junction communication in chemical carcinogenesis. Drug Metab. Rev. **33:** 117–124.
6. LOEWENSTEIN, W. 1981. Junctional intercellular communication: the cell to cell exchange channel. Physiol. Rev. **61:** 829–913.
7. PITTS, J. & M. FINBOW. 1986. The gap junction. J. Cell Sci. Suppl. **4:** 239–266.
8. BEYER, E. 1993. Gap junctions. Int. Rev. Cytol. **137C:** 1–37.
9. BENNETT, M.V.L. & D.C. SPRAY. 1987. Gap Junctions. Cold Spring Harbor Laboratory. Cold Spring Harbor, NY.
10. KALIMI, G., L. HAMPTON, J. TROSKO, et al. 1992. Homologous and heterologous gap-junctional intercellular communication in v-raf-, v-myc-, and v-raf/v-myc-transduced rat liver epithelial cell lines. Mol. Carcinog. **5:** 301–310.
11. FERNANDEZ-SARABIA, M. & J. BISHOP. 1993. Bcl-2 associates with the ras related protein R-ras p23. Nature **36:** 274–277.
12. LOWE, S., E. SCHMITT, S. SMITH, et al. 1993. p53 is required for radiation induced apoptosis in mouse thymocytes. Nature **362:** 847–849.
13. TOMEI, L., P. KANTER & C. WENNER. 1988. Inhibition of radiation-induced apoptosis *in vitro* by tumor promoters. Biochem. Biophys. Res. Commun. **155:** 324–331.
14. ALLES, A. & K. SULIK. 1989. Retinoic acid-induced lymb-reduction defects: perturbation of zones of programmed cell death as a pathogenetic mechanism. Teratology **40:** 163–171.
15. ROSE, B., P. METHA & W. LOEWENSTEIN. 1993. Gap junction protein gene suppresses tumorigenicity. Carcinogenesis **14:** 1073–1075.
16. ZHU, W., N. MIRONOV & H. YAMASAKI. 1997. Increased genetic stability of HeLa cells after connexin 43 gene transfection. Cancer Res. **57:** 2148–2150.
17. TROSKO, J. & J. GOODMAN. 1994. Intercellular communication may facilitate apoptosis: implication for tumor promotion. Mol. Carcinog. **11:** 8–12.
18. BELLO, D., M. WEBBER, H. KLEINMAN, et al. 1997. Androgen responsive adult human prostatic epithelial cell lines immortalized by human papillomavirus 18. Carcinogenesis **18:** 1215–1223.
19. TSAO, M., J. SMITH, K. NELSON, et al. 1984. A diploid epithelial cell line from normal adult rat liver with phenotypic properties of oval cells. Exp. Cell Res. **154:** 38–52.
20. WEBBER, M., D. BELLO, H. KLEINMAN, et al. 1997. Acinar differentiation in non-malignant immortalized human prostatic cells and its loss by malignant cells. Carcinogenesis **18:** 1225–1231.
21. BELLO-DEOCAMPO, D., H. KLEINMAN, N. DEOCAMPO, et al. 2001. Laminin-1 and $\alpha6\beta1$ integrin regulate acinar morphogenesis of normal and malignant human prostate epithelial cells. Prostate **46:** 142–153.
22. SUZUKI, H., A. KOMIYA, S. AIDA, et al. 1996. Detection of human papillomavirus DNA and p53 gene mutations in human prostate cancer. Prostate **28:** 318–324.
23. WEBBER, M., D. BELLO & S. QUADER. 1997. Immortalized and tumorigenic adult human prostatic epithelial cell lines: characteristics and applications Part 2. Tumorigenic cell lines. Prostate **30:** 58–64.
24. EL FOULY, M., J. TROSKO & C. CHANG. 1987. Scrape-loading and dye transfer: A rapid and simple technique to study gap junctional intercellular communication. Exp. Cell Res. **168:** 422–430.

25. WADE, M., J. TROSKO & M. SCHINDLER. 1986. A fluorescence photobleaching assay of gap junction-mediated communication between human cells. Science **232:** 525–528.
26. PAUL, D. 1995. New functions for gap junctions. Curr. Opin. Cell Biol. **7:** 665–672.
27. BRUZZONE, R., T. WHITE & D. PAUL. 1996. Connections with connexins: the molecular basis for direct intracellular signaling. Eur. J. Biochem. **238:** 1–27.
28. BAUKAUSKAS, F., C. ELFGANG, K. WILLECKE, et al. 1995. Heterotypic gap junction channels (connexin26-connexin32) violate the paradigm of unitary conductance. Pflüger's Arch. **429:** 870–872.
29. WOLBURG, H. & A. ROHLMAN. 1995. Structure function relationship in gap junctions. Int. Rev. Cytol. **157:** 315–373.
30. CRUCIANI, V., O. KAALHUS & S. MIKALSEN. 1999. Phosphatases involved in modulation of gap junctional intercellular communication and dephosphorylation of connexin43 in hamster fibroblasts: 2B or not 2B? Exp. Cell Res. **252:** 449–463.
31. LAMPE, P., E. TENBROEK, J. BURT, et al. 2000. Phosphorylation of connexin43 on serine368 by protein kinase C regulates gap junctional communication. J. Cell Biol. **149:** 1503–1512.
32. SWENSON, K., H. PIWNICA-WORMS, H. MCNAMEE, et al. 1990. Tyrosine phosphorylation of the gap junction protein connexin43 is required for the pp60v-src-induced inhibition of communication. Cell Regul. **1:** 989–1002.
33. HABERMANN, H., W. CHANG, L. BIRCH, et al. 2001. Developmental exposure to estrogens alters epithelial cell adhesion and gap junction proteins in the adult rat prostate. Endocrinology **142:** 359–369.
34. METHA, P., B. LOKESHWAR, P. SCHILLER, et al. 1996. Gap-junctional communication in normal and neoplastic prostate epithelial cells and its regulation by cAMP. Mol. Carcinog. **15:** 18–32.
35. CARRUBA, G., R. FARRUGGIO, M.D. MICELI, et al. 1998. Estrogen regulation of cAMP levels and growth of cultured human prostate cancer cells. 1012s of the First International Meeting on Rapid Response to Steroid Hormones. Mannheim, Germany.
36. MEDINA, D., M. LI, C. OBORN, et al. 1987. Casein gene expression in mouse mammary epithelial cell lines: dependence upon extracellular matrix and cell type. Exp. Cell Res. **172:** 192-203.
37. ALBINI, A., Y. IWAMOTO, H. KLEINMAN, et al. 1987. A rapid *in vitro* assay for quantitating the invasive potential of tumor cells. Cancer Res. **47:** 3239–3245.
38. NICOSIA, R. & A. OTTINETTI. 1990. Growth of microvessels in serum-free matrix culture of rat aorta. A quantitative assay of angiogenesis *in vitro*. Lab. Invest. **63:** 115–122.
39. BELLO-DEOCAMPO, D., H. KLEINMAN & M. WEBBER. 2001. The role of α6β1 integrin and EGF in normal and malignant acinar morphogenesis of human prostatic epithelial cells. Mutat. Res. **480/481:** 209–217.
40. TILL, J. 1982. Stem cells in differentiation and neoplasia. J. Cell Physiol. **1:** 3–11.
41. KONDO, S. 1983. Carcinogenesis in relation to the stem cell mutation hypothesis. Differentiation **24:** 1–8.
42. POTTER, V. 1978. Phenotypic diversity in experimental hepatomas: the concept of partially blocked ontogeny. Br. J. Cancer **38:** 1–23.
43. TROSKO, J. & R. RUCH. 1998. Cell-cell communication in carcinogenesis. Front. Carcinog. **3:** 208–236.
44. TROSKO, J., V. RICCARDI, C. CHANG, et al. 1985. Genetic predisposition to initiation or promotion phases in human carcinogenesis. *In* Biomarkers, Genetics and Cancer. H. Anton-Guirgis & H. Lynch, eds. :13–37. Van Nostrand Reinhold Co. New York.
45. QUADER, S., D. BELLO-DEOCAMPO, D. WILLIAMS, et al. 2001. Evaluation of chemopreventive potential for retinoids using a novel *in vitro* human prostate carcinogenesis model. Mutat. Res. **496:** 153–161.
46. SHARP, R., D. BELLO-DEOCAMPO, S. QUADER, et al. 2001. *N*-(4-hydroxy phenyl)retinamide (4-HPR) decreases neoplastic properties of human prostate cells: an agent for prevention. Mutat. Res. **496:** 163–170.

Precancerous Lesions and Conditions of the Prostate

From Morphological and Biological Characterization to Chemoprevention

RODOLFO MONTIRONI, ROBERTA MAZZUCCHELLI, AND MARINA SCARPELLI

Institute of Pathological Anatomy and Histopathology, University of Ancona, Ancona, Italy

ABSTRACT: Prostatic intraepithelial neoplasia (PIN) is composed of dysplastic cells with a luminal cell phenotype, expressing the androgen receptor as well as prostate-specific antigen. PIN is characterized by progressive abnormalities of phenotype that are intermediate between normal prostatic epithelium and cancer, indicating impairment of cell differentiation and regulatory control with advancing stages of carcinogenesis. High-grade PIN is considered the most likely precursor of prostatic carcinoma, according to virtually all available evidence. Androgen deprivation decreases the prevalence and extent of PIN and the degree of capillary vascularization (e.g., angiogenesis) in the surrounding stroma via suppression of vascular endothelial growth factor production. Prostatic carcinoma is also likely to arise from precursor lesions other than high-grade PIN such as low-grade PIN, atypical adenomatous hyperplasia, malignancy-associated foci, and atrophy.

KEYWORDS: prostate; prostatic intraepithelial neoplasia; intraductal dysplasia; intraductal carcinoma; atypical adenomatous hyperplasia; prostatic adenocarcinoma; chemoprevention

INTRODUCTION

Prostate cancer is usually heterogeneous and multifocal, with diverse clinical and morphological manifestations. Current understanding of the molecular basis of this heterogeneity is limited, particularly for prostatic intraepithelial neoplasia, the only putative precursor that can be identified according to morphological criteria.

Initial references to prostatic intraepithelial neoplasia (PIN) were made by Orteil,[1] Andrews,[2] and Kastendieck and Helpap,[3] but these investigators did not distinguish these findings from those mimicking PIN. In 1965, McNeal[4] emphasized the possible premalignant nature of proliferative changes in prostatic epithelium, but

---

Address for correspondence: Prof. Rodolfo Montironi, M.D., FRCPath., Institute of Pathological Anatomy and Histopathology, University of Ancona School of Medicine, Ospedale Regionale, I-60020 Torrette, Ancona, Italy. Fax: +39071889985.
r.montironi@popcsi.unian.it

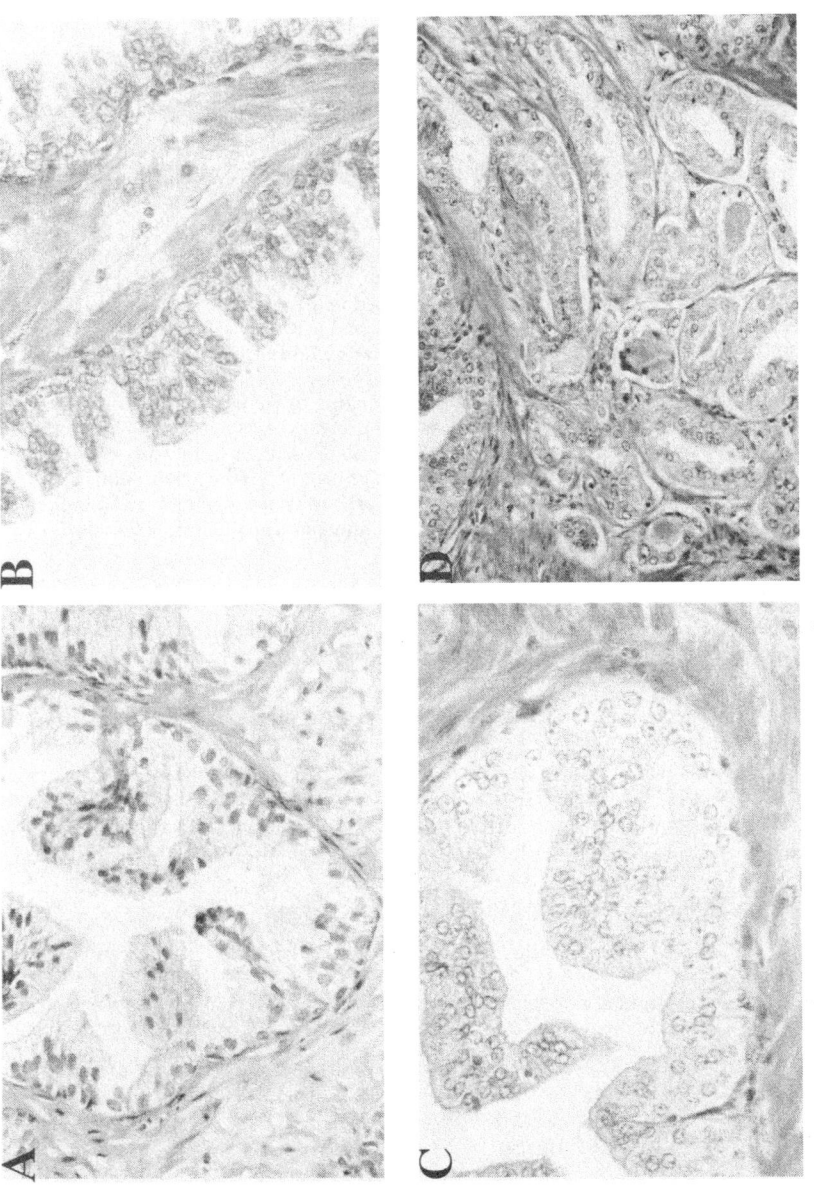

FIGURE 1. (**A**) Normal prostate; (**B**) low-grade prostatic intraepithelial neoplasia (PIN); (**C**) high-grade PIN; and (**D**) invasive prostatic adenocarcinoma.

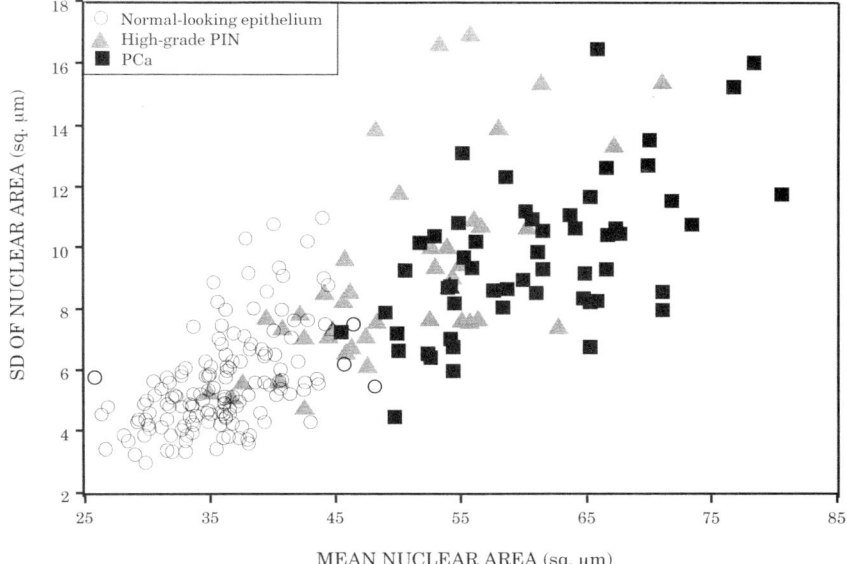

FIGURE 2. Scattergram obtained with mean and SD of the nuclear area of each sector. There is a continuum from normal-looking epithelium to prostatic intraepithelial neoplasia (PIN) and prostatic cancer (PCa). A certain degree of overlap exists between the values of normal-looking epithelium and those of PIN.

his description included a variety of morphological findings. Twenty-one years later, McNeal and Bostwick[5] first described reproducible criteria for the recognition of what they referred to as "intraductal dysplasia" and introduced a three-grade classification system. The following year, Bostwick and Brawer[6] proposed the term prostatic intraepithelial neoplasia as a replacement for intraductal dysplasia, and this new term was promulgated in 1989 at a workshop on prostate preneoplastic lesions sponsored by the American Cancer Society and National Cancer Institute.[7] The 1989 conference recommended compression of the PIN classification into two grades: low-grade and high-grade PIN (FIG. 1A-D). The clinical significance of high-grade PIN was considered substantial at that time, whereas low-grade PIN was considered largely inconsequential. Evidence supporting the relation of high-grade PIN to prostatic carcinoma (PCa) has been found in immunohistochemical, morphometric (FIG. 2), molecular, and genetic studies.[8–12]

HIGH-GRADE PROSTATIC INTRAEPITHELIAL NEOPLASIA

Prostatic intraepithelial neoplasia is characterized by a spectrum of atypical cytologic features, ranging from minimal changes to those that are indistinguishable from carcinoma cells.[8] A basal cell layer consistently envelops this intraduct/acinar proliferation. The classification of PIN into low grade and high grade is chiefly based on the cytologic characteristics of the cells. The nuclei of cells composing

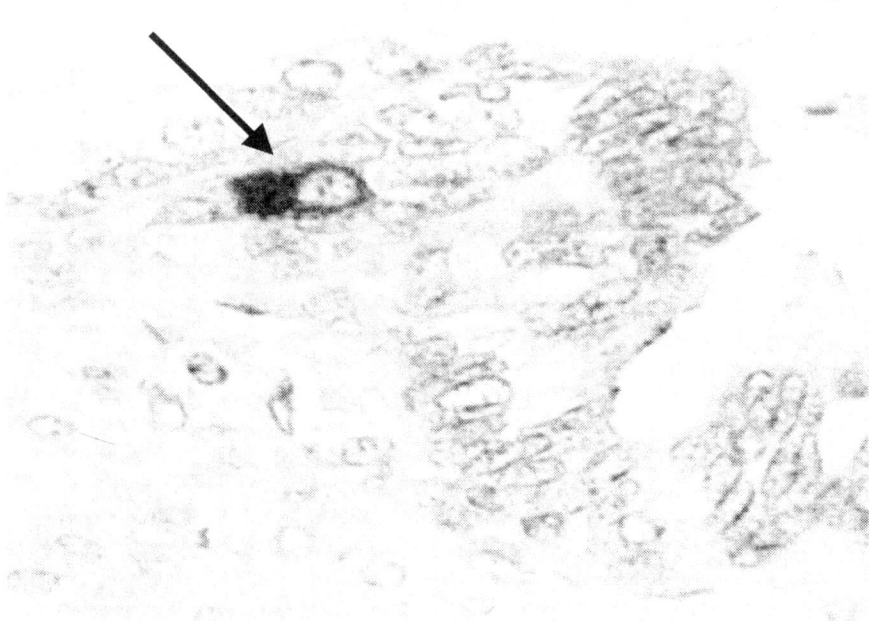

FIGURE 3. High-grade prostatic intraepithelial neoplasia (PIN). The intensely stained cell of neuroendocrine phenotype (*arrow*). The histologic section was incubated with chromogranin A.

low-grade PIN are enlarged, vary in size, have a normal or slightly increased chromatin content, and possess small or inconspicuous nucleoli. High-grade PIN is characterized by cells with large nuclei of relatively uniform size, an increased chromatin content, which may be irregularly distributed, and prominent nucleoli that are similar to those of carcinoma cells. Although the cytologic features of low-grade and high-grade PIN are fairly constant, the architecture shows a spectrum varying from a flattened epithelium to a florid cribriform proliferation. Four basic patterns that often coexist were described by Bostwick *et al.*[9]: flat, tufting, micropapillary, and cribriform. Familiarity with this diverse architectural spectrum may facilitate the histologic recognition of PIN, even though these various architectural patterns have no apparent clinicopathologic significance.

Neuroendocrine differentiation occurs in high-grade PIN, where it is intermediate in degree between normal prostate (NP) (which has the most cells with neuroendocrine differentiation) and carcinoma.[13,14] Paneth cell-like change of the prostatic epithelium (neuroendocrine cells with large eosinophilic granules) is considered a distinct form of neuroendocrine differentiation characterized by isolated cells or small groups of cells with prominent eosinophilic cytoplasmic granules (FIG. 3). The neuroendocrine products of these cells have local growth-promoting and possibly antiapoptotic activity on epithelial and endothelial cells. These findings raise the possibility that neuroendocrine differentiation is involved in the transition from PIN to invasive carcinoma.[15–17]

The PIN lesion is composed of dysplastic cells with a luminal cell phenotype, expressing the androgen receptor as well as prostate-specific antigen. PIN lesions undergo regressive changes under conditions of low androgen levels. By contrast, basal cells generally lack an androgen receptor,[18] they do not show regressive changes after androgen deprivation, and their proliferation is not driven by androgen.

Her-2-neu is a receptor tyrosine kinase that belongs to the epidermal growth factor receptor family. Overexpression of the Her-2-neu receptor tyrosine kinase has been associated with progression to androgen independence in prostate cancer cells. Preliminary data suggest that cells with increased expression of Her-2-neu receptor tyrosine kinase are already present in the intraepithelial phase of prostate neoplasia.[19]

Relation of High-Grade PIN to Prostate Cancer

Several studies[20,21] indicate that high-grade PIN is related more closely to PCa than to benign epithelium:

- Cell proliferation and death (apoptosis) are greater with high-grade PIN and PCa than with NP.
- High-grade PIN and PCa are phenotypically similar.
- High-grade PIN and PCa are morphometrically similar.
- High-grade PIN and PCa have common genetic alterations, the most common of which are: gain, deletion, and translocation of 7q22-q31; loss of 8p and gain of 8q; and loss of 10q, 16q, and 18q. Inactivation of tumor suppressor genes or overexpression of oncogenes in these regions may be important in the initiation and progression of prostate neoplasia. This strongly supports the hypothesis that PIN is the most likely precursor of PCa.[22–31]
- The basal cell layer is disrupted in high-grade PIN and absent in PCa.
- Neovascularization is greater in PIN and PCa than in NP. The available data indicate that angiogenesis has an important role in the progression of prostate neoplasia.

Several investigators reported the increasing frequency of high-grade PIN with advancing age and its association with prostate cancer. Bostwick and Brawer[6] demonstrated significantly greater frequency of high-grade PIN in prostates with cancer than in those without cancer. McNeal and Bostwick[5] showed that high-grade PIN was present in 82% of step-sectioned autopsy prostates with cancer, but only in 43% of benign prostates from patients of similar age. Qian et al.[28] found that 86% whole-mount radical prostatectomy specimens with cancer contained high-grade PIN, usually within 2 mm of the cancer. The extent of high-grade PIN was also increased in prostates with cancer than in those without cancer. High-grade PIN was more extensive in small cancers than in large cancers, presumably because of "overgrowth" or obliteration of high-grade PIN by larger cancers.

Most foci of high-grade PIN are exclusively located in the peripheral zone (or nontransition zone, where PCa is most frequently found; in one study, it was found in 63% of cases) or simultaneously in the peripheral and transition zones (36%), and only rare cases (1%) are exclusively in the transition zone.[32–34] Other investigators reported a higher frequency of high-grade PIN in the transition zone, with a range of 2–37% of cases.[34–37] Kovi and Jackson[38] reported that the highest frequency of involvement of the transition zone (37%) was in prostatectomy specimens with cancer.

PIN as Predictor of Malignancy in Needle Biopsy Specimens

High-grade PIN is identified in 2–16.5% of needle biopsy specimens. Its incidence probably varies according to the patient population under consideration (screening population versus urology office population). As an example, the American Cancer Society National Cancer Detection Project identified high-grade PIN and cancer in 5.2 and 15.8% of men, respectively, in a series of 330 biopsy specimens from men participating in an early detection project.[39] Lee et al.[40] studied 256 ultrasound-guided biopsies of hypoechoic lesions in a urology practice setting and identified high-grade PIN and cancer in 10.5 and 40.2% of patients. Interestingly, those with high-grade PIN had a mean age of 65 years, whereas those with cancer had a mean age of 70 years. High-grade PIN is encountered in up to 16.5% of contemporary needle biopsy specimens in urology office practice.[41]

High-grade PIN has a high predictive value as a marker of adenocarcinoma, and its identification in biopsy specimens warrants further search for concurrent invasive carcinoma. Davidson et al.[42] found adenocarcinoma in 35% of subsequent biopsy specimens from patients with a previous diagnosis of PIN compared with 13% in a control group without high-grade PIN. High-grade PIN, patient age, and serum PSA concentration were all highly significant predictors of cancer, but high-grade PIN alone increased the risk 15-fold more than those without PIN and provides the highest risk ratio. Others have reported a high-predictive value of high-grade PIN for cancer, ranging from 38–100%.[43–51] Approximately 50% of men with high-grade PIN on biopsy will be found to have carcinoma on repeat biopsy within 2 years of follow-up. These data underscore the strong association of high-grade PIN and adenocarcinoma and indicate that diagnostic follow-up is needed. The cancer detection rate in patients with low-grade PIN is identical to that in patients who underwent repeat biopsy because of persistent elevated serum PSA or an abnormal digital rectal examination.[47,52]

Identification of PIN in a prostate biopsy should not influence or dictate therapeutic decisions other than follow-up or chemoprevention. Whether a finding of high-grade PIN warrants further investigation depends on factors such as age, general physical condition, and the preferences of the patient. Only patients who may be subject to curative treatment for localized cancer should be further investigated for a PIN finding. Follow-up is suggested at 3- or 6-month intervals for 2 years and thereafter at 12-month intervals for life.

Chemoprevention in High-Grade PIN and Androgen Manipulation

The most desirable way of eliminating the impact of cancer in humans is prevention, provided it can be done with minimal risk or inconvenience. Although not without controversy, it follows that if high-grade PIN is indeed a precursor to invasive cancer, then the elimination, retardation, or reduction of high-grade PIN would lead to a parallel reduction in cancer incidence.

Chemoprevention in premalignant prostatic lesions such as high-grade PIN is a strategy designed to inhibit or reverse the process of carcinogenesis by administering

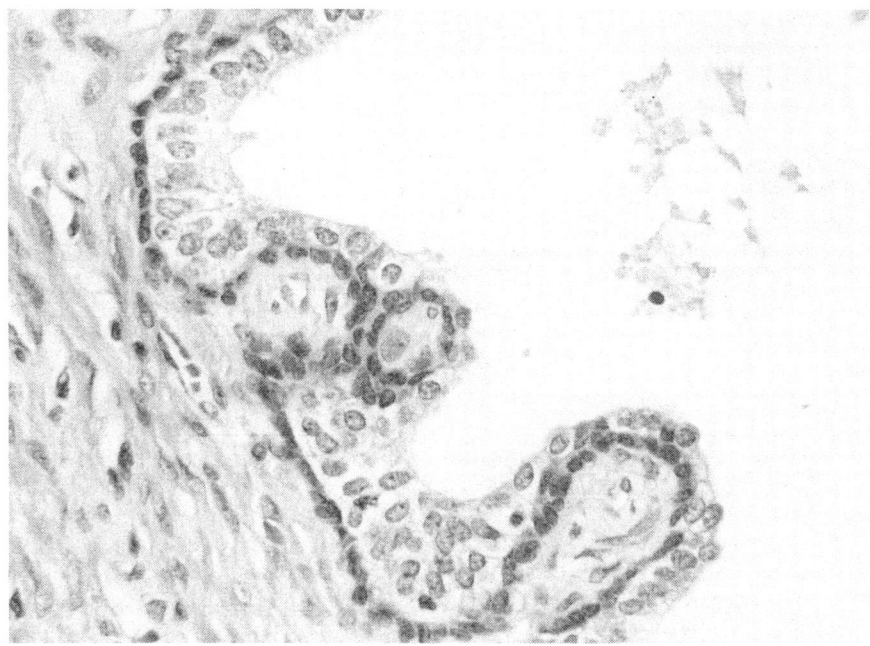

FIGURE 4. Prostatic intraepithelial neoplasia (PIN) following androgen ablation.

one or several noncytotoxic chemical compounds. A major pathway of chemoprevention unique to the prostate is the inhibition of androgen-induced effects on prostate growth. In fact, overwhelming evidence suggests that androgens play an important role in the development and progression of prostate cancer. (For more details on prostate cancer chemoprevention see Ref. 53.)

Several reports have dealt with the effect of androgen manipulation on high-grade PIN.[54–58] A degree of secretory cell type stratification is always present. However, crowding is less evident than in untreated high-grade PIN. The cells show cytoplasmic clearing and enlargement by coalescence of vacuoles and rupture of cell membranes. The nuclei have different degrees of chromatin changes, ranging from mild condensation, which barely allows the distinction between coarse chromatin granules (corresponding to heterochromatin) and finely dispersed chromatin (corresponding to euchromatin), to a tightly condensed state close to that observed in apoptosis.[54] Similar to treated PCa, apoptotic bodies are easily identifiable in all epithelial cell layers.[55] The hallmark of all untreated high-grade PIN is the frequently multinucleolated nuclei, the nucleoli being prominent and marginated and having a perinucleolar halo. In treated cases the nucleoli become inconspicuous, without margination, and have a decreased diameter[57] (FIG. 4). The duct and acinar lumen are always rich in cells; some are macrophages, some sloughed secretory cells with degenerative features, whereas others correspond to apoptotic cells. The basal cell layer is easily recognizable in most instances. In fact, basal cells generally lack an androgen receptor, they do not show regressive changes after androgen deprivation, and their proliferation is not driven by androgen.[18]

Some correspondence seems to exist between the type of treatment and the degree of regressive changes. Following total androgen ablation the morphological changes are more pronounced than after hormonal monotherapy, that is, LHRH analog or antiandrogen used alone. Chronic treatment with finasteride affects, only to a small extent, the cells composing high-grade PIN.[56]

A marked decrease in the prevalence and extent of high-grade PIN occurs in prostates after androgen deprivation therapy as compared with untreated prostates. Ferguson et al.[59] reported that the incidence of high-grade PIN was reduced from 83% in the prostatectomy-only group to 50% in patients who received preoperative androgen deprivation therapy. Also, PIN was present in greater than 2 high-power fields in only 21% of treated patients compared with untreated patients in whom 67% had greater than 2 high-power fields. Similar results were reported by Vaillancourt et al.[57] These findings indicate that the dysplastic prostatic epithelium is hormone dependent. The two basic effects of androgen ablation on epithelial cells consist of reducing proliferation and enhancing apoptosis.[11,60–62]

Androgen deprivation modifies the pattern of vascularization and downregulates vascular endothelial growth factor (VEGF) expression in normal tissue, PIN, and PCa and decreases the degree of vascularization except in cell areas with neuroendocrine features.[63] This indicates that androgens regulate VEGF content in normal tissue as well as in premalignant and malignant lesions of the prostate, as demonstrated experimentally in animals by Joseph et al.[64] This might indicate that inhibition of the action of an angiogenic factor produced by tumor cells might contribute to suppression of tumor growth *in vivo*.[65] Understanding the events controlling angiogenesis could lead to the development of new therapeutic approaches to prevent neoplastic progression as well as to induce the regression of cancers and their precursors. The rapid pace of research in this field suggests that this aspect of tumor biology will soon have an increasingly important role in evaluation and treatment.

HIGH-GRADE PROSTATIC INTRAEPITHELIAL NEOPLASIA VERSUS INTRADUCTAL CARCINOMA

The cribriform pattern of Gleason grade 3 acinar PCa is histologically anomalous relative to the rest of the architectural scheme for grading invasive PCa.[66] Like the other well differentiated and moderately differentiated (grade 1–3) carcinomas in the Gleason system, it is composed of individual glandular units separated by stroma. However, in all other grade 3 cancers, the neoplastic cells of each acinar unit typically have one pole abutting the stroma and an apical pole facing a single gland lumen. This pattern mimics normal glandular architecture. By contrast, in the cribriform grade 3 pattern, the potential lumen of each glandular unit is filled by a cell mass perforated by tiny lumens. This cribriform pattern of cancer cells is identical to that which characterizes one variant of Gleason grade 4 PCa, a pattern whose only distinguishing feature from grade 3 is that the cancer cells form large sheets with invasive borders.

Evidence has been presented that the histologic features of cribriform grade 3 pattern represent cancer growing within preexisting ducts and acini. Intraductal location is identified by recognition of the normal duct-acinar branching pattern. Further confirmation is provided by the demonstration of a partially intact basal cell layer using high molecular weight keratin immunostaining (34βE12). The topographic analysis by McNeal et al.[67] indicates that the incipient lesion may spread rather rapidly and widely throughout the duct segment of origin, judging by the frequent involvement in the continuity of lumens from near the urethra to the gland capsule. The same investigators postulate that intraductal neoplasia affects the natural history of PCa by giving rise to (or being associated with) an unusual aggressive variant of invasive tumor, probably grade 4 or 5 in histologic pattern.

This lesion was designated "intraductal carcinoma" by McNeal et al.[67] Other investigators adopted the term, high-grade cribriform PIN,[68–70] based on guidelines for the definition of high-grade PIN.

According to McNeal et al.,[67] intraductal carcinoma usually arises within established invasive cancer, perhaps often from the same dysplastic focus that was previously the source of that cancer. A consistent evolutionary sequence was traced in some of their cases. This included the initial step, gradual transition between normal epithelium and dysplasia. The next stage beyond dysplasia was focal epithelial accumulation into tufts, which developed into elongated pseudopapillations extending into the lumen. Fusion of pseudopapillations into trabeculae or narrow septa composed of cuboidal cells in orderly arrangement is then seen near the center of the lumen, thus dividing the gland lumens into multiple elongated spaces. Finally, increased cellularity of the trabeculae reduced the lumens to small round cribriforms. What is lacking in this last stage is the so-called "maturation phenomenon," a feature considered characteristic of high-grade PIN lesions; the perimeter cells have features of clearly dysplastic cells, whereas, from the periphery to the center, the nuclei become smaller, the nucleoli becoming less apparent. Mitoses and pleomorphism are infrequent in the cribriform pattern of high-grade PIN and frequent in the cribriform pattern of acinar carcinoma. Comedo necrosis is extremely infrequent in high-grade cribriform PIN and frequent in the cribriform pattern of acinar carcinoma.

In recent years also, other patterns of cytologically malignant intraductal proliferations have been identified: comedo, solid, and papillary.[71,72] Wilcox et al.[72] found that these patterns are associated with clinically aggressive PCa. These patterns, among which cribriform must be included, are usually associated with prostatic ductal carcinoma (formerly endometrioid carcinoma) arising predominantly in large periurethral primary prostatic ducts (FIG. 5) and with acinar PCa with focal ductal differentiation. Amin et al.[73] attempted to identify distinctive criteria for the cribriform intraductal proliferation seen in ductal carcinoma:

- Mitoses are frequent.
- Pleomorphism is prominent.
- Comedo necrosis is very frequent.

There is no agreement in the literature as to whether these patterns should be called high-grade PIN or intraductal carcinoma or intraductal spread of carcinoma. Ductal intraepithelial neoplasia of the prostate shows close morphological similarities with those of the breast.

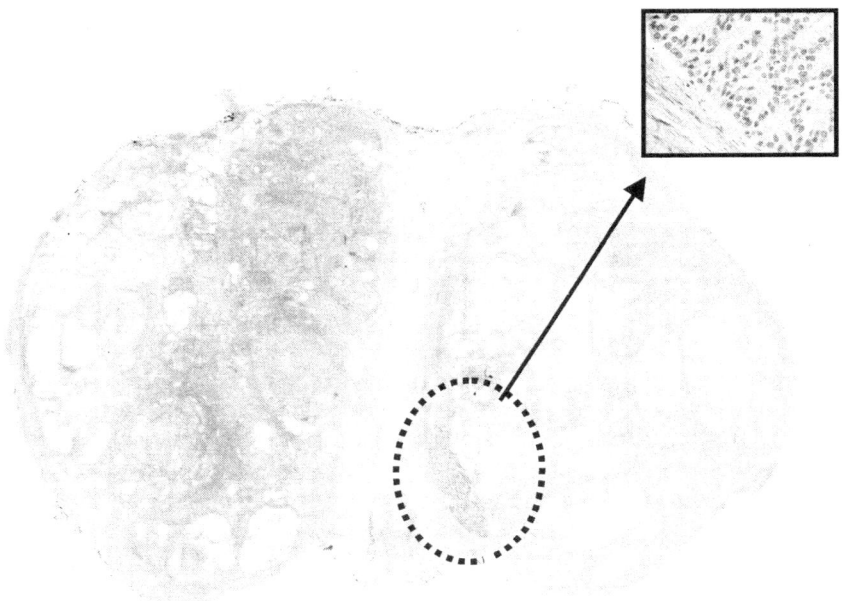

FIGURE 5. Whole mount section with malignant intraductal proliferation (cribriform pattern; see enlargement) in association with prostatic ductal carcinoma.

OTHER PROPOSED PRECANCEROUS LESIONS (OR CONDITIONS)

Other possible findings in the prostate (low-grade PIN, atypical adenomatous hyperplasia, malignancy-associated foci, and atrophy) may be premalignant, but the data for these are much less convincing than those for high grade PIN. Some of these findings might represent precancerous conditions, such as a state associated with a significant increased risk of cancer.

Atypical adenomatous hyperplasia (AAH) is characterized by circumscribed proliferation of closely packed small glands that, rather than appearing invasive, tend to merge with the surrounding, histologically benign glands.[74] AAH frequently demonstrates budding acini from adjacent foci of benign hyperplastic glands, and the cells have clear cytoplasm with variable intraluminal secretions. Architecturally, AAH resembles well differentiated adenocarcinoma, and most cases of Gleason primary pattern 1 cancer are now considered within the spectrum of AAH.[75] Recognition of the basal cell layer excludes the diagnosis of carcinoma. Unfortunately, identification of the basal epithelium is often difficult, as it is usually attenuated and may be discontinuous in AAH. Recognition of the basal cell layer may be facilitated by the use of an antibody to high molecular weight cytokeratin. Nuclear and nucleolar morphology is the key differentiating feature between AAH and carcinoma. Cancer cells contain enlarged clear nuclei with a fine or irregular chromatin pattern and thick chromatinic rim. Most cases of AAH (86%) are located in the transition zone. The incidence of AAH in prostate specimens varies from 2.2–23%.[76,77]

Atypical adenomatous hyperplasia is considered a premalignant lesion on the basis of several findings including an increased association with carcinoma (15% in 100 prostates without carcinoma at autopsy and 31% in 100 prostates with cancer at autopsy), topographic relation with small-acinar prostate cancer, and rare cases of genetic abnormalities.[78] However, some investigators claim that the link between cancer and AAH is an epiphenomenon and that data are insufficient to conclude that AAH is a premalignant lesion. In particular, a direct transition from AAH to cancer, as observed between PIN and cancer, has not been documented. The term adenosis is discouraged, as it is not entirely synonymous with AAH.

Malignancy-associated changes refer to abnormalities in epithelial cells that are not usually distinguishable by routine light microscopic examination.[79] Scant data

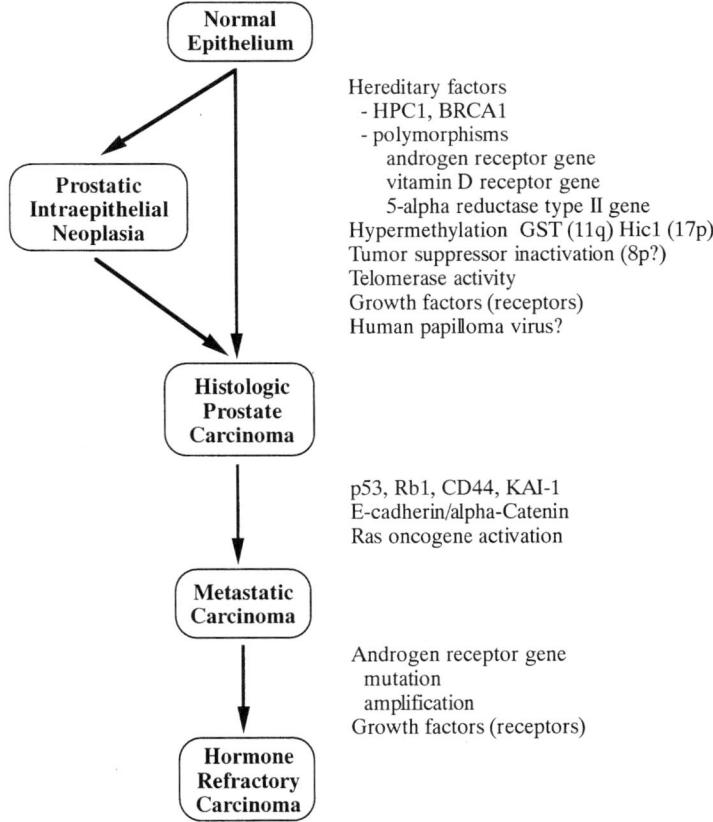

FIGURE 6. Transition from normal epithelium to prostate cancer with and without an intermediate morphological stage identifiable as prostatic intraepithelial neoplasia (PIN) (modified from Ref. 81).

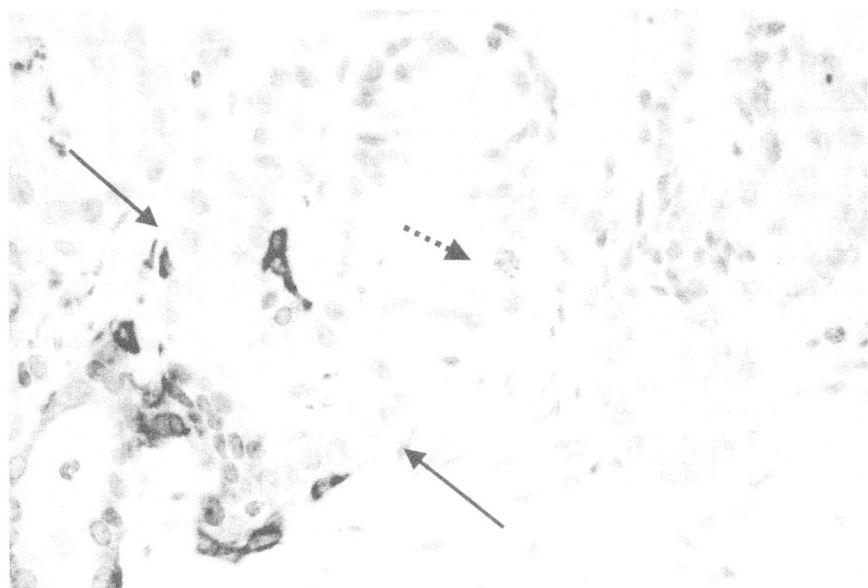

FIGURE 7. Prostate cancer originating from atrophic acini. Dark stained cells (result of immunohistochemistry reaction with an antibody against 34βE12 followed by a light counterstain with hematoxylin) are basal cells in the atrophic acini. The basal cell layer is a fragment at the point of emergence of cancer (indicated by *solid arrows*). Cancer is devoid of basal cells. *Dotted arrow* indicates a mitotic figure in the cancer acini.

on the prostate are available; benign prostatic epithelium may show some genetic abnormalities in GST-π and telomerase similar to those in cancer (malignancy-associated foci), but this recent report has not yet been confirmed. Changes also occur in the microvasculature of stroma. These changes are intermediate in degree between the pattern in normal epithelium from prostates devoid of cancer and that associated with PIN and cancer[21,80,81] (FIG. 6).

A recent report[82] suggested that atrophy may be causally linked to PIN and prostate cancer (FIG. 7). This hypothesis was based on recognition of increased proliferative activity, albeit low, in the secretory cells that persist within atrophic acini. Autopsy studies of atrophy by McNeal[20] in the 1960s rejected this concept, and data supporting reconsideration at this time are limited.

CONCLUSIONS

In this report, the current state of knowledge of the cell biological and genetic basis for linking PIN and prostatic adenocarcinoma is summarized. It is conceivable that a stem cell of basal phenotype, or an amplifying cell, is the target of prostatic carcinogenesis. Prominent genetic heterogeneity is characteristic of both high-grade PIN and carcinoma, and multiple foci of high-grade PIN arise independently within the same prostate. This observation suggests that a field effect probably underlies prostatic neoplasia. Multiple foci of cancer also often arise independently, lending additional support to this hypothesis. The strong genetic similarities between high-grade PIN and cancer strongly suggest that evolution and clonal expansion of PIN, or other precursor lesions, may account for the multifocal etiology of carcinoma. Uncertainties with respect to identification of the precursor lesions that are most likely to progress to invasive and metastatic prostate cancer reinforce the requirement for objective immunohistochemical or molecular biological markers of the aggressive phenotype.

REFERENCES

1. ORTEIL, H. 1926. Involutionary changes in prostate and female breast cancer in relation to cancer development. Can. Med. Assoc. J. **16:** 237.
2. ANDREWS, G.S. 1949. Latent carcinoma of the prostate. J. Clin. Pathol. **2:** 197.
3. KASTENDIECK, H. 1980. Correlation between atypical primary hyperplasia and carcinoma of the prostate. Histological study of 180 total prostatectomies. Pathol. Res. Pract. **169:** 366–387.
4. MCNEAL, J.E. 1965. Morphogenesis of prostatic carcinoma. Cancer **18:** 1659–1666.
5. MCNEAL, J.E. & D.G. BOSTWICK. 1986. Intraductal dysplasia: a premalignant lesion of the prostate. Hum. Pathol. **17:** 64–71.
6. BOSTWICK, D.G. & M.K. BRAWER. 1987. Prostatic intra-epithelial neoplasia and early invasion in prostate cancer. Cancer **59:** 788–794.
7. BOSTWICK, D.G. 1989. Prostatic intraepithelial neoplasia (PIN). Urology **34:** 16–22.
8. AMIN, M.B. *et al.* 1993. Putative precursor lesions of prostatic adenocarcinoma: fact or fiction? Mod. Pathol. **6:** 476–483.
9. BOSTWICK, D.G. *et al.* 1993. Architectural patterns of high grade prostatic intraepithelial neoplasia. Hum. Pathol. **24:** 298–310.
10. MCNEAL, J.E., O. HAILLOT & C. YEMOTO. 1995. Cell proliferation in dysplasia of the prostate: analysis by PCNA immunostaining. Prostate **27:** 258–268.
11. MONTIRONI, R., D. THOMPSON & P.H. BARTELS. 1999. Premalignant lesions of the prostate. *In* Recent Advances in Histopathology. D.G. Lowe & J.C.E. Underwood, eds. :147–172. Churchill Livingstone. Edinburgh.
12. QIAN, J., R.B. JENKINS & D.G. BOSTWICK. 1997. Detection of chromosomal anomalies and c-myc gene amplification in the cribriform pattern of prostatic intraepithelial neoplasia and carcinoma by fluorescence in situ hybridization. Mod. Pathol. **10:** 1113–1119.
13. BOSTWICK, D.G. *et al.* 1994. Neuroendocrine differentiation in prostatic intraepithelial neoplasia and adenocarcinoma. Am. J. Surg. Pathol. **18:** 1240–1246.
14. DI SANT'AGNESE, P.A. 1996. Neuroendocrine differentiation in the precursors of prostate cancer. Eur. Urol. **30:** 185–190.
15. BONKHOFF, H., U. STEIN & K. REMBERGER. 1994. Multidirectional differentiation in the normal, hyperplastic, and neoplastic human prostate: simultaneous demonstration of cell-specific epithelial markers. Hum. Pathol. **25:** 42–46.
16. DI SANT'AGNESE, P.A. 1994. Neuroendocrine differentiation in prostatic adenocarcinoma does not represent true Paneth cell differentiation. Hum. Pathol. **25:** 115–116.
17. NOORDZIJ, M.A. *et al.* 1995. Neuroendocrine cells in the normal, hyperplastic and neoplastic prostate. Urol. Res. **22:** 333–341.
18. FOSTER, C. *et al.* 2000. Cellular and molecular pathology of prostate cancer precursor. Scand. J. Urol. Nephrol. (suppl) **205:** 19–43.
19. SIGNORETTI, S. *et al.* 2000. Her-2-neu expression and progression toward androgen independence in human prostate cancer. J. Natl. Cancer. Inst. **92:** 1918–1925.
20. BOSTWICK, D., R. MONTIRONI & I. SESTERHENN. 2000. Diagnosis of prostatic intraepithelial neoplasia. Scand. J. Urol. Nephrol. (suppl) **205:** 3–10.
21. MONTIRONI, R. *et al.* 2000. Morphological identification of the patterns of prostatic intraepithelial neoplasia and their importance. J. Clin. Pathol. **53:** 655–665.

22. ALERS, J.C. *et al.* 1995. Interphase cytogenetics of prostatic adenocarcinoma and precursor lesions: analysis of 25 radical prostatectomies in 17 adjacent prostatic intraepithelial neoplasias. Genes Chromosomes Cancer **12:** 241–250.
23. BERGERHEIM, U.S.R. *et al.* 1991. Deletion mapping of chromosomes 8, 10 and 16 in human prostatic carcinoma. Genes Chromosomes Cancer **3:** 215–220.
24. BOVA, G.S. *et al.* 1993. Homozygous deletion and frequent allelic loss of chromosome 8p22 loci in human prostatic cancer. Cancer Res. **53:** 3869–3873.
25. CUNNINGHAM, J.M. *et al.* 1996. Allelic imbalance and microsatellite instability in prostatic adenocarcinoma. Cancer Res. **56:** 4475–4482.
26. EMMERT-BUCK, M.R. *et al.* 1995. Allelic loss on chromosome 8p12-21 in microdissected prostatic intraepithelial neoplasia (PIN). Cancer Res. **55:** 2959–2962.
27. MACGROGAN, D. *et al.* 1994. Loss of chromosome 8p loci in prostate cancer: mapping by quantitative allelic balance. Genes Chromosomes Cancer **10:** 151–159.
28. QIAN, J. *et al.* 1995. Chromosomal anomalies in prostatic intraepithelial neoplasia and carcinoma detected by fluorescence in situ hybridization. Cancer Res. **55:** 5408–5414.
29. QIAN, J., R.B. JENKINS & D.G. BOSTWICK. 1996. Potential markers of aggressiveness in prostatic intraepithelial neoplasia detected by fluorescence in situ hybridization. Eur. Urol. **30:** 177–184.
30. SAKR, W.A. *et al.* 1994. Allelic loss in locally metastatic, multisampled prostate cancer. Cancer Res. **54:** 3273–3277.
31. TAKAHASHI, S. *et al.* 1994. Potential markers of prostate cancer aggressiveness detected by fluorescence in situ hybridization in needle biopsies. Cancer Res. **54:** 3574–3579.
32. EPSTEIN, J.I., K.R. CHO & B.D. QUINN. 1990. Relationship of severe dysplasia to stage A (incidental) adenocarcinoma of the prostate. Cancer **65:** 2321–2327.
33. QUINN, B.D., K.R. CHO & J.I. EPSTEIN. 1990. Relationship of severe dysplasia to stage B adenocarcinoma of the prostate. Cancer **65:** 2328–2337.
34. SAKR, W.A. *et al.* 1996. Age and racial distribution of prostatic intraepithelial neoplasia. Eur. Urol. **30:** 138–144.
35. GAUDIN, P.B. *et al.* 1997. Incidence and clinical significance of high-grade prostatic intraepithelial neoplasia in TURP specimens. Urology **49:** 558–563.
36. HARVEI, S. *et al.* 1998. Is prostatic intraepithelial neoplasia in the transition/central zone a true precursor of cancer? A long-term retrospective study in Norway. Br. J. Cancer **78:** 46–49.
37. PACELLI, A. & D.G. BOSTWICK. 1997. Clinical significance of high-grade prostatic intraepithelial neoplasia in transurethral resection specimens. Urology **50:** 355–359.
38. KOVI, J., M.A. JACKSON & M.Y. HESHMAT. 1985. Ductal spread in prostatic carcinoma. Cancer **56:** 1566–1573.
39. METTLIN, C. *et al.* 1991. The American Cancer Society National Prostate Cancer Detection Project. Findings on the detection of early prostate cancer in 2425 men. Cancer **67:** 2949–2958.
40. LEE, F. *et al.* 1989. Use of transrectal ultrasound and prostate-specific antigen in diagnosis of prostatic intraepithelial neoplasia. Urology **24:** 4–12.
41. HADDAD, F.S. 1990. Risk factors for perineal seeding of prostate cancer after needle biopsy. J. Urol. **143:** 587–588.
42. DAVIDSON, D. *et al.* 1995. Prostatic intraepithelial neoplasia is a risk factor for adenocarcinoma: predictive accuracy in needle biopsies. J. Urol. **154:** 1295–1299.
43. ABOSEIF, S. *et al.* 1995. The significance of prostatic intra-epithelial neoplasia. Br. J. Urol. **76:** 355–359.
44. BERNER, A. *et al.* 1993. DNA distribution in the prostate. Normal gland, benign and premalignant lesions, and subsequent adenocarcinomas. Anal. Quant. Cytol. Histol. **15:** 247–252.
45. BOSTWICK, D.G. & K.A. ICZKOWSKI. 1997. Minimal criteria for the diagnosis of prostate cancer on needle biopsy. Ann. Diagn. Pathol. **1:** 104–129.
46. BRAWER, M.K. *et al.* 1991. Significance of prostatic intraepithelial neoplasia on prostate needle biopsy. Urology **38:** 103–107.

47. KEETCH, D.W. et al. 1995. Morphometric analysis and clinical follow-up of isolated prostatic intraepithelial neoplasia in needle biopsy of the prostate. J. Urol. **154:** 347–351.
48. LANGER, J.E. et al. 1996. Strategy for repeat biopsy of patients with prostatic intraepithelial neoplasia detected by prostate needle biopsy. J. Urol. **155:** 228–231.
49. MARKHAM, C.W. 1989. Prostatic intraepithelial neoplasia. Detection and correlation with invasive cancer in fine-needle biopsy. Urology **24:** 57–61.
50. RAVIV, G. et al. 1996. Does prostate specific antigen and prostate-specific antigen density enhance the detection of prostate cancer in patients initially diagnosed to have prostatic intraepithelial neoplasia? Cancer **77:** 2103–2108.
51. SHEPHERD, D. et al. 1996. Repeat biopsy strategy in men with isolated prostatic intraepithelial neoplasia on prostate needle biopsy. J. Urol. **156:** 460–463.
52. RAVIV, G. et al. 1996. Prostatic intraepithelial neoplasia: influence of clinical and pathological data on the detection of prostate cancer. J. Urol. **156:** 1–6.
53. MONTIRONI, R. et al. 1999. Prostate cancer prevention: review of target populations, pathological biomarkers, and chemopreventive agents. J. Clin. Pathol. **52:** 793–803.
54. AKAKURA, K. et al. 1993. Effects of intermittent androgen suppression on androgen-dependent tumors. Cancer **71:** 2782–2790.
55. MAGI-GALLUZZI, C. et al. 1993. Prostatic invasive adenocarcinoma. Effect of combination endocrine therapy (LHRH agonist and flutamide) on the expression and location of proliferating cell nuclear antigen (PCNA). Pathol. Res. Pract. **189:** 1154–1160.
56. MONTIRONI, R. et al. 1996. Prostatic intraepithelial neoplasia following six-month treatment with a 5-α-reductase inhibitor (finasteride). Anal. Quant. Cytol. Histol. **18:** 461–471.
57. VAILLANCOURT, L. et al. 1996. Effect of neoadjuvant endocrine therapy (combined androgen blockade) on normal prostate and prostatic carcinoma. Am. J. Surg. Pathol. **20:** 86–93.
58. VAN DER KWAST, T., F. LABRIE & B. TETU. 1999. Persistence of high-grade prostatic intra-epithelial neoplasia under combined androgen blockade therapy. Hum. Pathol. **30:** 1503-1507.
59. FERGUSON, J. et al. 1994. Decrease of prostatic intraepithelial neoplasia following androgen deprivation therapy in patients with stage T3 carcinoma treated by radical prostatectomy. Urology **44:** 91–95.
60. ARMAS, O.A. et al. 1994. Clinical and pathobiological effects of neoadjuvant total androgen ablation therapy on clinically localized prostatic adenocarcinoma. Am. J. Surg. Pathol. **18:** 979–991.
61. JOHNSON, M.I. et al. 1998. Expression of Bcl-2, p53 in high-grade prostatic intraepithelial neoplasia and localized prostate cancer: relationship with apoptosis and proliferation. Prostate **37:** 223–229.
62. MONTIRONI, R. & C.C. SCHULMAN. 1998. Pathological changes in prostate lesions after androgen manipulation. J. Clin. Pathol. **51:** 5–12.
63. MAZZUCCHELLI, R. et al. 2000. Vascular endothelial growth factor expression and capillary architecture in high-grade PIN and prostate cancer in untreated and androgen-ablated patients. Prostate **45:** 72–79.
64. JOSEPH, I.B. et al. 1997. Androgens regulate vascular endothelial growth factor content in normal and malignant prostatic tissue. Clin. Cancer Res. **3:** 2507–2511.
65. KIM, K.J. et al. 1993. Inhibition of vascular endothelial growth factor-induced angiogenasis suppresses tumor growth *in vivo*. Nature **362:** 841–844.
66. KRONZ, J., A. SHAIKH & J.I. EPSTEIN. 2001. Atipical cribriform lesions on prostate biopsy. Am. J. Surg. Pathol. **25:** 147–155.
67. MCNEAL, E.J. et al. 1986. Cribriform adenocarcinoma of the prostate. Cancer **58:** 1714–1719.
68. ALGABA, F. et al. 1995. Working standards in prostatic intraepithelial neoplasia and atypical adenomatous hyperplasia. Pathol. Res. Pract. **191:** 836–837.
69. ALGABA, F. & I. TRIAS. 1996. Diagnostic limits in precursor lesions of prostate cancer. Eur. Urol. **30:** 212–221.

70. RUBIN, M.A. et al. 1998. Cribriform carcinoma of the prostate and cribriform prostatic intraepithelial neoplasia. Incidence and clinical implication. Am. J. Surg. Pathol. **22:** 840–848.
71. SAMARATUNGA, H. & M. SINGH. 1997. Distribution pattern of basal cells detected by cytokeratin 34 beta E12 in primary prostatic duct adenocarcinoma. Am. J. Surg. Pathol. **21:** 435–440.
72. WILCOX, G. et al. 1998. Patterns of high-grade prostatic intraepithelial neoplasia associated with clinically aggressive prostate cancer. Hum. Pathol. **29:** 1119–1123.
73. AMIN, M.B., D.S. SCHULTZ & R.J. ZARBO. 1994. Analysis of cribriform morphology in prostatic neoplasia using antibody to high-molecular-weight cytokeratins. Arch. Pathol. Lab. Med. **118:** 260–264.
74. MONTIRONI, R. et al. 1999. Subtle morphological and molecular changes in normal-looking epithelium in prostates with prostatic intraepithelial neoplasia or cancer. Eur. Urol. **35:** 468–473.
75. BOSTWICK, D.G. & L. CHENG. 1999. Overdiagnosis of prostatic adenocarcinoma. Semin. Urol. Oncol. **17:** 199–205.
76. BOSTWICK, D.G. et al. 1993. Atypical adenomatous hyperplasia of the prostate: morphologic criteria for its distinction from well-differentiated carcinoma. Hum. Pathol. **24:** 819–832.
77. HELPAP, B. et al. 1997. Relationship between atypical adenomatous hyperplasia (AAH), prostatic intraepithelial neoplasia (PIN), and prostatic adenocarcinoma. Pathologica **89:** 288–300.
78. CHENG, L. et al. 1998. Atypical adenomatous hyperplasia of the prostate: a premalignant lesion? Cancer Res. **58:** 389–391.
79. PRETLOW, T.G., M. NAGABHUSHAN & T.P. PRETLOW. 1995. Prostatic intraepithelial neoplasia and other changes during promotion and progression. Path. Res. Pract. **191:** 842–849.
80. MONTIRONI, R. et al. 2000. Expression of π-class glutathione S-transferase: two populations of high-grade prostatic intraepithelial neoplasia with different relationship to carcinoma. Mol. Pathol. **53:** 122–128.
81. RUIJTER, E. et al. 2001. Molecular changes associated with prostate cancer development. Analyt. Quant. Cytol. Histol. **23:** 67–88.
82. DE MARZO, A. et al. 1999. Proliferative inflammatory atrophy of the prostate. Implications for prostatic carcinogenesis. Am. J. Pathol. **155:** 1985–1992.

Src Is an Initial Target of Sex Steroid Hormone Action

A. MIGLIACCIO, G. CASTORIA, M. DI DOMENICO, A. DE FALCO, A. BILANCIO, AND F. AURICCHIO

Istituto di Patologia Generale e Oncologia, Seconda Università di Napoli, 80138 Naples, Italy

ABSTRACT: Recent observations that steroids use pathways universally known to be regulated by growth factors and interleukins highlight the following points: (1) Steroid stimulation of the canonical pathway Src/Ras/Erk signaling from membrane to nuclei or its single members has been observed in different cell types including human cancer-derived cells, neurons, osteoblasts, osteocytes, and endothelial cells. This stimulation has been reconstituted and analyzed in transiently transfected cells. (2) Cellular context and intracellular localization of receptors are crucial in determining the biological effects evoked by this hormonal stimulation: proliferation, protection from apoptosis, and vasorelaxation. (3) Classical steroid receptors localized in the extranuclear compartment directly and, in some cases, simultaneously interact with Src. They are capable of unexpected cross talks responsible for the observed effects. (4) Other signaling pathways including PI3K/AKT are also stimulated by steroids. The aim of future work will be to arrive at an integrated general view of the different signaling pathways activated by steroids and to analyze the concert between these pathways and the hormonal transcriptional action. This general view should be simultaneously verified in different cell contexts, under different physiologic and pathologic conditions. We expect that the new technologies, above all gene and protein microarray, will make this goal feasible.

KEYWORDS: Src; sex steroids; nongenomic action

INTRODUCTION

Src is a 60-kDa protein with intrinsic tyrosine kinase activity involved in different aspects of cell regulation and transformation. Myristylation of the N-terminal sequences causes membrane localization. Src presents an SH3 domain that interacts with proline-rich sequences and an SH2 domain that binds phosphotyrosine. Autophosphorylation on tyrosine 416 in the kinase domain increases enzyme activity, whereas under basal conditions, phosphorylation on tyrosine 527 represses this activity through two distinct intramolecular interactions. Binding of the SH2 domain to C-terminal phosphorylated tyrosine locks the molecule in an inhibited conformation. Such an interaction is stabilized by the SH3 domain, which contacts the linker

---

Address for correspondence: Ferdinando Auricchio, M.D., Dipartimento di Patologia Generale, Seconda Università di Napoli, Via De Crecchio, 7, 80138 Naples, Italy. Voice: +39-081-5665676; fax: +39-081-291327.
ferdinando.auricchio@unina2.it

Ann. N.Y. Acad. Sci. 963: 185–190 (2002). © 2002 New York Academy of Sciences.

between SH2 and the kinase domain. Displacement of the intramolecular interactions by higher affinity sequences present in other proteins will cause kinase activation. Src is activated by membrane receptors, such as receptor tyrosine kinase, integrins, and G-protein–coupled receptors.[1] We have accumulated evidence that Src is downstream of classical sex-steroid receptors, which lack intrinsic kinase activity and belong to the large family of nuclear receptors. These findings are presented and discussed in terms of signaling pathway activation, a new frontier in nontranscriptional steroid hormone action.

SRC ACTIVITY IS STIMULATED BY STEROIDS

The initial finding of steroid action on Src showed that under strict conditions of hormone-stimulated growth, 10 seconds of estradiol treatment of MCF-7 cells derived from human mammary cancer leads to strong stimulation of Src tyrosine phosphorylation and kinase activity.[2] After this treatment, only a small percentage of the total endogenous receptor is ligand occupied.[3] The stimulation occurs in the absence of changes in Src expression and vanishes after 60 minutes. The antiestrogen ICI 164 384 prevents hormone-induced kinase stimulation, suggesting that an estradiol receptor (ER) mediates estradiol effects. The increase in Src tyrosine phosphorylation parallels the enzymic activation and is likely due to autophosphorylation of the 416 tyrosine residue of Src. The "Src family" has eight members; three (Src, Fyn, and Yes) are ubiquitously expressed; the others are more tissue restricted.[1] We observed that estradiol stimulates the growth of subconfluent Caco-2 cells derived from human colon carcinoma.[6] Under the same conditions the hormone stimulates the activity not only of Src but also of Yes with similar, rapid kinetics. Because members of the Src family share similar structural features, such as SH2 and SH3 domains, these domains are likely involved in hormonal activation of the two kinases. This point is addressed in the *in vitro* association section.

In addition to being stimulated by estradiol, Src activity is activated by progestins in human mammary cancer-derived T47D cells[7] and androgens in human prostate cancer-derived LNCaP cells[8] under strict conditions of hormone-dependent cell growth. With these steroids, stimulation is also rapid and transient, and no change of Src expression occurs during stimulation of activity. It is worth stressing that progestin stimulation of Src in T47D cells is comparable in intensity and kinetics to stimulation of Src in the same cells by a typical growth factor such as EGF.

CLASSIC STEROID RECEPTORS ACTIVATE SRC

The surprising finding that estradiol stimulates a nonreceptor tyrosine kinase usually expressed at the membrane raises the question of ER identity. To approach this problem, Cos cells were transiently transfected with a plasmid encoding the human ER_α. The cells become estradiol responsive in terms of Src activation only after expression of this receptor, and the antiestrogen ICI 182 780 prevented this effect.[3] These and similar findings show that in Cos cells transfected with ER_β, PR-B, and androgen receptor (AR), these "classical" sex-steroid receptors can activate Src. Our view is supported by findings by other groups. Recently, an extranuclear steroid receptor, the xPR of the *Xenopus laevis* oocyte, was cloned. This receptor in *Xenopus* is only expressed outside the nucleus and stimulates the MAP kinase; nevertheless, when the same receptor is targeted to nuclei of Cos cells, it functions as a transcription activator.[4] In addition, nontranscriptional activity of steroid receptors is undetectable when these receptors are exclusively targeted to nuclei of HeLa cells through nuclear localization sequences.[5] From these findings it appears that intracellular localization of identical steroid receptors dictates the type of hormonal effect (transcriptional or nontranscriptional) evoked.

ASSOCIATION OF STEROID RECEPTORS WITH SRC AND CROSS TALKS BETWEEN STEROID RECEPTORS

Association in Whole Cells

T47D cells are endowed with PR-B, PR-A and ER_α. Strictly following the kinetics of Src activation by the progestin R5020 or estradiol, stimulated T47D cells were lysed and the lysates were immunoprecipitated with anti-PR, anti-ER, or anti-Src antibodies. Results show that PR-B (but not PR-A!) and ER_α are preassociated, and Src associates with ER_α only after progestin R5020 or estradiol treatment. No association of PR-B with Src was detected under all the conditions employed. Similar findings were observed in Cos cells cotransfected with hPR-B and hER_α cDNA. Surprisingly, the presence of ER_α is required to observe Src stimulation by R5020. The cross talk between PR-B and ER_α is confirmed by the Src-ER_α association prevented by antiestrogens when T47D cells are treated with progestin.

In Cos cells a transcriptionally inactive hRP-B was fully active in stimulating Src activity when coexpressed with ER_α, indicating that nontranscriptional receptor activity is separated from transcriptional activity. Altogether, our findings show that estradiol induces ER_α association with Src and triggers its activation; progestin also leads to ER_α-Src association after binding to PR-B. This association is also followed by Src activation.[7] We speculate that when progestin binds to PR-B, ER_α dissociates from PR-B and interacts with Src (FIG. 1).

LNCaP cells are endowed with hER_β and a mutant of hAR. Estradiol or the androgen R1881 induces a ternary complex formed by AR/ER/Src in LNCaP cells as well as in Cos cells cotransfected with AR and ER_β or ER_α. The cross talk between AR and

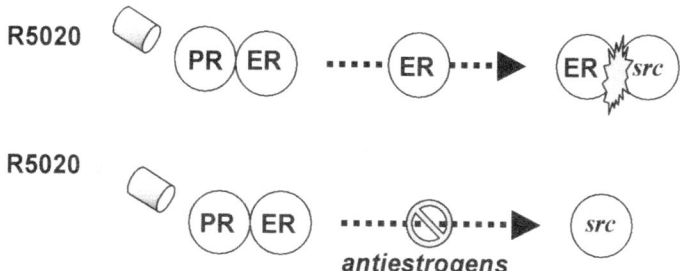

FIGURE 1. Cross talk between PgR-B and ER_α, leading to Src activation. Antiestrogens prevent progestin-triggered Src activation.

ER_α or ER_β is confirmed by the finding that this ternary complex, like Src activity stimulation, is prevented by either ICI 182,780 or the antiandrogen Casodex independently of the agonist (estradiol or R1881) used to stimulate the cells.[8]

In Vitro *Association of ER_α and AR with Src*

Interaction of ER_α with Src was initially observed using Src-Sepharose and bovine uterus cytosol ER.[3] Because a crude ER preparation was employed, it was not clear from this experiment if the observed interaction is direct. The following findings have clarified this point. Chimeric GST-Src interacts with [^{35}S]-labeled human ER_α or ER_β synthesized in reticulocyte lysate. Use of deleted mutants of Src shows that SH2 domains are required for this interaction. Phosphotyrosine 537 of ER_α, the only phosphotyrosine of this receptor, interacts with the SrcSH2 domain. Similar experiments show that AR interacts with the SrcSH3 domain through a proline-rich sequence.[8]

The combined association of the two receptors with Src induced in either LNCaP cells or transfected Cos cells by estradiol or androgen triggers activation of Src stronger than that evoked by a single receptor. We speculate that in the ternary complex Src assumes a conformation more active than that in the binary complex.

SRC-DEPENDENT SIGNALING ACTIVATION AND ITS ROLE IN CELL PROLIFERATION

Findings presented in the previous sections show that activation of Src follows interaction of this kinase with ER_β or ER_α induced by either estradiol or the agonist-occupied PR-B. AR, like ER, directly interacts with Src. When ER and AR are both present in cells, the agonist-induced association of one receptor with Src also leads to interaction of the other receptor with Src. Therefore, the cross talk between PR-B and ER is one way (from PR-B to ER), whereas that between AR and ER is reciprocal. Once activated by steroids, Src phosphorylates a 46-kDa Shc protein and the GAP-associated proteins, increasing the level of Ras-GTP and the activity of the Ras-dependent Raf-1/MEK/Erk_s cascade.[3,6,7,8] The role of Src and Src-dependent signaling has been analyzed in detail. Nuclei of quiescent MCF-7 cells and T47D cells were microinjected with constructs expressing SrcK$^-$ or Src wild type, cells were stimulated by estradiol or R5020, respectively, and DNA synthesis was measured by BrdU incorporation. Although expression of wild-type Src did not affect the strong hormonal stimulation, it was almost abolished by SrcK$^-$. Similar findings were obtained when cells were microinjected with anti-Ras mAb or treated with the MEK-1 inhibitor PD98059.[9] Use of a transcriptionally inactive mutant of ER in NIH fibroblast in parallel with SrcK$^-$ and PD98059 shows that transcriptional activity of the receptor is not required for the Src-dependent S-phase entry of cells stimulated by estradiol.[9] This finding, in addition to showing the prevalent role of the nontranscriptional action of steroids in stimulating the cell S-phase entry, supports the view of the separation of transcriptional and nontranscriptional action of receptors. This point has been confirmed and extended in a study on osteoblasts and osteocytes[5] and *Xenopus* oocytes.[4] A model of the nontranscriptional proliferative action of estradiol is summarized in FIGURE 2.

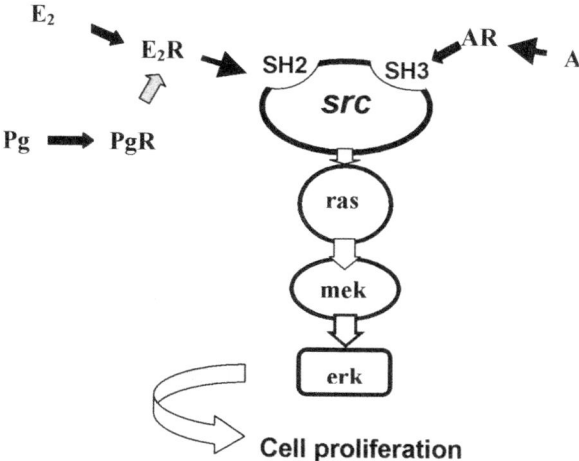

FIGURE 2. Nontranscriptional, receptor-dependent proliferative action of estrogens. ER refers to the α^3 and β^8 isoforms. Agonist-occupied androgen receptor[8] and progesterone receptor-B[7] also trigger cell proliferation of prostate and mammary cancer cell lines through the Src/Ras/Erk$_s$ pathway.

Use of PP1, an Src inhibitor, or expression of SrcK⁻ strongly reduces the proliferative activity of either estradiol or androgen in LNCaP cells. Similar inhibition is observed when MEK-1 is inhibited by either PD98059 or expression of an MEK-1 dominant negative.[8]

From all these experiments we conclude that Src activation by steroids leads to DNA synthesis and cell proliferation through stimulation of the Shc/Ras/Erk pathway.

OTHER EFFECTS OF SRC ACTIVATION BY STEROIDS

After our observations on Src/Ras/Erk$_s$ activation by estradiol, progestins, and androgens and its role in cell proliferation, other groups focused their interest on steroid effects on the same or other signaling pathways in different cellular contexts. We present some of these findings on the basis of the hormonal effects observed.

Antiapoptotic Action

MCF-7 cells. Erk activation contributes to the estrogen-dependent antiapoptotic effect.[10]

Primary cortical neurons. Estrogen stimulates tyrosine kinase activity and Erk$_s$. Src kinase and MEK-1 inhibitors abolish the estrogen-dependent neuroprotection.[11]

Murine osteoblastic and osteocyte cells. Estradiol and androgens activate the Src/Shc/Erk pathway. Activation of this pathway in these cells is responsible for the protective effect against apoptosis.[5]

Activation of Nitric Oxide Synthase (NOS)

Endothelial cells. Estradiol through the tyrosine kinase/Erk pathway activates endothelial nitric oxide synthase (NOS).[12] It is noteworthy that in human endothelial cells the NOS activation depends on activation of the phosphatidylinositol-3-OH kinase and protein kinase B (AKT) pathway.[13] Activation of the same pathway by estradiol triggers cell proliferation.[14]

ACKNOWLEDGMENTS

This research was supported by grants from Associazione Italiana della Ricerca sul Cancro and Ministero dell'Università e della Ricerca Scientifica.

REFERENCES

1. ABRAM, C.L. & S.A. COURTNEIDGE. 2000. Src family tyrosine kinase and growth factor signalling. Exp. Cell Res. **254:** 1–13.
2. MIGLIACCIO, A., M. PAGANO & F. AURICCHIO. 1993. Immediate and transient stimulation of protein tyrosine phosphorylation by estradiol in MCF-7 cells. Oncogene **8:** 2183–2191.
3. MIGLIACCIO, A., M. DI DOMENICO, G. CASTORIA, *et al.* 1996. Tyrosine kinase/p21ras/MAP-kinase pathway activation by estradiol-receptor complex in MCF-7 cells. EMBO J. **15:** 1292–1300.
4. BAYAA, M., R.A. BOOTH, Y. SHENG & X.J. LIN. 2000. The classical progesterone receptor mediates Xenopus oocyte maturation through a nongenomic mechanism. Proc. Natl. Acad. Sci. USA **97:** 12607–12612.
5. KOUSTENI, S., T. BELLIDO, L.I. PLOTKIN, *et al.* 2001. Nongenotropic, sex-nonspecific signaling through the estrogen or androgen receptors: dissociation from transcriptional activity. Cell **104:** 719–730.
6. DI DOMENICO, M., G. CASTORIA, A. BILANCIO, *et al.* 1996. Estradiol activation of human colon carcinoma-derived Caco-2 cell growth. Cancer Res. **56:** 4516–4521.
7. MIGLIACCIO, A., D. PICCOLO, G. CASTORIA, *et al.* 1998. Activation of the Src/p21ras/Erk pathway by progesterone receptor via cross-talk in the estrogen receptor. EMBO J. **17:** 2008–2018.
8. MIGLIACCIO, A., G. CASTORIA, M. DI DOMENICO, *et al.* 2000. Steroid-induced androgen receptor-oestradiol receptor β-Src complex triggers prostate cancer cell proliferation. EMBO J. **19:** 5406–5417.
9. CASTORIA, G., M.V. BARONE, M. DI DOMENICO, *et al.* 1999. Non-transcriptional action of oestradiol and progestin triggers DNA synthesis. EMBO J. **18:** 2500–2510.
10. RAZANDI, M., A. PEDRAM & E.R. LEVIN, 2000. Plasma membrane estrogen receptors signal to antiapoptosis in breast cancer. Mol. Endocrinol. **14:** 1434–1447.
11. SINGER, C.A., X.A. FIGUEROA-MASOT, R.H. BATCHELOR & D.M. DORSA. 1999. The mitogen-activated protein kinase pathway mediates estrogen neuroprotection after glutamate toxicity in primary cortical neurons. J. Neurosci. **19:** 2455–2463.
12. CHEN, Z., I.S. YUHANNA, Z. GALCHEVA-GARCOVA, *et al.* 1999. Estrogen receptor alpha mediates the nongenomic activation of endothelial nitric oxide synthase by estrogen. J. Clin. Invest. **103:** 401–406.
13. SIMONCINI, T., A. HFEZI-MOGHADAM, D.P. BRAZIL, K. LEY, W.W. CHIN & J.K. LIAO. 2000. Interaction of oestrogen receptor with the regulatory subunit of phosphatidylinositol-3-OH kinase. Nature **407:** 538–541.
14. CASTORIA, G., A. MIGLIACCIO, D. BILANCIO, *et al.* 2001. P13-kinase in concert with Src promotes the S-phase entry of oestradiol-stimulated MCF-7 cells. EMBO J. **20:** 6050–6059.

From Castration-Induced Apoptosis of Prostatic Epithelium to the Use of Apoptotic Genes in the Treatment of Prostate Cancer

YE ZHANG,[a] BICHENG NAN,[a] JIANG YU,[a] TITHI SNABBOON,[a] FRANCESCA ANDRIANI,[a] AND MARCO MARCELLI[a,b]

Departments of [a]Medicine and [b]Molecular and Cellular Biology, Baylor College of Medicine and VA Medical Center, Houston, Texas 77030, USA

ABSTRACT: Current knowledge of the mechanisms regulating androgen-ablation–induced apoptosis is reviewed, and our efforts to develop a system in which genes of the apoptotic pathway are used to induce therapeutic apoptosis in experimental models of prostate cancer are described.

KEYWORDS: apoptosis; prostate cancer; castration; epithelium; genes

INTRODUCTION

Understanding the mechanisms regulating androgen-ablation (AA)–induced apoptosis of prostatic epithelium is extremely important, because it is the only form of treatment conferring unequivocal, but temporary, benefit in patients with metastatic prostate cancer. Unfortunately, this form of treatment eventually becomes ineffective because of the development of resistance to AA-induced apoptosis. Current knowledge of the mechanisms regulating AA-induced apoptosis is reviewed, and our efforts to develop a system in which genes of the apoptotic pathway are used to induce therapeutic apoptosis in experimental models of prostate cancer are described.

THE PROSTATE AS AN ANDROGEN- AND ANDROGEN-RECEPTOR–DEPENDENT ORGAN

The prostate is composed of a mixture of stromal cells with a structural function interspersed with epithelial cells, which form the secretory exocrine portion. Interactions between the two compartments are essential for normal progression into the mature gland. Exocrine prostatic secretions are critical during reproductive years, in that they provide nourishment and protection of sperm before and after coitus. During aging, the prostate is a common site of chronic disease, such as chronic prostati-

---

Address for correspondence: Marco Marcelli, M.D., Department of Medicine, Baylor College of Medicine and VA Medical Center, 2002 Holcombe Blvd., Houston, Texas 77030. Voice: 713 794 7945; fax: 713 794 7771.
marcelli@bcm.tmc.edu

tis, benign prostatic hyperplasia, and prostatic adenocarcinoma (CaP). The high prevalence of these diseases in elderly men and the morbidity and mortality associated with them are the main reasons for the biomedical community's interest in the prostate. The prostate gland is possibly the best-characterized androgen target organ. Normal levels of circulating androgens and a functioning androgen receptor (AR) are necessary for the development and maintenance of this gland throughout the life span of a male individual. The major circulating androgen is testosterone, which is released in the systemic circulation by the Leydig cells. Testosterone functions as a pro-hormone, as in the prostate it is converted to dihydrotestosterone by the enzyme 5α-reductase. Consequently, dihydrotestosterone is the main androgenic ligand interacting with AR within the prostate. AR is a transcription factor belonging to the steroid receptor superfamily. Immunocytochemical studies have identified its expression both in prostatic epithelium and in the stromal compartment. Abnormal steroidogenesis, or inactivating mutations of AR during embryologic development, are associated with lacking or inappropriate prostatic development. Lack of testosterone surge at puberty is associated with development of a rudimental gland. Lack of testosterone after successful completion of puberty is associated with progressive involution of the gland. Thus, a functioning androgen-androgen receptor axis is a *conditio sine qua* for the normal development and function of the prostate. Androgens not only regulate proliferation and differentiation of the prostate, but also prevent prostate cell apoptosis. This concept is of critical importance, as induction of apoptosis after androgen ablation has been the basis of treatment for advanced prostate cancer since the 1940s.[1]

ANDROGEN RECEPTOR ACTION, APOPTOSIS, AND PROSTATE CANCER

The classic mechanism of action of androgenic steroids and AR was elucidated at the molecular level after AR was cloned approximately 13 years ago. Upon ligand binding, the receptor dissociates from heat shock proteins and undergoes posttranslational changes, which include phosphorylation, dimerization, and nuclear translocation. After becoming intranuclear, the AR-ligand complex binds DNA, interacts with response elements located in the promoter region upstream of androgen-dependent genes, and regulates their transcription. Transcription of androgen-responsive genes is further modulated by coactivators or corepressors, which function as docking molecules between AR and the general transcription apparatus. Although AR is a prototypical transcription factor, an alternative, nongenotropic mechanism of action was recently formulated for this molecule, after similar observations were made with other steroid receptor family members.[2,3] According to this, AR regulates cellular functions, such as proliferation and prevention of apoptosis, by setting in motion intracellular pathways, such as MAP kinase[4-6] and possibly other kinase signaling pathways. Although it is not known if this nongenotropic pathway has biological significance in the prostate, preliminary evidence suggests that it has a significant anabolic effect in the bone (Manolagas, personal communication).

The main form of systemic treatment of metastatic prostate cancer is AA. AA is thought to work by inducing apoptosis of prostate cancer cells, which depend on androgen for their survival.[7] Unfortunately, this form of treatment selects a population of androgen-independent cells,[8] which continue to proliferate even in the androgen-depleted environment of these patients,[9] producing overwhelming disease and death.[10] The form of prostate cancer generated after AA failure is known as androgen-independent (AI) disease. Typically AI prostate cancer is resistant to apoptosis induced by additional hormonal manipulation or by other forms of cytotoxic treatment. AI prostate cancer is viciously aggressive, accounting for 30,000 new deaths per year in the United States.[11] The development of AI CaP is, for all practical purposes, simultaneous with the development of resistance to AA-induced apoptosis; therefore, the mechanisms causing these two events may share some similarities. Understanding the molecular switches causing androgen independence and apoptosis resistance in CaP is the most critical question for basic scientists, whereas identifying new effective therapies to effectively defeat AI CaP is the most urgent issue for clinicians.

MITOCHONDRIAL PATHWAY OF APOPTOSIS

Two major apoptotic pathways originating from two separate subcellular compartments have been identified.[12] The receptor-mediated (or extrinsic) pathway originates at the level of the plasma membrane[13] after interaction of death receptors with their ligands. The mitochondrial (or intrinsic) pathway originates from the mitochondria after their functional incapacitation by pro-apoptotic Bcl-2 family members.[14] Although each pathway is initially centered around unique events and each activates a specific apical caspase (i.e., caspase-8 is activated by the extrinsic pathway and caspase-9 by the intrinsic pathway), the final phase of apoptosis is thought to be common[12] and consists in the activation of the executioner caspases (caspase-3 and caspase-7) and in their dismantling of substrates critical for cell survival.[15] It is not completely clear which of these two pathways is activated during castration-induced apoptosis, although observations by Buttyan and collaborators[16] strongly suggest involvement of the mitochondrial pathway (to be discussed). Three major phases have been described for the mitochondrial pathway. In the premitochondrial phase there is disruption of survival pathways that inactivate proapoptotic molecules[17–20] or facilitate the formation of new anti-apoptotic factors.[21,22] In the mitochondrial phase, proapoptotic members of the Bcl-2 family of factors (such as Bak and Bax) become mitochondrial bound,[23–26] cause loss of mitochondrial transmembrane potential,[27] and release to the cytosol apoptotic molecules, such as cytochrome c,[28] the apoptosis-inducing factor (AIF),[29] Smac,[30] and endonuclease-G.[31] Finally, in the postmitochondrial phase there is the assembling of the apoptosome,[32] activation of caspase-9 and then of the executioner caspases,[15] disintegration of cellular contents, and subsequent absorption by neighboring cells.

MECHANISMS OF ANDROGEN ABLATION-INDUCED APOPTOSIS

A complete understanding of the molecular basis of AA-induced apoptosis has been hampered by the lack of a cell-line based model. Although treatment with androgens induces proliferation or differentiation in cell lines derived from prostatic epithelium,[33–35] androgen removal is usually not associated with induction of apoptosis in these models. Thus, the leading model to study AA-induced apoptosis has been that of the rat ventral prostate harvested before and after castration.[36] With the advent of ddPRC and microarray technology, investigators identified a significant number of genes regulated by the addition or removal of androgens in various AR-positive (AR+) cell lines or AR+ CaP-derived xenografts. Although manipulation of the androgen level in these experimental models is not followed by apoptosis, some of the genes identified using these approaches were subsequently found to regulate apoptotic function, and this has furthered our understanding of the possible mechanisms regulating androgen-ablation–induced apoptosis.

Contribution of Rat Ventral Prostate Model to Understanding Androgen-Ablation–Induced Apoptosis

From a temporal point of view, epithelial cells with apoptotic features appear at 24 hours postcastration and peak at 48–72 hours postcastration.[37] By 2 weeks postcastration the wet weight of the ventral prostate is dramatically decreased, and approximately 85% of the cells have undergone apoptosis.[38] From a morphological point of view, the events associated with AA-induced apoptosis of the ventral prostate secretory epithelium have carefully been described by Buttyan and his group.[39] They reflect the general features observed by others in other models of apoptosis and include early blebbing of the apical membrane followed by cell shrinkage, chromatin condensation, formation of apoptotic bodies, and detachment from the basal membrane and neighboring cells.

From a biochemical point of view, a number of genes induced or repressed during castration-induced apoptosis have been identified. Genes upregulated in the ventral prostate after castration are testosterone-repressed prostate message-2 (TRPM-2 or clusterin),[40] transforming growth factor-β (TFG-β),[41] c-fos,[42] c-myc,[42] the 70-kDa heat shock protein,[42] fas,[43] rat ventral prostate gene 1 (RVP.1),[44] matrix carboxyglutamic acid protein,[44] glutathione S-transferase,[45] and Nur77/TR3.[46] A pro-apoptotic role has clearly been defined for some of these molecules (i.e., fas, TFG-β, c-myc, c-fos, and Nur77); however, others, such as clusterin, are presumed to work by protecting prostatic epithelial cells from undergoing apoptosis,[47] indicating the complex interaction of androgen with the survival and death machinery of a cell. The relation between the other genes upregulated by castration and AA-induced apoptosis has not yet been established. Among the prostatic genes downregulated by castration, EGF (epidermal growth factor)[48] is of potential interest. EGF is a mitogenic factor, and its absence in the prostate, combined with TGF-β–increased expression, may be one of the mechanisms though which castration induces apoptosis in prostatic epithelium. Subsequent studies have also addressed changes in the expression of various pro- and anti-apoptotic Bcl-2 family members.[16] These studies showed the importance of the Bax/Bcl-2 ratio as a determinant of apoptosis. When the ratio was in favor of Bax, usually immediately after castration, cells were undergoing apoptosis. By contrast, no apoptosis was evident after longer intervals, and this was associated with a Bax/Bcl-2 ratio in favor of Bcl-2. Evidence for an upregulated Bax/Bcl-2 ratio supports the concept that castration activates the mitochondrial pathway of apoptosis, as Bax is one of the most powerful inducers of this pathway. In addition, an imbalance among pro- and anti-apoptotic Bcl-2 family members also plays a role in AI CaP, in which many investigators have reported increased expression of Bcl-2,[49,50] and in AI CaP cell lines such as PC-3, in which the anti-apoptotic factor Bcl-x_L is overexpressed and protects the mitochondria from functional incapacitation.[51]

The ventral prostate of castrated animals regenerates after androgen replacement. Sampling the regenerating prostate before and after androgen replacement is an additional useful model in which to study the identity and function of genes that are induced, or repressed, following treatment with androgens. Because these genes are identified in regenerating tissue, we assume that they are involved in antiapoptotic and possibly proliferative function. Using a polymerase chain reaction-based cDNA subtraction method from rat ventral prostates harvested at base line and after androgen stimulation, Wang et al.[52] identified 25 upregulted and 4 downregulated transcripts. One of these, calreticulin, is an important modulator of apoptosis. Calreticulin protects the cell from apoptosis induced by calcium overload. The importance of calreticulin as an antiapoptotic factor was demonstrated in LNCaP cells. In this cell line, calreticulin prevents apoptosis due to intracellular calcium load induced by the Ca^{2+} ionophore A23187 by increasing intracellular Ca^{2+}-buffering activities. By contrast, downregulation of this protein following use of antisense primers resumes A23187-induced apoptosis.[53] That a calcium-binding protein is androgen stimulated in prostatic epithelium is a potentially important observation, as AA-induced apoptosis was described after perturbations of intracellular calcium levels.[54] In addition, known inducers of apoptosis of prostatic epithelium, such as thapsigargin, work by disregulating the intacellular levels of calcium.[55,56] On this basis, we could speculate that under normal circumstances androgen stimulates calreticulin production and, with it, maximal ability to buffer changes in intracellular Ca^{2+} and to prevent apoptosis. By contrast, calreticulin levels fall in response to castration. Consequently, the ability to buffer changes in intracellular Ca^{2+} decreases, and the cell becomes more prone to undergo apoptosis.

Another important change occurring in the prostate of castrated rats is a significant decrease in blood flow (50% within the initial 24 hours postcastration).[57] Interestingly, castration was not associated with blood flow changes of other androgen-dependent tissues, and replacement of testosterone in the castrated animal prevented castration-induced blood flow changes in the prostate.[57] As castration-induced blood flow changes are associated with apoptosis of the vascular endothelium, and because this occurs earlier than in secretory epithelium, some investigators have formulated the hypothesis that prostatic epithelium loss occurs because hypoxic/ischemic conditions develop within the prostate after castration.[58] This novel hypothesis was preliminarily validated after observing that hypoxic biomarkers, such as the presence of hydroxyprobe 1 adducts or increased expression of the hypoxia-inducible factor 1 α, were present in prostatic epithelium soon after castration.[59]

Contribution of Prostatic Cancer Cell Lines to Understanding Androgen-Ablation Induced Apoptosis

As LNCaP cells contain AR and secrete prostate-specific antigen (PSA) in response to androgen stimulation, they are widely used as an androgen-dependent (and well-differentiated) *in vitro* model of CaP. LNCaP cells undergo growth arrest but not apoptosis in response to androgen deprivation; however, on androgen removal they are more likely to undergo apoptosis when treated with a variety of apoptotic substances. Use of LNCaP cells has been instrumental in the detection of several

AR-regulated genes. Many of these were subsequently characterized and found to be involved in the regulation of apoptosis. Chang et al.[60] used differential display polymerase chain reaction (dd-PCR) analysis of AI and androgen-dependent LNCaP sublines and identified a novel gene, GC79, that is expressed to a higher degree in androgen-dependent cells. GC79 was repressed by physiologic levels (0.1 nM) of androgens only in the androgen-dependent LNCaP-FGC cell line. This molecule seems to have many features of a potentially important factor regulating apoptosis in the prostate, because its expression was increased in the regressing rat ventral prostate after castration, and its transfection and induction in both COS-1 and LNCaP cells led to an apoptotic index eightfold higher than that observed in uninduced transfected cells.

Further experimental models to study the mechanisms of apoptosis prevention by androgens were recently developed. Essential to this was the observation that androgens support survival of androgen-dependent CaP cell lines treated with apoptotic stimuli. For instance, LNCaP cells growing in medium devoid of serum and treated with the PI3K inhibitor LY294002 were rescued from apoptosis by concomitant treatment with androgens.[61] Dissection of the apoptotic pathway in these cells showed that androgen treatment decreased cytocrome c translocation to the cytosol compared to that in cells treated with LY294002 alone. The authors of this paper concluded that the site of androgen-mediated survival is located upstream of mitochondrial cytochrome c release and caspase activation and downstream of PI3K-AKT inhibition. The observation that PI3K inhibition and androgen removal from the medium leads to apoptosis of LNCaP cells is important. Through its downstream effector AKT, the PI3K pathway induces cell survival by inhibiting proapoptotic molecules, such as Bad and Nur77,[17,20] and turns on AR activity,[62] possibly through phosphorylation of serines 213 and 791.[63] Due to inactivation of the tumor suppressor gene PTEN, the PI3K pathway is frequently constitutively active in prostate cancer. This can lead to a situation in which AR acts unopposed and possibly sustains antiapoptosis and cell proliferation. Other models of androgen-mediated survival were examined by Kimura et al.[64] These investigators observed that androgens rescue cells treated with TNF-α and Fas (± irradiation) by inhibiting both intrinsic (through inhibition of caspase-8 activation) and extrinsic (through inhibition of Bax activation, mitochondrial release of cytochrome c, and activation of caspase-9) pathways. Additionally, they described that androgens inhibit ceramide-induced apoptosis with mechanisms downstream of ceramide production. The foregoing data suggest that androgens suppress apoptosis induced by a variety of cytotoxic stimulations by interfering with various steps of the extrinsic and possibly the intrinsic pathways. Research is needed to unravel the antiapoptotic/survival signals that become dominant and prevent completion of the apoptotic pathway in men treated with AA who developed AI disease.

Contribution of New Technologies to Understanding Castration-Induced Apoptosis

Using microarray technology with LNCaP cell lines[65] and the CWR22 xenograft[66] harvested before and after the addition of androgen to the medium, or specimens of prostate cancer obtained at different stages of the disease from a variety of patients,[67] additional androgen-regulated genes were identified. Although these technological breakthroughs have made it possible to identify many novel genes of potential interest, the precise contribution of these molecules to understanding the mechanisms of induction or prevention of apoptosis after AA is still uncertain and will become clear only once their biology is understood.

USE OF APOPTOTIC MOLECULES TO INDUCE THERAPEUTIC APOPTOSIS OF PROSTATE CANCER

Because AI prostate cancer is so prevalent and incurable, the community of investigators is under significant pressure to identify novel forms of treatment. The approach of our group has been to use genes of the apoptotic pathway as therapeutic agents. These genes provide the advantage that once active, they will set in motion an irreversible and efficient endogenous suicide program and therefore should be perceived as potential therapeutic targets. Our initial attempts to identify molecules of the apoptotic pathway essential to mediate death of prostatic epithelium using AA to induce apoptosis were unsuccessful, because we were unable to identify a reproducible and efficient *in vitro* model of AA-induced apoptosis. Using alternative tactics we identified two groups of molecules whose activity is required for prostate cancer cells to die by an apoptotic mechanism (to be described). We proceeded to study if manipulation of the expression/activity of these molecules can be exploited therapeutically to induce apoptosis of prostate cancer cells growing *in vitro* and *in vivo*. The general approach of this project is schematically presented in TABLE 1.

Several *in vitro* models of apoptosis using CaP cell lines and the apoptotic agents staurosporine (STS), lovastatin, and sodium phenyl acetate[68–70] were established in our laboratory to identify the events required for the induction of programmed cell death in prostatic epithelium. For the purpose of brevity, we concentrate most of this discussion to findings with LNCaP and PC-3 cells, which represent two established models of androgen-dependent (LNCaP) and androgen-independent (PC-3) CaP, and our positive (LNCaP) and negative (PC-3) models of apoptotic death after the addition of the protein kinase inhibitor STS.[70] In response to STS, LNCaP cells die by essentially activating the mitochondrial pathway of apoptosis. Chronologically, the first identified event consisted in the translocation of proapoptotic Bcl-2 family members Bax and Bad to the mitochondrial membrane.[51] This was followed by loss of mitochondrial transmembrane potential,[70] egress of cytotoxic factors such as cytochrome c,[69,70] SMAC,[30] and endonuclease G[31] to the cytosol, by activation of the caspase pathway, and by disintegration of cellular contents through cleavage of substrates that are essential for survival.[69,70] In LNCaP cells, STS-induced apoptosis could be prevented by: (1) overexpression of the anti-apoptotic protein Bcl-2, which protects the mitochondria from functional incapacitation and from releasing cytochrome c to cytosol[69]; and (2) use of the pan-capase-inhibitor z-VAD-FMK.[69] Our negative control PC-3 cells did not undergo apoptosis after STS. Similar to LNCaP cells, Bax and Bad became mitochondrial bound when STS was added to the PC-3 cells.[51] However, as this cell line naturally overexpresses the anti-apoptotic Bcl-2 family member Bcl-x_L, mitochondrial incapacitation did not occur, the caspase pathway was not activated, and apoptosis was prevented.[70] We extended these studies to DU-145 and TsuPr(1) cells, and their response to STS was similar to that of PC-3 and LNCaP, respectively.[70] In conclusion, these initial studies identified two steps

TABLE 1. Establishment of *in-vitro* models of apoptosis using prostate cancer cell lines and investigating the events leading to apoptosis in these model

Establishment of *in-vitro* models of apoptosis using prostate cancer cell lines

Investigating the events leading to apoptosis in these models

Manipulation of the expression/activity of these molecules to induce apoptosis in these cell lines

Development of reagents inducing therapeutic apoptosis of prostate cancer cells in *in-vivo* models

---

necessary for the completion of the intrinsic apoptotic pathway in CaP cell lines: (1) the functional incapacitation of the mitochondria and their release to the cytosol of cytochrome c; and (2) the activation of the caspase pathway. In the absence of the first, as in LNCaP overexpressing Bcl-2[69] or in PC-3 which naturally overexpress Bcl-x_L,[51,70] or of the second, as in LNCaP treated with the pancaspase inhibitor zVAD-FMK,[69] apoptosis did not occur. Thus, these two steps of the apoptotic pathway were identified as attractive therapeutic targets.

MANIPULATION OF THE EXPRESSION/ACTIVITY OF APOPTOTIC MOLECULES TO INDUCE PROGRAMMED CELL DEATH IN PROSTATE CANCER CELL LINES

We attempted to force CaP cells to undergo apoptosis by inducing activation of the caspase pathway (one of the two therapeutic targets mentioned above). We developed adenoviral constructs to manipulate the activity of two pro-caspases (pro-caspase-3 and pro-caspase–7). The decision to use this approach was based on data discussed herein and on reports showing that plasmid-mediated overexpression of various pro-caspases is associated with their autocatalytic activation in a variety of systems.[71–73] The adenoviruses for pro-caspase-3 and pro-caspase–7 (AvC3[74] and AvC7[69]) were first generation vectors under the control of the powerful rous sarcoma virus (RSV) promoter. A dramatic overexpression of pro-caspase-3 and pro-caspase–7 was observed in every cell line used. Disappointingly, overexpressed pro-caspase-3 did not undergo autocatalytic activation and did not induce apoptosis in any cell line.[75] Overexpressed pro-caspase-7 underwent autocatalytic activation and induced apoptosis only in LNCaP and LNCaP-Bcl-2 cells.[69,75] Autocatalytic activation of the pro-caspase of interest or apoptosis was not present in any of the remaining cells that were infected with AvC7.[69,75] In synthesis, we observed that massive apoptosis occurred when the zymogen became active (as in the case of pro-caspase-7 in LNCaP and LNCaP-Bcl-2). By contrast, apoptosis was not observed when the zymogen remained an inactive pro-caspase (as in pro-caspase-3 with every cell line, and pro-caspase-7 with PC-3, TsuPr(1), and DU-145).[69,75]

Searching for a therapeutic target more effective than pro-caspase overexpression, we attempted to induce therapeutic apoptosis by forcing mitochondrial incapacitation (the second therapeutic target identified). To do so, we used a binary system that overexpresses Bax,[76] and consists of two adenoviruses. The first (Ad/

PGK/GV16) produces a GAL4-VP16 fusion protein under the control of the constitutively active PGK promoter. The second (Ad/GT-Bax) contains a Bax cDNA under the control of a GAL/TATA minipromoter. Transcription of Bax is therefore induced by the fusion protein (a powerful transactivator) interacting with the minipromoter. We decided to use this system based on data demonstrating that plasmid-mediated Bax overexpression causes Bax to localize inside the mitochondria. This is followed by loss of mitochondrial transmembrane potential, cytosolic release of cytochrome c, activation of the caspase pathway, and apoptosis.[77,78] The binary system induced Bax overexpression and apoptosis in every CaP cell line. As expected, this was achieved by forcing mitochondrial incapacitation, cytochrome c release from the mitochondria, and activation of the caspase pathway.[75]

DEVELOPMENT OF REAGENTS INDUCING THERAPEUTIC APOPTOSIS OF PROSTATE CANCER CELLS IN *IN VIVO* MODELS

In additional experiments, we treated PC-3 tumors growing subcutaneously in nu/nu mice with the binary Bax system and appropriate controls and demonstrated that growth was inhibited in tumors receiving the binary system overexpressingg Bax. Three injections of the Bax overexpression system into PC-3 cell tumors in nude mice *in vivo* caused 25% regression in tumor size (p <0.0006) corresponding to 90% reduction (p <0.00005) relative to continued tumor growth in animals injected with the control binary system expressing Lac-Z. These data, therefore, supported the concept that the apoptotic pathway can be manipulated *in vitro* and *in vivo* for therapeutic purposes by overexpressing the apoptotic factor Bax.[75]

DEVELOPMENT OF A CONSTRUCT EXPRESSING BAX UNIQUELY IN PROSTATIC EPITHELIUM

Other investigations have shown that adenoviral-mediated Bax overexpression can be lethal in many cell types.[76,79] Thus, development of a system specific for the expression of genes in prostatic epithelium was mandatory for keeping this lethal molecule from accumulating in extraprostatic tissue and causing life-threatening side effects. To direct Bax overexpression uniquely in AR+ CaP cell lines, this gene was placed under the control of ARR_2PB,[80] an artificial androgen-responsive and prostate-specific promoter developed in Matusik's laboratory. The resulting first generation adenovirus Av-ARR_2PB-Bax expressed Bax only in AR-positive cells of prostatic origin, but not in AR-positive cells of nonprostatic origin or AR-negative cells of any origin. Injection of Av-ARR_2PB-Bax into AR-positive prostate cancer tumor xenografts in nu/nu mice resulted in an increase in the percentage of apoptotic cells and a decrease in tumor size compared to that in control treated tumors.[81]

FUTURE DIRECTIONS

Initial trials of adenoviral-mediated transduction of therapeutic genes in the treatment of primary CaP have already been completed,[82,83] and these patients have experienced some benefit and minimal side effects. Development of powerful prostate-specific promoters such as ARR_2PB linked to pancytotoxic genes such as Bax, represent significant steps towards safely treating and eliminating primary CaP. Gene therapy for CaP is currently at its dawn, and in the end it may possibly evolve into a mainstream form of treatment integrated with other mainstream forms of treatment such as chemotherapy and radiation therapy. In addition, a combination of therapeutic genes, instead of only one, will likely be given to simultaneously target several cellular pathways. Nevertheless, new technology needs to be developed to successfully defeat metastatic CaP using gene therapy, and at this purpose investigators are working to develop prostate-specific conditionally replicating vectors. In the end, and like with any other disease, complete understanding of the basic biology of transition to AI CaP as well as to AA-resistant disease will be instrumental in developing novel therapeutic interventions on disease-specific mechanisms.

ACKNOWLEDGMENTS

The original studies were supported by grants from the Department of Defense Prostate Cancer Research Program and the VA Merit Review Program to M.M.

REFERENCES

1. HUGGINS, C. & C.V. HODGES. 1941. The effect of castration, of estrogens and androgen injection on serum phosphatase in metastatic carcinoma of the prostate. Cancer Res. **1:** 293–297.
2. MIGLIACCIO, A. *et al.* 1998. Activation of the Src/p21ras/Erk pathway by progesterone receptor via cross-talk with estrogen receptor. Embo J. **17:** 2008–2018.
3. BOONYARATANAKORNKIT, V. *et al.* 2001. Progesterone receptor contains a proline-rich motif that directly interacts with SH3 domains and activates c-Src family tyrosine kinases. Mol. Cell. **8:** 269–280.
4. PETERZIEL, H. *et al.* 1995. Mutant androgen receptors in prostatic tumors distinguish between amino-acid-sequence requirements for transactivation and ligand binding. Int. J. Cancer **63:** 544–550.
5. MIGLIACCIO, A. *et al.* 2000. Steroid-induced androgen receptor-oestradiol receptor beta-Src complex triggers prostate cancer cell proliferation. Embo J. **19:** 5406–1547.
6. KOUSTENI, S. *et al.* 2001. Nongenotropic, sex-nonspecific signaling through the estrogen or androgen receptors: dissociation from transcriptional activity. Cell **104:** 719–730.
7. KYPRIANOU, N. *et al.* 1990. Programmed cell death during regression of PC-82 human prostate cancer following androgen ablation. Cancer Res. **50:** 3748–3753.
8. ISAACS, J.T. 1999. The biology of hormone refractory prostate cancer. Why does it develop? Urol. Clin. North Am. **26:** 263–273.
9. LAUFER, M. *et al.* 2000. Complete androgen blockade for prostate cancer: what went wrong? J. Urol. **164:** 3–9.
10. EISENBERGER, M.A. & P.C. Walsh. 1999. Early androgen deprivation for prostate cancer? [editorial; comment]. N. Engl. J. Med. **341:** 1837–1848.
11. GREENLEE, R.T. *et al.* Cancer statistics, 2000. CA Cancer J. Clin. **50:** 7–33.
12. MEHMET, H. 2000. Caspases find a new place to hide [news]. Nature **403:** 29–30.
13. ASHKENAZI, A. & V. DIXIT. 1998. Death receptors: signaling and modulation. Science **281:** 1305–1308.
14. GREEN, D. & J. REED. 1998. Mitochondria and apoptosis. Science **281:** 1309–1312.
15. THORNBERRY, N. & Y. LAZEBNICK. 1998. Caspases: enemies within. Science **281:** 1312–1316.

16. PERLMAN, H. *et al.* 1999. An elevated bax/bcl-2 ratio corresponds with the onset of prostate epithelial cell apoptosis. Cell Death Differ. **6:** 48–54.
17. ZHA, J. *et al.* 1996. Serine phosphorylation of death agonist BAD in response to survival factor results in binding to 14-3-3 not Bcl-xl. Cell **87:** 619–628.
18. BRUNET, A. *et al.* 1999. Akt promotes cell survival by phosphorylating and inhibiting a Forkhead transcription factor. Cell **96:** 857–868.
19. CARDONE, M.H. *et al.* 1998. Regulation of cell death protease caspase-9 by phosphorylation. Science **282:** 1318–1321.
20. PEKARSKY, Y. *et al.* 2001. Akt phosphorylates and regulates the orphan nuclear receptor Nur77. Proc. Natl. Acad. Sci. USA **98:** 3690–3694.
21. ZONG, W.X. *et al.* 1999. The prosurvival Bcl-2 homolog Bfl-1/A1 is a direct transcriptional target of NF-kappaB that blocks TNFalpha-induced apoptosis. Genes Dev. **13:** 382–387.
22. WANG, C.Y. *et al.* 1998. NF-kappaB antiapoptosis: induction of TRAF1 and TRAF2 and c-IAP1 and c- IAP2 to suppress caspase-8 activation. Science **281:** 1680–1683.
23. GOPING, I.S. *et al.* 1998. Regulated targeting of BAX to mitochondria. J. Cell Biol. **143:** 207–215.
24. DESAGHER, S. *et al.* 1999. Bid-induced conformational change of Bax is responsible for mitochondrial cytochrome c release during apoptosis. J. Cell Biol. **144:** 891–901.
25. ESKES, R. *et al.* 2000. Bid induces the oligomerization and insertion of Bax into the outer mitochondrial membrane. Mol. Cell Biol. **20:** 929–935.
26. GRIFFITHS, G.J. *et al.* 1999. Cell damage-induced conformational changes of the pro-apoptotic protein Bak *in vivo* precede the onset of apoptosis. J. Cell Biol. **144:** 903–014.
27. ZAMZAMI, N. *et al.* 1995. Sequential reduction of mitochondrial transmembrane potential and generation of reactive oxygen species in early programmed cell death. J. Exp. Med. **182:** 367–377.
28. LIU, X. *et al.* 1996. Induction of apoptotic program in cell-free extracts: requirement for dATP and cytochrome c. Cell **86:** 147–157.
29. SUSIN, S. *et al.* 1999. Molecular characterization of mitochondrial apoptosis-inducing factor. Nature **397:** 441–446.
30. DU, C. *et al.* 2000. Smac, a mitochondrial protein that promotes cytochrome c–dependent caspase activation by eliminating IAP inhibition. Cell **102:** 33–42.
31. LI, L.Y. *et al.* 2001. Endonuclease G is an apoptotic DNase when released from mitochondria. Nature **412:** 95–99.
32. LI, P. *et al.* 1997. Cytochrome c and dATP-dependent formation of Apaf-1/caspase-9 complex initiates an apoptotic protease cascade. Cell **91:** 479–489.
33. GECK, P. *et al.* 2000. Androgen-induced proliferative quiescence in prostate cancer cells: the role of AS3 as its mediator. Proc. Natl. Acad. Sci. USA **97:** 10185–1090.
34. LEE, C. *et al.* 1995. Regulation of proliferation and production of prostate specific antigen in androgen-sensitive prostate cancer cells, LNCaP, by dihydrotestosterone. Endocrinology **136:** 796–803.
35. SONNENSCHEIN, C. *et al.* 1989. Negative controls of cell proliferation: human prostate cancers and androgens. Cancer Res. **49:** 3474–3481.
36. KYPRIANOU, N. & J. ISAACS. 1988. Activation of programmed cell death in the rat ventral prostate after castration. Endocrinology **122:** 552–562.
37. SANDFORD, N.L. *et al.* 1984. Successive waves of apoptosis in the rat prostate after repeated withdrawal of testosterone stimulation. Pathology **16:** 406–410.
38. ENGLISH, H.F. *et al.* 1985. Cellular response to androgen depletion and repletion in the rat ventral prostate: autoradiography and morphometric analysis. Prostate **7:** 41–51.
39. COLOMBEL, M.C. & R. BUTTYAN. 1995. Hormonal control of apoptosis: the rat prostate gland as a model system. Methods Cell Biol. **46:** 369–385.
40. LEGER, J.G. *et al.* 1987. Characterization and cloning of androgen-repressed mRNAs from rat ventral prostate. Biochem. Biophys. Res. Commun. **147:** 196–203.
41. KYPRIANOU, N. & J.T. ISAACS. 1989. Expression of transforming growth factor-b in the rat ventral prostate during castration-induced programmed cell death. Mol. Endocrinol. **3:** 1515–1522.
42. BUTTYAN, R. *et al.* 1988. Cascade induction of *c-fos*, *c-myc*, and heat shock 70K transcripts during regression of the ventral prostate gland. Mol. Endocrinol. **2:** 650–657.

43. SUZUKI, A. *et al.* 1996. Down regulation of Bcl-2 is the first step on Fas-mediated apoptosis of male reproductive tract. Oncogene **13:** 31–37.
44. BRIEHL, M.M. & R.L. MIESFELD. 1991. Isolation and characterization of transcripts induced by androgen withdrawal and apoptotic cell death in the rat ventral prostate. Mol. Endocrinol. **5:** 1381–1388.
45. CHANG, C.S. *et al.* 1987. Identification of glutathione S-transferase Yb1 mRNA as the androgen-repressed mRNA by cDNA cloning and sequence analysis. J. Biol. Chem. **262:** 11901–1193.
46. UEMURA, H. & C. CHANG. 1998. Antisense TR3 orphan receptor can increase prostate cancer cell viability with etoposide treatment. Endocrinology **139:** 2329–2334.
47. SENSIBAR, J.A. *et al.* 1995. Prevention of cell death induced by tumor necrosis factor alpha in LNCaP cells by overexpression of sulfated glycoprotein-2 (clusterin). Cancer Res. **55:** 2431–2437.
48. NISHI, N. *et al.* 1996. Changes in gene expression of growth factors and their receptors during castration-induced involution and androgen-induced regrowth of rat prostates. Prostate **28:** 139–152.
49. MCDONNELL, T.J. *et al.* 1992. Expression of the protooncogene *bcl-2* in the prostate and its association with emergence of androgen-independent prostate cancer. Cancer Res. **52:** 6940–6944.
50. COLOMBEL, M. *et al.* 1993. Detection of the apoptosis suppressing oncoprotein bcl-2 in hormone refractory human prostate cancers. Am. J. Pathol. **143:** 390–400.
51. LI, X.-Y. *et al.* 2001. Overexpression of BCL-X_L underlies the molecular basis for resistance to staurosporine-induced apoptosis on PC-3 cells. Can. Res. **61:** 1699–1706.
52. WANG, Z. *et al.* 1997. Genes regulated by androgen in the rat ventral prostate. Proc. Natl. Acad. Sci. USA **94:** 12999–13004.
53. ZHU, N. & Z. WANG. 1999. Calreticulin expression is associated with androgen regulation of the sensitivity to calcium ionophore-induced apoptosis in LNCaP prostate cancer cells. Cancer Res. **59:** 1896–1902.
54. MARTIKAINEN, P. *et al.* 1991. Programmed death of nonproliferating androgen-independent prostatic cancer cells. Cancer Res. **51:** 4693–4700.
55. FURUYA, Y. *et al.* 1994. The role of calcium, pH, and cell proliferation in the programmed (apoptotic) death of androgen-independent prostatic cancer cells induced by thapsigargin. Cancer Res. **54:** 6167–6175.
56. WERTZ, I.E. & V.M. DIXIT. 2000. Characterization of calcium release-activated apoptosis of LNCaP prostate cancer cells. J. Biol. Chem. **275:** 11470–11477.
57. SHABSIGH, A. *et al.* 1998. Rapid reduction in blood flow to the rat ventral prostate gland after castration: preliminary evidence that androgens influence prostate size by regulating blood flow to the prostate gland and prostatic endothelial cell survival. Prostate **36:** 201–206.
58. BUTTYAN, R. *et al.* 1999. Regulation of Apoptosis in the Prostate Gland by Androgenic Steroids. Trends Endocrinol. Metab. **10:** 47–54.
59. SHABSIGH, A. *et al.* 2001. Biomarker analysis demonstrates a hypoxic environment in the castrated rat ventral prostate gland. J. Cell Biochem. **81:** 437–444.
60. CHANG, G.T. *et al.* 2000. Characterization of a zinc-finger protein and its association with apoptosis in prostate cancer cells. J. Natl. Cancer Inst. **92:** 1414–1421.
61. CARSON, J.P. *et al.* 1999. Antiapoptotic signaling in LNCaP prostate cancer cells: a survival signaling pathway independent of phosphatidylinositol 3'-kinase and Akt/protein kinase B. Cancer Res. **59:** 1449–1453.
62. LI, P. *et al.* 2001. Antagonism between PTEN/MMAC1/TEP-1 and androgen receptor in growth and apoptosis of prostatic cancer cells. J. Biol. Chem. **276:** 20444–20450.
63. WEN, Y. *et al.* 2000. HER-2/neu promotes androgen-independent survival and growth of prostate cancer cells through the Akt pathway. Cancer Res. **60:** 6841–6845.
64. KIMURA, K. *et al.* 2001. Androgen blocks apoptosis of hormone-dependent prostate cancer cells. Cancer Res. **61:** 5611–5618.
65. VAARALA, M.H. *et al.* 2000. Differentially expressed genes in two LNCaP prostate cancer cell lines reflecting changes during prostate cancer progression. Lab. Invest. **80:** 1259–1268.

66. AMLER, L.C. et al. 2000. Dysregulated expression of androgen-responsive and nonresponsive genes in the androgen-independent prostate cancer xenograft model CWR22-R1. Cancer Res. **60:** 134–141.
67. DHANASEKARAN, S.M. et al. 2001. Delineation of prognostic biomarkers in prostate cancer. Nature **412:** 822–826.
68. MARCELLI, M. et al. 1998. Caspase-7 is activated during lovastatin-induced apoptosis of the prostate cancer cell line LNCaP. Cancer Res. **58:** 76–83.
69. MARCELLI, M. et al. 1999. Signaling pathway activated during apoptosis of the prostate cancer cell line LNCaP: overexpression of caspase-7 as a new gene therapy strategy for the treatment of prostate cancer. Cancer Res. **59:** 398–406.
70. MARCELLI, M. et al. 2000. Heterogeneous apoptotic responses of prostate cancer cell lines identify an association between sensitivity to staurosporine-induced apoptosis, expression of Bcl-2 family members, and caspase activation. Prostate **42:** 260–273.
71. MIURA, M. et al. 1993. Induction of apoptosis in fibroblasts by IL-1β-converting enzyme, a mammalian homolog of the C elegans cell death gene ced-3. Cell **75:** 653–660.
72. DUAN, H. et al. 1996. ICE-LAP6, a novel member of the ICE/Ced-3 gene family, is activated by the cytotoxic T cell protease granzyme B. J. Biol. Chem. **271:** 16720–16724.
73. SRINIVASULA, S. et al. 1998. Generation of constitutively active recombinant caspases-3 and -6 by rearrangment of their subunit. J. Biol. Chem. **273:** 10107–10111.
74. MARCELLI, M. et al. 2000. Induction of apoptosis in BPH stromal cells by adenoviral-mediated overexpression of caspase-7. J. Urol. **164:** 518–525.
75. LI, X.-Y. et al. 2001. Adenoviral-mediated Bax overexpression for the induction of therapeutic apoptosis in prostate cancer. Can. Res. **61:** 186–191.
76. KAGAWA, S. et al. 2000. A binary adenoviral vector system for expressing high levels of the proapoptotic gene bax. Gene Ther. **7:** 75–79.
77. XIANG, J. et al. 1996. Bax-induced cell death may not require interleukin 1beta-converting enzyme-like proteases. Proc. Natl. Acad. Sci. USA **93:** 14559–14563.
78. GROSS, A. et al. 1998. Enforced dimerization of BAX results in its translocation, mitochondrial dysfunction and apoptosis. Embo J. **17:** 3878–3885.
79. KAGAWA, S. et al. 2000. Antitumor effect of adenovirus-mediated Bax gene transfer on p53- sensitive and p53-resistant cancer lines. Cancer Res. **60:** 1157–1161.
80. ZHANG, J.F. et al. 2000. A small composite probasin promoter confers high levels of prostate-specific gene expression through regulation by androgens and glucocorticoids in vitro and in vivo. Endocrinology **141:** 4698–4710.
81. ANDRIANI, F. et al. 2001. Use of the probasin promoter ARR(2)PB to express bax in androgen receptor-positive prostate cancer cells. J. Natl. Cancer Inst. **93:** 1314–1324.
82. HERMAN, J.R. et al. 1999. In situ gene therapy for adenocarcinoma of the prostate: a phase I clinical trial. Hum. Gene Ther. **10:** 1239–1249.
83. BELLDEGRUN, A. et al. 2001. Interleukin 2 gene therapy for prostate cancer: phase I clinical trial and basic biology. Hum. Gene Ther. **12:** 883–892.

Biological Selection Criteria for Radical Prostatectomy

GIOVANNI MUZZONIGRO AND ANDREA B. GALOSI

Institute of Urology, Azienda Ospedaliera Umberto 1st, University of Ancona, Ancona, Italy

ABSTRACT: Tumors clinically confined to the prostate gland (T1-2) are heterogeneous with respect to pathological staging and outcome after definitive radical surgery (radical prostatectomy). The preoperative prognostic factors that could predict pathological stage and outcome of individual patients with clinically localized prostate cancer are reviewed. New preoperative factors have been identified by histological analysis of needle biopsy prostate specimens in addition to Gleason grading score, serum markers (PSA), and clinical staging. These factors are related to tumor volume, zonal origin of the tumor, and spread into the gland and surrounding tissues. Other biological factors are identified by molecular and immunohistochemical analysis (neuroendocrine differentiation, DNA content, microvessel density, and perineural invasion). Biomolecular factors can also be assessed preoperatively on serum samples (free/total PSA ratio, PSA RT-PCR). Although only a few of these factors have a role in predicting treatment failure and/or disease recurrence, the neural network analysis seems to be the most important tool for identifying patients with more aggressive disease. A combination of these new factors, also using neural networks, could be relevant in the preoperative management of patients with prostate cancer to identify those with confined disease and to select those suitable for a "nerve sparing radical prostatectomy" to preserve sexual function and to achieve definitive cancer control.

KEYWORDS: prostate neoplasms; prognostic factors; therapy; biopsy; staging

INTRODUCTION

Prostate cancer is a leading cause of morbidity and mortality in males, accounting for ~30% of all new cases of cancer and ~14% of cancer deaths.[1] Despite the high prevalence (~27%) of prostate cancer in autopsy series in 30–40-year-old patients,[2] the lifetime probability of being diagnosed with prostate cancer is 8%, whereas the probability of dying of prostate cancer is 3%.[3] Therefore, screening programs detect clinically confined tumors of the prostate gland (T1-2) that are heterogeneous with respect to pathological staging and outcome.[4]

Address for correspondence: Giovanni Muzzonigro, M.D., Institute of Urology, University of Ancona, Umberto 1st Hospital, Piazza Cappelli 1, I-60121 Ancona, Italy. Voice: +39.071.202642; fax: +39.071.2070501.
g.muzzonigro@popcsi.unian.it

Modern surgical approaches to localize prostate cancer have contributed significantly to cancer control and preservation of patients' quality of life. Despite considerable advances in the surgical treatment of prostate cancer, no significant corresponding decreases have been noted in disease recurrence and mortality after definitive treatment, mostly due to positive surgical margins and clinical understaging of extraprostatic tumor in 30–40% of cases.[5]

Radical prostatectomy is the most effective form of treatment of patients with tumor confined to the prostatic capsule (pT2, TNM 1997), whereas in patients with extraprostatic tumor (pT3a) or seminal vesicle invasion, the disease-free survival is poor.

Two main clinical issues are: (1) In patients with clinically localized prostate cancer, actually diagnosed in younger patients, and potential candidates for radical prostatectomy, do we have preoperatively the biological prognostic factors that could predict treatment failure and/or disease recurrence? (2) Do we preoperatively have factors or criteria to select the patient for radical prostatectomy, using the nerve-sparing technique to preserve sexual function? In others words, are there available prognostic factors to stratify patients with different risk of treatment failure or success?

PROGNOSTIC FACTORS IN PROSTATE CANCER

We discuss the preoperative prognostic factors that could accurately predict outcome in individual patients with prostate cancer. The goal is to tailor the therapeutic approach to the clinical, morphological, and molecular features of each patient. Classic radiological procedures, such as transrectal ultrasound, endorectal MRI, and computerized tomography (CT)/magnetic resonance (MR) of the abdomen and pelvis, failed to significantly improve the staging of localized prostate cancer.[6]

Many clinically important predictive factors in prostate cancer are derived from the serum prostate-specific antigen (PSA) level and light microscopic examination of biopsy tissue specimens by pathologists.

PROSTATE-SPECIFIC ANTIGEN

Prostate-specific antigen is a glycoprotein produced by epithelial cells. Serum total PSA levels depend on tumor volume and differentiation. PSA rises 3.5 ng/ml per gram of prostatic tumor; in benign hypertrophy, the PSA level is elevated only 0.3 ng/ml per gram of benign prostate tissue.

Prostate-specific antigen has been used successfully to improve clinical staging. If PSA is less than 4 ng/ml, the probability of cancer being confined to the gland after pathological stage pT2 and negative pelvic lymph nodes (pN0) is 64 and 99%, respectively. If PSA is >50 ng/ml, probability decreases, respectively, to 9% (for pT2) and 63% (for pN0). PSA predictive value is less satisfactory at 4–10 ng/ml, which represents about half the men with prostate cancer.[7]

BIOPSY FEATURES AND PARAMETERS

To provide diagnostic tissue for pathologic study to detect cancer and identify the precise tumor location it is necessary to know the zonal anatomy of the prostate gland with its site of anatomic weakness and site of origin of prostate cancer. These factors may influence the prognostic significance of biopsy features.[8,9] Factors that determine the biological aggressiveness, other than clinical staging, are Gleason score, cancer zonal origin (transition zone or peripheral zone),[10,11] and tumor volume (in relation to percentage of cancer in biopsy specimens,[12] side,[13] and number and percentage of positive biopsies[14,15]), perineural invasion,[16] and microvessel density (angiogenesis).[17]

Other prognostic factors can be identified using additional prostatic biopsies to stage the tumor: (1) to assess local spread of prostate cancer in the gland, in seminal vesicles, and in extraprostatic tissues (fat, bladder neck, and external sphincter) or capsular perforation on biopsy;[18,19] (2) to improve the accuracy of prediction of Gleason grading;[20] and (3) to detect perineural invasion.[16,21]

The finding of a small number of positive biopsies depends on the total prostate volume and the distribution of tumor in the gland. Also, a biopsy can detect low-volume tumors depending on the prevalence of these tumors in the population studied and the sites and numbers of prostatic biopsies performed (e.g., a site of origin is the lateral subcapsular area of the peripheral zone). Sebo et al.[14] showed that pT2 prostate cancer was found in 94% of patients with only one positive biopsy out of six sextant biopsies, whereas it was identified in 64% of patients with two or more positive cores for prostate cancer.[14]

Some of their features are used routinely alone or in combination with PSA and digital rectal examination to predict the final pathological stage of tumor (pT). These biological and biopsy parameters are correlated with tumor foci, grading, extraprostatic extension, seminal vesicle invasion, positive margin, and lymph node metastases on surgical specimens after prostatectomy and pelvic lymph node dissection.[22]

Identifying the anatomic zone of a positive biopsy has a clinical relevance: cancer arising in the transition zone is different from those arising in the peripheral zone. Noguchi et al.[10] reported that 25% of impalpable tumors were located in the transition zone. The biochemical cure rate is 72% in transition zone cancer versus 49% in peripheral zone cancer ($p < 0.01$) after radical prostatectomy and 5 years of follow-up. Anatomic differences (anterior fibromuscular stroma overlying the transition zone is frequently invaded, but rarely perforated; posterolaterally they are confined by the transition zone boundary, which is made of compressed fibromuscular tissue) and biological differences (high PSA levels in relation to high tumor volumes) explain the better prognosis of transition zone cancer. Therefore, transition zone cancer should be considered separately. Transition zone biopsies can be used to make this important distinction preoperatively.[10]

INTERNATIONAL CONSENSUS CONFERENCES

The contemporary status of the prognostic factors was addressed in two recent international consensus conferences, the 1999 College of American Pathologists

(CAP) Conference[23] and the 1999 World Health Organization (WHO) Second International Consultation on Prostate Cancer.[24]

A multidisciplinary group of clinicians, pathologists, and statisticians analyzed the existing predictive factors and separated them into categories, reflecting the strength of published evidence and taking into account the opinions of the Prostate Working Group members of the CAP.[23] Factors were ranked according to the previous CAP categorical ranking: *category I,* factors proven to be of prognostic importance and useful in clinical patient management; *category II,* factors that have been extensively studied biologically and clinically, but whose importance remains to be validated in statistically robust studies; and *category III,* all other factors not sufficiently studied to demonstrate their prognostic value.

The CAP categorical ranking was fully endorsed by the WHO conference, whose emphasis was mainly on biopsy-derived predictive factors. In particular, the adoption of all pathology factors grouped in category I was recommended; the factors grouped in category II may be included, based on local discretion; and adoption of any of the factors in category III was not recommended.[24]

Factors ranked in category I include preoperative serum prostate-specific antigen level, TNM stage grouping, histologic grade, and surgical margin status. In particular, when considering the histologic grade, the Gleason system is recommended as the standard for grading prostate cancer. Gleason score should be reported as the composite score and its component patterns, for example, Gleason $7 = 4 + 3$. The first reported pattern is the most frequent and the second reported pattern is the second most frequent. The highest-grade pattern should also be reported, regardless of frequency. If the sample is a needle biopsy, the Gleason score of the entire sample should be reported as a composite score. If Gleason scores must be compressed for reporting purposes, the groups should be 2–5, 6, 7, and 8–10, or 2–6, 7, and 8–10. The WHO conference additionally recommends the use of WHO nuclear grade, pathologic effects of treatments, and location of cancer within the prostate.

Category II factors include tumor volume, histologic type, and DNA ploidy. There is a fair to good correlation between the amount of cancer reported in the biopsy specimens and that subsequently found in radical prostatectomy specimens. This correlation is greatest for large cancers. For this reason, pathologists must include in the report the total percentage of cancer in the total number of needle biopsy segments. Although the volume of cancer in radical prostatectomy specimens was shown to have predictive value in only some studies. Also, including this determination may be of value until further data are available.

Factors in category III include perineural invasion, neuroendocrine differentiation, microvessel density (angiogenesis), nuclear roundness, chromatin texture, other karyometric factors, proliferation markers, prostate-specific antigen derivatives (complexed PSA and free to total PSA ratio [f/t PSA]), and other factors (oncogenes, tumor suppressor genes, and apoptosis genes).

Serum-Free Prostate-Specific Antigen

The serum free to total PSA ratio (f/t PSA) is the percentage of free PSA unbound to serum proteins. To date, its clinical significance as a staging marker is still under investigation. Recently, Catalona *et al.*[25] reported a statistically significant increase in probability of intraprostatic disease (pT2) as the f/t PSA ratio increased.

Biomolecular Factors

Recently, the relevance of biomolecular methods (PSA RT-PCR) to determine the presence of PSA-positive cells in the blood stream, which could indicate early metastatic disease, has raised great interest; however, long-term clinical trial is needed for evaluation. Molecular staging up to now has to be considered as investigational without clinical relevance.[26] Serum levels of human glandular kallikrein-2 (hK-2), which is secreted by prostate epithelial cells, seems to have high specificity (100%) for intraprostatic cancer (pT2) with low sensitivity (37%).

Neuroendocrine differentiation and angiogenesis are two factors in category III that are considered among the most promising from a practical point of view.[27,28] prostate cancer may show divergent differentiation towards a neuroendocrine phenotype in the form of neuroendocrine small cell carcinoma or carcinoid-like tumors.[27] Much more common is focal neuroendocrine differentiation in prostate cancer, which may be pronounced in approximately 10% of carcinomas. The prognostic significance of focal neuroendocrine differentiation in prostate cancer is controversial, but current evidence suggests an influence on prognosis related to hormone-resistant tumors and/or a role in the conversion to a hormone-resistant phenotype. Chromogranin A appears to be the best overall tissue and serum marker of neuroendocrine differentiation. Chromogranin A serum levels may be useful in assessing the emergence of and/or progression of hormone-resistant cancer.

Recent studies have demonstrated that angiogenesis is a potent prognostic indicator of patients with prostate cancer and that evaluation of endothelial growth factors is useful in assessing angiogenic phenotype in prostate cancer.[28]

Oncogenes such as *c-myc, c-erb-B2*, and *bcl-2* are potential candidate markers, as are various tumor suppressor genes such as *p27(Kip1), pp32r1/2,* and *PTEN,* following findings that implicate their involvement in controlling the development and progression of prostate cancer. Several metastasis suppressor or anti-invasion genes are also implicated in the progression of prostate cancer and are considered potential future prognostic markers, but they need to be tested for clinical relevance.[29]

Combined Staging (Partin's Table, Artificial Neural Network)

Several investigators have combined individual staging parameters to construct models for predicting intraprostatic cancer (pT2).[30] Partin's table is the most commonly used model for predicting prostate cancer stage. Partin combined three clinical variables (biopsy Gleason grading, PSA, and clinical stage) using a multinomial log-linear analysis.[31] Partin's table has an estimated accuracy of prediction of 67% (confidence interval 95%) for determining organ-confined disease (pT2), 59% for extracapsular disease (pT3-4), 79% for seminal vesicle invasion (pT3b), and 83% for lymph node metastases (pN+). The screening program selects a great number of patients with serum PSA levels between 4 and 10 ng/ml and with Gleason Score 7; therefore, they fall into the intermediate risk group. In this wide group of patients it is difficult to predict stage, because each patient has a 25% chance of being categorized into more than one group, limiting the use of the table for the individual.

An alternate method for integrating preoperative parameters and biological factors is the neural network analysis.[32,33] Preliminary results are promising, and current accuracy for predicting tumor extracapsular extension is 79%. Further research is ongoing.[34,35] For example, the application of the Bayesian Believes Network was tested in our experience.[36] To date, we have obtained encouraging results (unpublished data). The additional use of artificial neural networks is expected to improve the accuracy of diagnosis, staging, and treatment outcomes for prostate cancer.

CLINICAL SELECTION CRITERIA FOR RADICAL PROSTATECTOMY

A wealth of clinical information is available in even the smallest tissue specimens of the prostate, including biopsy specimens. Clinical, biological, and pathological criteria have to be identified for target therapy, because different treatment options are available. A major challenge faced by the clinician is to identify the individual patients who will benefit from radical prostatectomy.

Radical prostatectomy combines a primary oncological procedure with reconstructive surgery, including nerve sparing for potency and continence. However, a nerve-sparing procedure for potency is secondary to the primary oncological aim of prostatectomy. The oncological goal of radical prostatectomy is cancer control, confirmed by negative surgical margins and undetectable levels of serum prostate-specific antigen (PSA, ≤ 0.1 ng/ml) after surgery.

The ability to predict accurately the final pathological stage from preoperative variables is the key element in proper patient selection for radical surgery with the nerve-sparing technique.

From a review of the literature, the well-assessed selection criteria for identifying patients suitable for nerve-sparing surgery are: (1) negative digital rectal examination of the prostate, (2) preoperative PSA level <10 ng/ml, (3) Gleason's score of <7 on biopsy, (4) intracapsular disease according to Partin's table, (5) intracapsular disease on imaging studies (TRUS or endorectal/body coil RMI), and (6) staging biopsy: <30% of core length biopsy with cancer in biopsy, single positive biopsy, with no bilaterality.[37–39]

Biopsy parameters and features add important elements to the therapeutic decision-making process, because they contribute considerably to estimating the risk of extraprostatic tumor extension and PSA failure after radical prostatectomy. Patients who are suitable for radical surgery have initial PSA levels <15 ng/ml, Gleason's scores ≤ 6 or 3+4. Patients who are not suitable for surgery because of a high risk of extracapsular disease have PSA levels >15 ng/ml, Gleason's score >8, and more than two thirds of positive biopsies and cancer in more than 30% of the biopsy core length.

The retropubic approach is the most common way to perform radical prostatectomy. Although the perineal route is still used, recently the use of the laparoscopic approach (either transperitoneal or retropubic [extraperitoneal]) is emerging. In the last few years, surgery rates continue to increase dramatically in younger men in relation to the PSA screening program, whereas surgical treatment for prostate cancer has declined in men over 65 years. In older patients (over 65–70 years) new treatment options are now available.

The treatment option for radical surgery is definitive radiation therapy. Mini-invasive and alternative treatment options including brachytherapy ± external beam radiotherapy, cryoablation, and high-intensity focused ultrasound (HIFU), need to be tested on large randomized trials with long-term follow-up.

In addition to the standard criteria, these new parameters can be tested preoperatively and evaluated to guide our patients through a series of informed choices and treatment options (surgery, radiation therapy, brachytherapy, cryosurgery, plus neoadjuvant and/or adjuvant androgen ablation).[40,41]

CONCLUSIONS

Selection criteria should be used to guide patients through a series of informed choices and treatment options. Biological criteria to determine risk of treatment failure or success are under investigation, especially for managing young patients with early prostatic cancer.

In conclusion, only a few biological features for classifying patients with aggressive disease are promising and need to be tested in clinical trial. Several clinical criteria (serum PSA and biopsy features) are now available for preoperatively selecting patients with prostatic cancer suitable for nerve-sparing radical prostatectomy and those with definitive cancer.

REFERENCES

1. LIJOVIC, M., M.E. FABIANI, J. BADER & A.G. FRAUMAN. 2000. Prostate cancer: are new prognostic markers on the horizon? Prostate Cancer P.D. **3:** 62–65.
2. SAKR, W.A., G.P. HAAS, B.F. CASSIN, et al. 1993. The frequency of carcinoma and intraepithelial neoplasia of the prostate in young male patients. J. Urol. **150:** 379–382.
3. SURVEILLANCE, EPIDEMIOLOGY AND END RESULTS PROGRAM. 1981. Incidence and mortality data: 1973–77. In National Cancer Institute Monograph. Vol. 57. NIH 81–2330. Bethesda, MD.
4. HOEDEMAEKER, R.F., J.B.W. RIETBERGEN, R. KRANSE, et al. 2000. Histopathological prostate cancer characteristics at radical prostatectomy after population based screening. J. Urol. **164:** 411–415.
5. PARTIN, A.W., J. YOO, H.B. CARTER, et al. 1993. The use of PSA, clinical stage and Gleason score to predict pathological stage in men with localized prostate cancer. J. Urol. **149:** 1478–1481.
6. ENGLEBRECHT, M.R.W., J.O. BARENTSZ, G.J. JAGER, et al. 2000. Prostate cancer staging using imaging. Br. J. Urol. Int. **86:** 123–134.
7. PARTIN, A.W., M.V. KATTAN, E.N.P. SUBONG, et al. 1997. Combination of PSA, clinical stage and Gleason score to predict pathological stage of localized prostate cancer. J.A.M.A. **277:** 1445–1451.
8. NARAYAN, P. & A. TEWARI. 1998. Systematic biopsy-based staging of prostate cancer: scientific background, individual variables combination of parameters and current investigative models. Semin. Urol. Oncol. **16:** 172–181.
9. GALOSI, A.B., M. DELLABELLA, M. YEHIA, et al. 2000. Intraprostatic spread of prostate cancer: graphical representation based on TRUS and biopsy findings. Arch. Ital. Urol. Androl. **72:** 264–269.
10. NOGUCHI, M., T.A. STAMEY, J.E. MCNEAL & C.E. YEMOTO. 2000. An analysis of 148 consecutive transition zone cancers: clinical and histological characteristics. J. Urol. **163:** 1751–1755.
11. MAI, K.T., M. MOAZIN, C. MORASH & J.P. COLLINS. 2001. Transition zone and anterior peripheral zone of the prostate. Urol. Int. **66:** 191–196.

12. TERRIS, M.K., D.J. HANEY, I.M. JOHNSTONE, et al. 1995. Prediction of prostate cancer volume using PSA levels, transrectal ultrasound and systematic sextant biopsies. Urology **45**: 75–80.
13. HULAND, H., D. HUBNER & R.P. HANKE. 1994. Systematic biopsies and digital rectal examination to identify the nerve-sparing side for radical prostatectomy without risk of positive margin in patient with clinical stage T1, T2 No prostatic carcinoma. Urology **44**: 211–214.
14. SEBO, T.J., B.J. BOCK, J.C. CHEVILLE, et al. 2000. The percent of cores positive for cancer in prostate needle biopsy specimens is strongly predictive of tumor stage and volume at radical prostatectomy. J. Urol. **163**: 174–178.
15. DJAVAN, B., A.R. ZLOTTA, S. EKANE, et al. 2000. Is one set of sextant biopsies enough to rule out prostate cacer? Influence of transition and total prostate volume on prostate cancer yeld. Eur. Urol. **38**: 218–224.
16. D'AMICO, A.V., Y. WU, M.H. CHEN, et al. 2001. Perineural invasion as a predictor of biochemical outcome following radical prostatectomy for select men with clinically localized prostate cancer. J. Urol. **165**: 126–129.
17. STROHMEYER, D., C. ROSSING, et al. 2000. Tumor angiogenesis is associated with progression after radical prostatectomy in pT2/pT3 prostate cancer. Prostate **42**: 26–33.
18. EGAWA, S., K. SUYAMA, K. MATSUMOTO, et al. 1998. Improved predictability of extracapsular extension and seminal vesicles involvement based on clinical and biopsy findings in prostate cancer in Japanese men. Urology **160**: 2407–2410.
19. SALIKEN, J.C., R.R. GRAY, B.J. DONNELLY, et al. 2000. Extraprostatic biopsy improves the staging of localized prostate cancer. Can. Assoc. Radiol. J. **51**: 114–120.
20. RUBIN, M.A., N.R. MUCCI, S. MANLEY, et al. 2001. Predictors of Gleason pattern 4/5 prostate cancer on prostatectomy specimens: can high grade tumor be predicted preoperatively ? J. Urol. **165**: 114–118.
21. LEE, F., D.K. BAHN, D.B. SIDERS & C. GREENE. 1998. The role of TRUS-guided biopsies for determination of internal and external spread of prostate cancer. Semin. Urol. Oncol. **16**: 129–136.
22. RAVERY, V., H.P. SCHIMID, M. TOUBLANC & L. BOCCON-GIBOD. 1996. Is the percentage of cancer in biopsy cores predictive of extracapsular disease in T1-2 prostate cancer? Cancer **78**: 1079–1084.
23. BOSTWICK, D.G., D. GRIGNON, E.H. HAMMOND, et al. 2000. Predictive factors in prostate cancer. College of American Pathologists Consensus Statements 1999. Arch. Pathol. Lab. Med. **124**: 996–1000.
24. BOSTWICK, D.G., C.S. FOSTER, F. ALGABA, et al. 2000. Prostate tissue factors. In Prostate Cancer. G.P. Murphy, S. Khoury, A. Partin & L. Denis, eds. :162–201. Second International Consultation on Prostate Cancer. Paris, France, June 27–29, 1999. Plymbridge Distributors Ltd.
25. CATALONA, W.J., P.C. SOUTHWICK, K.M. SLAWIN, et al. 2000. Comparison of percent free PSA, PSA density, and age-specific PSA cutoffs for prostate cancer detection and staging. Urology **56**: 255–260.
26. GRASSO, Y.Z., M.K. GUPTA, H.S. LEVIN, et al. 1998. Combined nested RT-PCR assay for PSA and prostate-specific membrane antigen in prostate cancer patients: correlation with pathological stage. Cancer Res. **58**: 1456–1459.
27. DI SANT'AGNESE, P.A. 2000. Divergent neuroendocrine differentiation in prostatic carcinoma. Semin. Diagn. Pathol. **17**: 149–161.
28. MAZZUCCHELLI, R., R. MONTIRONI, A. SANTINELLI, et al. 2000. Vascular endothelial growth factor expression and capillary architecture in high-grade PIN and prostate cancer in untreated and androgen ablated patients. Prostate **45**: 72–79.
29. BURTON, J.L., N. OAKLEY & J.B. ANDRESON. 2001. Recent advances in the histopathology and molecular biology of prostate cancer. Br. J. Urol. Int. **85**: 87–94.
30. KATTAN, M.W., A.M.F. STAPLETON, T.M. WHEELER & P.T. SCARDINO. 1997. Evaluation of nomogram used to predict the pathologic stage of clinically localized prostate carcinoma. Cancer **79**: 528–537.
31. BLUTE, M.L., E.J. BERGSTRAHL, A.W. PARTIN, et al. 2000. Validation of Partin tables for predicting pathological stage of clinically localized prostate cancer. J. Urol. **164**: 1591–1595.

32. BATUELLO, J.T., E.J. GAMITO, E.D. CRAWFORD, *et al.* 2001. Artificial neural network model for the assessment of lymph node spread inpatients with clinically localized prostate cancer. Urology **57:** 481–485.
33. MONTIE, J.E. & J.T. WEI. 2000. Artificial neural networks for prostate carcinoma risk assessment: an overview. Cancer **88:** 2655–2660.
34. BABAIAN, R.J., H. FRITSCHE, A. AYALA, *et al.* 2000 Performance of a neural network in detecting prostate cancer in the prostate-specific antigen reflex range of 2.5 to 4.0 ng/mL. Urology **56:** 1000–1006.
35. TEWARI, A. & P. NARAYAN. 1998. Novel staging tool for localized prostatic cancer: a pilot study using genetic adaptive neural networks. J. Urol. **160:** 430–436.
36. MONTIRONI, R., P.H. BARTELS, D. THOMPSON, *et al.* 1996. Androgen-deprived prostate adenocarcinoma: evaluation of treatment-related changes versus no distinctive treatment effect with a Bayesian belief network. Eur. Urol. **30:** 307–315.
37. EPSTEIN, J.E., A.W. PARTIN, S.R. POTTER & P.C. WALSH. 2000. Adenocarcinoma of the prostate invading the seminal vesicle: prognostic stratification based on pathologic parameters. Urology **56:** 283–288.
38. VAN POPPEL, H., H. GOETHUYS, *et al.* 2000. Radical prostatectomy can provide a cure for well selected clinical stage T3 prostate cancer. Eur. Urol. **38:** 372–379.
39. DELLABELLA, M., A.B. GALOSI, M. YEHIA, *et al.* 2000. Different techniques in prostate biopsy: individual and methodological variability: our opinion. Presented at the First International Meeting on Urology. Ancona, Italy, March 29.
40. POLITO, M., G. MUZZONIGRO, D. MINARDI & R. MONTIRONI. 1996. Effects of neoadjuvant androgen deprivation therapy on prostatic cancer. Eur. Urol. **30** (suppl 1): 26–31.
41. MINARDI, D., M. POLITO, JR., A.B. GALOSI, *et al.* 2000. Echoguided prostate cryosurgery: experience after short and medium term follow-up. Arch. Ital. Urol. Androl. **72:** 270–275.

Connexin Expression in Nonneoplastic Human Prostate Epithelial Cells

FRANCESCA SALADINO,[a] GIUSEPPE CARRUBA,[a] SALMAAN T.A. QUADER,[b] MARIA AMOROSO,[a] ANTONIETTA DI CRISTINA,[c] MUKTA M. WEBBER,[b] AND LUIGI A.M. CASTAGNETTA[a,c]

[a]*Department of Experimental Oncology and Clinical Application, University Medical School, Palermo, Italy*

[b]*Departments of Zoology and Medicine, Michigan State University, East Lansing, Michigan 48824, USA*

[c]*Unit of Experimental Oncology & Palermo Branch of IST-GE, Department of Clinical Oncology, "M. Ascoli" Cancer Hospital Centre, A.R.N.A.S., Civico, Palermo, Italy*

ABSTRACT: Expression of gap-junction proteins connexins (Cx), specifically Cx43, Cx32, and Cx26, in both nontumorigenic (RWPE-1) and tumorigenic (RWPE-2) human prostate epithelial cells as well as in two cell clones (WPEI-7 and WPEI-10) originating from the RWPE-1 cell line was investigated. The aim was to determine whether individual connexins are differentially expressed in cultured cells. Western blot analysis revealed striking differences in the expression of individual connexins in the cell lines studied. In particular, Cx43 is largely expressed in RWPE-1 and WPEI-10 cells, whereas Cx32 is expressed predominantly in RWPE-2 and WPEI-7 cells. In addition, both forskolin and estrone increase Cx43 expression levels in WPEI-10 cells, with no apparent effect on WPEI-7 cells. Conversely, forskolin and especially estrone induce a marked increase of Cx32 in WPEI-7 cells, whereas Cx32 expression is limitedly affected by both agents in WPEI-10 cells. Overall, expression levels of Cx43 and Cx32 appear to be inversely related, with RWPE-1 and WPEI-10 cells having a significantly higher Cx43 to Cx32 ratio than that observed in RWPE-2 and WPEI-7 cells. We recently reported that junctional communication could be rescued in RWPE-1 cells by either forskolin or estrone and that restoration of GJIC is associated with an increase of Cx43 or a decrease of Cx32, or both, eventually leading to a marked rise of the Cx43 to Cx32 ratio. Studies are currently ongoing in our laboratories to assess the potential effect of agents increasing the Cx43 to Cx32 ratio on GJIC activity in these systems.

KEYWORDS: connexin; prostate; epithelial cells

Address for correspondence: Dr. Francesca Saladino, Unit of Experimental Oncology, "M. Ascoli" Cancer Hospital Center, Via Parlavecchio 139, 90127 Palermo, Italy. Voice: +39 091 666-4346; fax: +39 091 666-4352.
lucashbl@unipa.it

INTRODUCTION

Connexins are a family of transmembrane proteins that are differentially expressed in a tissue-specific manner. Connexins have four transmembrane domains, with both N- and C-termini oriented in the cytoplasm. Differences in molecular weight among members of the connexin family primarily reflect differences in the length of their carboxy-terminal tail. Connexins self-assemble into hexameric structural units, called connexons; two connexons located on the membrane of coupled cells align end to end to give rise to intercellular channels that allow the diffusion of a variety of ions and small molecules below 2,000 daltons. These intercellular channels, called gap junction channels, may contain connexons composed of the same connexin (homotypic) or different connexins (heterotypic).[1] Formation of heterotypic intercellular channels has important functional consequences. First, it affects the unitary conductance and gating properties of channels; second, only certain combinations of connexins are compatible and may give rise to functional channels.[2]

The gap-junction–mediated intercellular communication (GJIC) plays an important role in both embryonic and adult life, being required for the regulation of cell growth and differentiaton, tissue homeostasis, and adaptive responses of differentiated cells.[3] Connexin proteins are encoded by a multifamily of highly conserved genes that are thought to behave as tumor suppressor genes.[4] Incorporation of the Cx43 gene in GJIC-deficient mouse-transformed cells results in a significant decrease in their growth and tumorigenicity and the rescue of junctional communication.[5] This suggests that deficient or disrupted GJIC may be implicated in carcinogenesis.[6]

The present work investigates connexin expression in immortalized, nontumorigenic and tumorigenic, human prostate epithelial cells to determine if differential expression of individual connexins may be associated with the biological characteristics of cells.

MATERIAL AND METHODS

Cell Cultures. Nontumorigenic RWPE-1 and tumorigenic RWPE-2 prostate epithelial cells were originally established from nonneoplastic human prostate tissue samples, obtained from a patient who underwent cystectomy for bladder cancer and then immortalized by using HPV18 for RWPE-1 cells or a combination of HPV18 and the Ki-MuSV containing the activated Ki-*ras* oncogene for RWPE-2 cells.[7] The two WPE1-10 and WPE1-7 cell clones were isolated from the RWPE-1 cells.[8] Cells were grown in keratinocyte–serum-free medium (K-SFM) containing 50 µg/ml of bovine pituitary extract and 5 ng/ml EGF plus antibiotic/antimycotic mixture. All cells were routinely tested for mycoplasma contamination.

Western Blot Analysis. Expression of various connexins (Cx43, Cx32, and Cx26) was examined by Western blot analysis, as recently described.[9] Connexin expression was investigated under both standard conditions and after exposure of cells for 48 hours to either 30 µM forskolin (FK) or 1 µM estrone (E1). Briefly, cells were lysed and proteins extracted by 2× Laemmli sample buffer containing 10% SDS and quantified by Biorad DC protein assay. The amount of protein loaded/lane was 16 µg. After separation by SDS-PAGE, proteins were transferred onto nitrocellulose

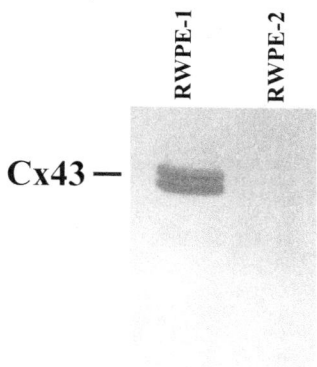

FIGURE 1. Connexin 43 levels in RWPE-1 and RWPE-2 cells. Autoradiograph of the immunoblot shows relative expression levels of Cx43 in cell lysates. Equal amounts of protein (16 µg) were loaded on each lane.

membrane by electrophoresis. The membranes were incubated for 18 hours in 5% nonfat dry milk in TBS-T with gentle agitation to prevent nonspecific binding. Incubation with the primary antibody was performed for 2 hours (monoclonal antibody against Cx43, Zymed) or overnight (polyclonal antibody against Cx32). Membranes were developed using an ECL detection system (Amersham Int.), according to the manufacturer's instructions.

RESULTS AND DISCUSSION

Western blot analysis of connexin expression was carried out on both nontumorigenic RWPE-1 cells and their tumorigenic, *ras*-transformed derivative, counterpart, RWPE-2 cells. In addition, WPE1-7 and WPE1-10 cells, the two clones derived from RWPE1 cells, were also investigated.

Results reveal striking differences in the expression of individual connexins in the cell lines studied. In particular, RWPE-1 cells showed markedly greater amounts of Cx43 when compared to RWPE-2 cells. In addition, differentially phosphorylated species of Cx43 were detected in RWPE-1 cells only (FIG. 1). Conversely, higher expression levels of Cx32 were observed in RWPE-2 cells with respect to RWPE-1 cells (not shown). Interestingly, WPE1-10 cells exhibited remarkably high amounts of Cx43, whereas Cx43 expression could not be observed in WPE1-7 cells (FIG. 2). By contrast, remarkably greater amounts of Cx32 were found in WPE1-7 than in WPE1-10 cells. Overall, expression levels of Cx43 and Cx32 appear to be inversely related, with RWPE-1 and WPE1-10 cells having a significantly higher Cx43 to Cx32 ratio than that observed in RWPE-2 and WPE1-7 cells.

We recently reported that both RWPE-1 and RWPE-2 immortalized human prostate epithelial cells have weak or absent GJIC activity.[9] Since immortalization is a necessary event in the multistep process of carcinogenesis, it is intriguing to speculate that a deficient or disrupted GJIC may play a role in malignant transformation

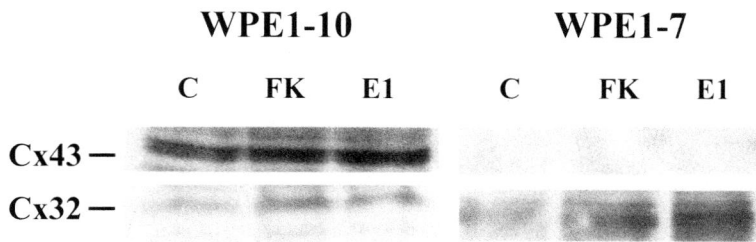

FIGURE 2. Connexin 32 and 43 expression and regulation in WPE1-10 and WPE1-7 cell clones. Autoradiograph of the immunoblot shows the relative expression levels of Cx32 and Cx43 in cell lysates. Equal amounts of protein (16 µg) were loaded in each lane. FK, forskolin; E1, estrone.

of prostatic epithelium. However, our recent studies revealed that junctional communication could be rescued in RWPE-1 cells only and that restoration of GJIC is associated with an increase in Cx43 or a decrease in Cx32, or both, eventually leading to a marked increase in the Cx43 to Cx32 ratio.[9] It should be emphasized that Cx43 and Cx32 are not compatible connexins and that heterotypic connexons composed of Cx43 and Cx32 could not give rise to functional channels.[1]

Cx43 is largely expressed in RWPE-1 and WPE1-10 cells, whereas RWPE-2 and WPE1-7 cells express predominantly Cx32. In addition, both forskolin (FK) and estrone (E1) increased Cx43 expression levels in WPE1-10 cells, with no apparent effect on WPE1-7 cells (FIG. 2). Conversely, FK and especially E1 induced a marked increase of Cx32 in WPE1-7 cells, whereas Cx32 expression was limitedly affected by both agents in WPE1-10 cells. Therefore, it is likely that, as in RWPE-1 cells, junctional activity can be restored in WPE1-10 cells by either FK or E1. Studies are currently ongoing in our laboratories to assess GJIC activity and its regulation in relation to the use of agents capable of increasing the Cx43 to Cx32 ratio.

ACKNOWLEDGMENT

These studies were partly supported by the Italian Association for Cancer Research (AIRC) and the National Research Council (CNR).

REFERENCES

1. BRUZZONE, R., T. WHITE & D. PAUL. 1996. Connections with connexins: the molecular basis for direct intracellular signaling. Eur. J. Biochem. **238:** 1–27.
2. WHITE, W.W. & R. BRUZZONE. 2000. Gap junctions: fates worse than death? Curr. Biol. **10:** R685–R688.
3. BEYER, E. 1993. Gap junctions. Int. Rev. Cytol. **137C:** 1–37.
4. ROSE, B., P. MEHTA & W. LOWENSTEIN. 1993. Gap junction protein gene suppresses tumorigenicity. Carcinogenesis **14:** 1073–1075.

5. MEHTA, P.P., C. PEREZ-STABLE, M. NADJI, et al. 1999. Suppression of human prostate cancer cell growth by forced expression of connexin genes. Dev. Gen. **24:** 91–110.
6. YAMASAKI, H., Y. OMORI, M. ZAIDAN-DAGLI, et al. 1999. Genetic and epigenetic changes of intercellular communication during multistage carcinogenesis. Cancer Detect. Prev. **23:** 273–279.
7. BELLO, D., M.M. WEBBER, H. KLEINMAN, et al. 1997. Androgen responsive adult human prostatic epithelial cell lines immortalized by human papillomavirus 18. Carcinogenesis **17:** 1641–1646.
8. SHARP, R.M., D. BELLO-DEOCAMPO, S.T.A. QUADER & M.M. WEBBER. 2001. N-(4-hydroxyphenyl)retinamide (4-HPR) decreases neoplastic properties of human prostate cells: an agent for prevention. Mut. Res. **496:** 163–170.
9. CARRUBA, G., M.M. WEBBER, S.T.A. QUADER, et al. 2002. Regulation of cell-to-cell communication in non-tumorigenic and malignant human prostate epithelial cells. Prostate **30:** 73–82.

Methods to Obtain More Clinical and Pathologic Information from Needle Core Biopsy of the Prostate Gland

ANDREA B. GALOSI AND GIOVANNI MUZZONIGRO

Institute of Urology, Azienda Ospedaliera Umberto 1st, University of Ancona, Ancona, Italy

ABSTRACT: Prostate needle biopsy can disclose important clinical information on tumor extension and grading, useful prognostic parameters for therapeutic choices and prognostic definition. To obtain more histopathologic information on specimens and clinical prognostic parameters, we used a new method to handle and embed tissue fragments of prostate biopsy as well as a new transrectal probe (TRUS) with an end-fire convex ultrasound transducer to guide ultrasonically precise needle placement in the prostate gland. In our experience these methods combined can be useful in obtaining reliable clinical and prognostic information in the management of patients with prostate cancer.

KEYWORDS: prostate neoplasms; biopsy; diagnosis; histopathology; embedding methods; prognostic factors

INTRODUCTION

Prostate needle biopsy can disclose important clinical information on tumor extension and grading, useful prognostic parameters for therapeutic choices and prognostic definition.[1] To date, different methods to perform needle biopsy and to improve histologic yield of prostatic biopsy have been described.[2,3]

To obtain more histopathologic information on specimens and clinical prognostic parameters, we used a new method to handle and embed tissue fragments of prostate biopsy. Furthermore, we used a new transrectal probe (TRUS) with an end-fire convex ultrasound transducer designed to ultrasonically guide precise needle placement in the prostate gland.

METHOD

Needle core biopsies were collected according to the following method. First, the end-fire ultrasound probe (EUB 6,000 Astro-Esaote, end-fire transrectal probe 5.0–

Address for correspondence: Andrea B. Galosi, M.D., Institute of Urology, Umberto 1st Hospital, University of Ancona, Piazza Cappelli 1, I-60121 Ancona, Italy. Voice: +39.071. 202642: fax: +39.071. 2070501.

Clinuro@popcsi.unian.it

7.5 MHz, Mitsubishi) was used to perform diagnostic and staging transrectal biopsy according to the six sextant lateral biopsies. Additional biopsies were taken at midgland and base level in the posterolateral sides and hypoechoic areas. If necessary (PSA >15 ng/ml, palpable lesion, or suspected cT3 tumor), biopsies of the neurovascular bundle, seminal vesicle, or bladder neck were taken to detect extraprostatic tumor extension.

Secondly, the pre-embedding method was the "Sandwich" technique,[4] a modified technique from that proposed by Rogatsch.[3,5] We used two foam rubber sponges (thin layer, 2.5 wide, 3 cm long; Bioptica, Milan, Italy) soaked with 10% buffered formalin and plastic tissue boxes (2.8 × 3.3 cm) in order to include each tissue fragment covered by two soaked sponges. Each single prostatic fragment was released from the needle (18 gauge, Bard MaxCore), and it fell flat on the buffered sponge. The tissue fragment was stretched to the full length of the sponge, oriented and covered with a soaked sponge, and then enclosed in a plastic tissue cassette (2.8 × 3.3 cm). Each box (labeled by a pencil) contained one core squeezed between two sponges. The proximal end (rectal extremity) of the biopsy specimen was inked with China ink. To allow it to fix on the tissue we washed the specimen with some drops of Bouin solution. All boxes were enclosed in a small jar containing 10% formalin and then sent to the pathologist. Cores were embedded in paraffin wax with one core per block. At least five to eight serial longitudinal sections per slide were made from every block.

Finally, each biopsy was separately labeled, stating and drawing the exact location from which it was taken on a graphic representation of the prostate that was enclosed and also sent to the pathologist. On this prostate map, the TRUS operator drew biopsy tracks of the needle and ultrasound abnormalities: side, areas, direction, and precise angle of entry of needle placement in the prostate. Data of 30 cases were correlated with the final histopathologic analysis of surgical specimens after radical prostatectomy.

RESULTS

Biopsy results were compared with pathologic analysis on whole-mount radical prostatectomy specimens; stage was predicted in 85% of cases and Gleason's grading in 80%. In five cases of atypical glands on the initial set of biopsies, it was possible to repeat a new set of biopsies in the same place on the gland. Tumor was diagnosed in three of five cases (60%). If a second set of biopsies was required, the advantages of the map were more evident in large prostate glands (volume >60 ml), reducing the number of biopsies needed for diagnosis (mean 7, range 5–11). It reduced the risk of unsampled areas related to variability linked to different operators and also related to the anatomy of large prostate glands.

This sandwich technique, a new method for handling fragments of prostatic tissue, has provided evident advantages for the pathologist, optimizing the visible area of the section plane compared to that obtained from free floating core biopsies. With this method, tissue fragments are stretched between two soaked sponges, and the full length (>80%) of the biopsy is within the section plane. Extremities of core biopsies, frequently broken, are available for histologic examination, whereas they are usually lost with the standard technique (free floating specimens). Accuracy in detecting the final grading of prostate cancer (Gleason's score) and perineural invasion was more reliable. Biopsy parameters such as side, area and number of positive biopsies, and percentage of involvement of tissue cores were accurately identified. These parameters are strictly correlated to tumor volume in the surgical specimen and to the final pathologic stage. Other prognostic parameters obtained from histopathologic analysis were extraprostatic spread including capsule invasion, fat invasion, or seminal vesicle infiltration, and smooth muscle infiltration identified in the bladder neck or anterior fibromuscular stroma). Biopsies of the posterolateral angle of the prostate gland were made easy and with high accuracy using the end-fire-probe. Cancer was found in 55% of cases in the posterolateral angle of the gland compared to 35% in the sextant biopsies. In 20% of cases, cancer was found only in biopsies of the posterolateral part of the peripheral zone, the most frequent location of prostate cancer.[6]

CONCLUSION

Routinely, application of the pre-embedding prostatic core biopsies could improve the accuracy of histopathologic examination and therefore provide more reliable data on tumor extension and grade. Intraprostatic and extraprostatic spread of prostate cancer using the graphic representation based on TRUS and biopsy findings could overcome the methodologic variables and operator-linked variables. It seems useful to repeat biopsy in the same area where atypical glands were observed. The end-fire ultrasound probe can be used to perform easy needle biopsy on the posterolateral angle of the peripheral zone and neurovascular boundles. In our experience, these methods, when combined, can give reliable clinical and prognostic information, useful in the management of patients with prostate cancer.

REFERENCES

1. MUZZONIGRO, G., A.B. GALOSI, G. MILANESE, et al. 2000. Fragments of prostatic biopsy: characteristics, dimensions, and number. Arch. Ital. Urol. Androl. **72:** 145–149.
2. SHAW, E.B., J.B. CARTER, B.W. DANIEL & E.D. WOFFORD. 1997. Adequate tissue sampling of prostate core needle biopsies. Am. J. Clin. Pathol. **107:** 26–29.
3. ROGATSCH, H., T. MAIRINGER, W. HORNINGER, et al. 2000. Optimized preembedding method improves the histologic yield of prostatic core needle biopsies. Prostate **42:** 124–129.
4. GALOSI, A.B., M. DELLABELLA, M. POLITO, JR., et al. 2001. A new method to embed fragments of prostate biopsy: the "sandwich" technique; preliminary experience. Urologia **68:** 170–174.
5. ROGATSCH, H. et al. 2000. Cancer detection rate increased by optimized per embedding procedure for prostate needle biopsies (abstr). Eur. Urol. **37:** 73.
6. AUS, G., S. BERGDAHL, J. HUGOSSON, et al. 2001. Outcome of laterally directed sextant biopsies of the prostate in screened males aged 50-66 years. Eur. Urol. **39:** 655–661.

Human Type 1 Estrogen Sulfotransferase

Catecholestrogen Metabolism and Potential Involvement in Cancer Promotion

FRÉDÉRIC FAUCHER, LUCILLE LACOSTE, AND VAN LUU-THE

Oncology and Molecular Endocrinology Research Center, Laval University Medical Center (CHUL) and Laval University, Quebec G1V 4G2, Canada

ABSTRACT: Using purified human type 1 estrogen sulfotransferase (hEST1), we show that the best substrate for this enzyme is 2-hydroxy-catecholestrogen. The enzyme also catalyzes the transformation of 4-hydroxy-estrogens and 16-hydroxy-estrogens, but with a lower affinity. We also present evidence to indicate that estrogen sulfotransferase may play a role in processes other than the detoxification and elimination of steroids. Indeed, hEST1 may also be involved in the production of stable precursors for local steroid biosynthesis or in the activation of promutagenic estrogen metabolites into carcinogens.

KEYWORDS: steroidogenesis; estrogen sulfotransferase; expression; transfection; estrogens; catecholestrogens

INTRODUCTION

Sulfotransferases catalyze the sulfonation of exogenous products, such as drugs and xenobiotics, as well as the sulfonation of endogenous compounds, such as steroids and bile acids, by transferring a sulfonate moiety from a cofactor, 3′-phosphoadenosine-5′-phosphosulfate (PAPS), to a hydroxyl group of the substrate. It is generally recognized that this process leads to detoxification or elimination, because sulfonation increases the hydrophilicity of chemical compounds and therefore their excretion.[1] Indeed, sulfonation is generally accepted as a mechanism for increasing solubility in water and excretion of the products of the phase I oxidation reactions. However, recent molecular studies of sulfotransferases revealed other interesting roles of sulfotransferases such as the production of steroid precursors[2] and the activation of promutagens to mutagens.[3]

SULFATED STEROIDS AS PRECURSORS FOR LOCAL STEROID BIOSYNTHESIS

The long half-life of steroid sulfates[1] and the widespread expression of steroid sulfatase, the enzyme that catalyzes the hydrolysis of the sulfate group, suggest that

---

Address for correspondence: Dr. Van Luu-The, Oncology and Molecular Endocrinology Research Center, Laval University Medical Center (CHUL), 2705 Laurier Boulevard, Quebec, (Quebec) G1V 4G2, Canada. Voice: 418-654-2296; fax: 418-654-2761.

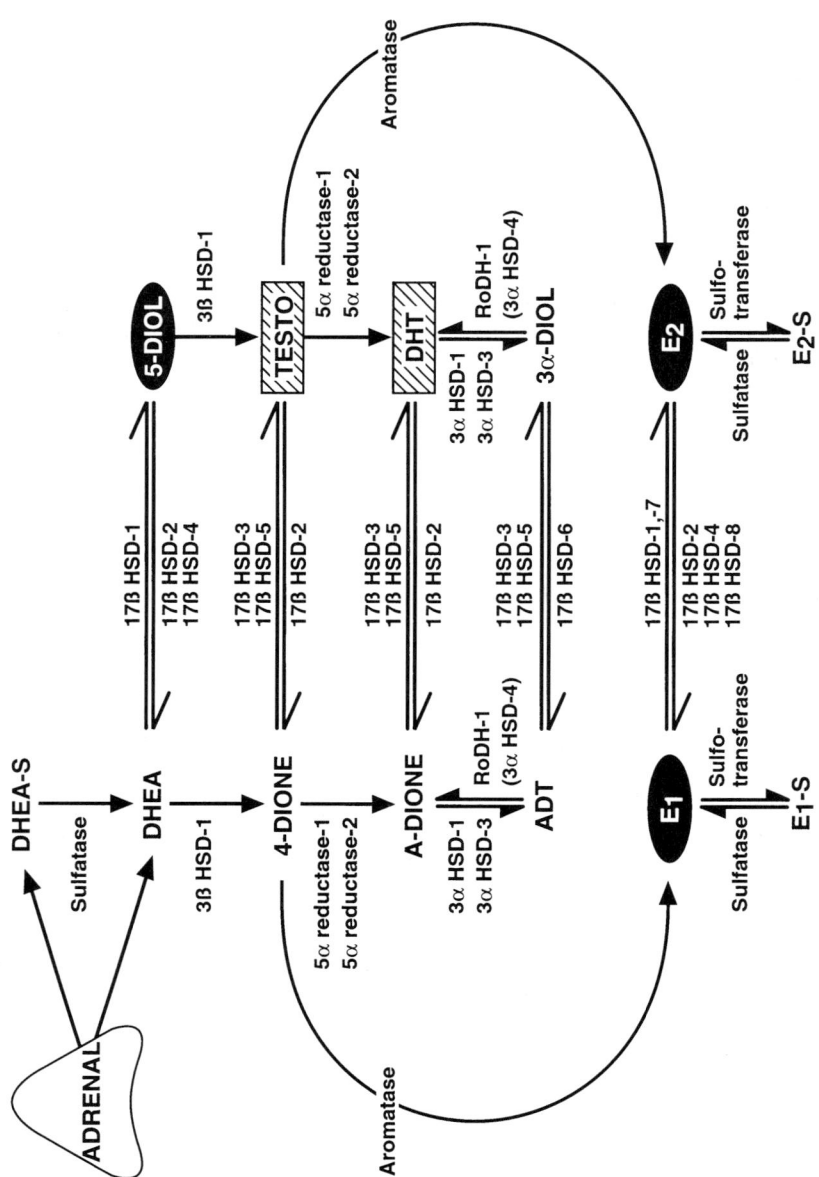

FIGURE 1. Biosynthetic pathway of steroid hormones from sulfoconjugated steroids.

sulfated compounds could play a role as precursors of steroid hormone synthesis in peripheral target tissues (FIG. 1). Indeed, there are many physiological examples showing that the sulfonation of steroids is not simply a process of elimination but also a process of storage under a more stable form.

One physiological example is the production of estrogens in the human placenta: because this organ does not possess the enzyme 17α-hydroxylase-17,20-lyase (CYP17), it cannot produce DHEA from pregnenolone. However, the fetus produces a large amount of stable DHEAS and delivers it to the mother. The placenta possesses a high level of sulfatase that transforms DHEAS into DHEA, which then, by the successive actions of 3β-hydroxysteroid dehydrogenase,[4,5] aromatase, and type 1 17β-hydroxysteroid dehydrogenase,[6,7] converts DHEA into estradiol required for the development of the pregnancy.

Another physiological example that illustrates the importance of the concerted roles of sulfotransferase and sulfatase is the regulation of the cholesterol and cholesterol-sulfate concentration in the skin. Indeed, it has been shown that the deficiency of steroid sulfatase leads to an accumulation of CholS in the skin, causing a disease called X-linked ichthyosis.[8]

Furthermore, estrogen sulfates have been shown to act as a reservoir for the formation of unconjugated estrogens via the action of sulfatase. As a matter of fact, the concentration of estrone sulfate (E1S) in the plasma and in breast tissues is much higher than that of unconjugated estrogens, and the half-life of conjugated estrogens is much longer than that of unconjugated ones.[1] The activity of sulfatase is much higher than that of aromatase in normal and malignant breast tissues.[9] In an experiment using tumor homogenates and appropriate substrate concentrations, as much as 10 times more estrone (E1) was found to be formed from E1S, via the sulfatase pathway, than from androstenedione via the aromatase route.[10] This local active estrogen production via the concerted action of estrogen sulfotransferase and of sulfatase is even more important in postmenopausal women in whom the ovaries' ability to produce sex steroids is dramatically decreased, whereas the prevalence of breast cancer is increased.

METABOLIC ACTIVATION OF CARCINOGENS BY SULFOTRANSFERASES

In parallel with the sulfonation reaction, which produces stable and long half-life products, sulfotransferases could also generate bioactive by-products that bind to nucleic acids and cause DNA damage.[3,11] Indeed, the sulfate group is "electron-withdrawing" and may, in certain classes of compounds, be cleaved off, leading to an electrophilic cation (FIG. 2). This cleavage of the sulfate group is facilitated if the resulting cation is stabilized by mesomerism, as is the case with sulfuric acid esters of benzylic and allylic alcohols or aromatic hydroxylamines and hydroxamic acids. Because of this isomeric stabilization, the cation does not necessarily bind to the nucleophil at the position where the sulfate group had been attached.

It is often assumed that the initial phase of the xenobiotic metabolism, which generally involves the hydroxylation step catalyzed by cytochromes P450, is responsible for the formation of reactive intermediates, whereas conjugation is more closely associated with detoxification. However, this view is probably biased because of the difficulties in detecting the effect of bioreactive by-products generated by sulfona-

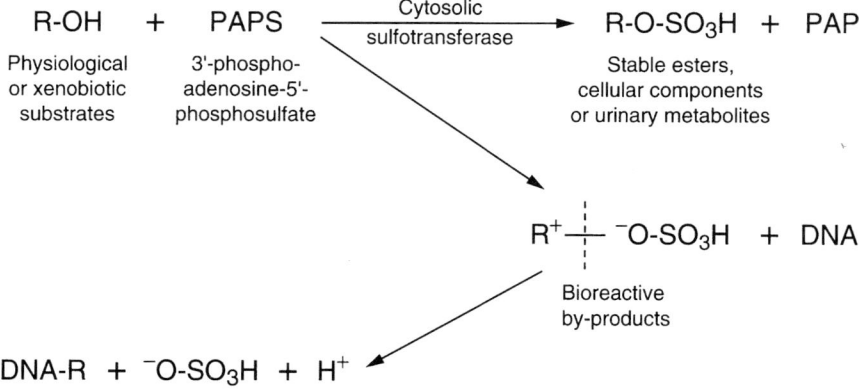

FIGURE 2. Scheme showing the sulfonation reaction producing stable products or bioreactive by-products that bind to nucleic acids and cause DNA damage (modified from Miller, J.A. 1994. Chem.-Biol. Interact. **92:** 329–341).

tion. Indeed, the reactive metabolites produced through the sulfonation reaction are short-lived and ionized and cannot readily penetrate the bacterial membrane. A recent improvement in the Ames test, using *Salmonella typhimurium* that is transformed with the enzyme of interest,[3] allows us to see the metabolic activation capability and stereoselectivity of sulfotransferases. Indeed, it has been shown that hEST1, hEST2, P-PST, and DHEAST can activate 1-hydroxymethylpyrene into mutagen; DHEAST is more active on hycanthone and 2-hydroxy-3-methylcholanthrene, P-PST on 1-hydroxy-3-methylcholanthrene, and hEST on 10-hydroxy-7,8,-9,10-tetrahydrobenzo[a]pyrene and 7-hydroxy-7,8,9,10-tetrahyrobeno[a]pyrene.

METABOLIZATION OF CATECHOLESTROGENS BY TYPE 1 hEST

Recently, using purified enzyme overexpressed in *Escherichia coli*, we showed that type 1 hEST selectively metabolizes 2-hydroxy-catecholestrogen.[12] A Lineweaver plot analysis (FIG. 3A, B, and C) showed that the enzyme catalyzes more efficiently 2-hydroxy-catecholestrogens than 4- and 16-hydroxy-catecholestrogens.

DISCUSSION

The role of estrogens in the initiation and promotion of breast and endometrial cancer has been clear for more than 100 years since Beatson[13] demonstrated that oophorectomy induced remissions in breast cancer. However, the details of these responses are still not clear. The best known model of metabolic activation of estrogens in the genesis of cancer is estrogen-induced tumors of the kidney in the Syrian hamster.[14] It has been demonstrated that 16α-hydroxy-estrogen is a genotoxic compound[15] and a promoting agent of tumor growth.[16] The exact mechanism leading to the formation of a bioreactive compound is not yet known. It is proposed that

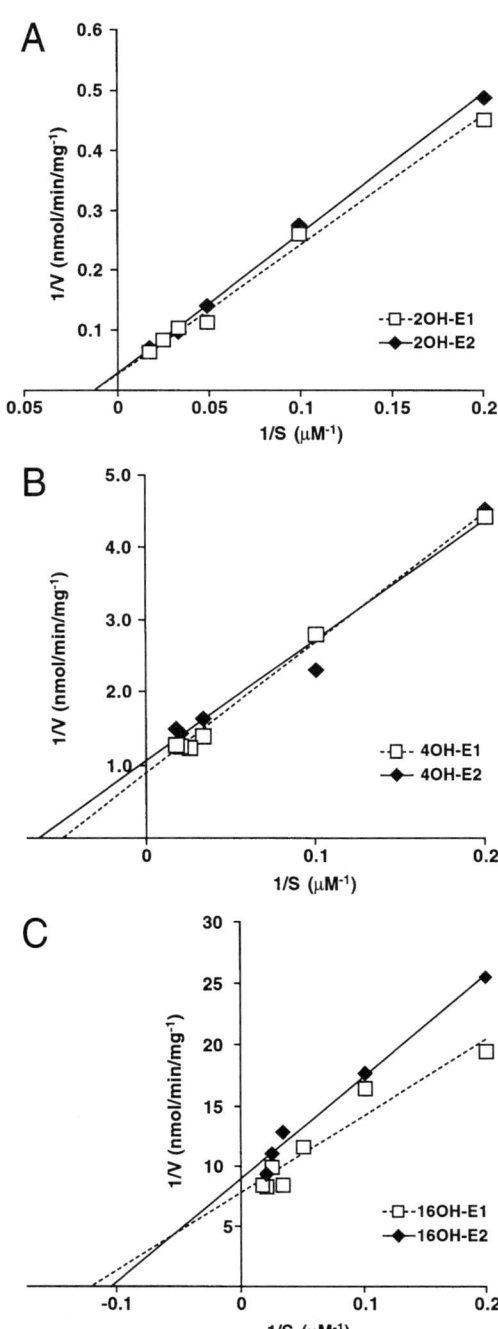

FIGURE 3. Lineweaver plots of the sulfonation of catecholestrogens. Purified hEST1 (prepared as described by Faucher et al., 2001) was incubated at 37°C with [^{35}S]PAPS for 2 hours, in the presence of 2-OH-estrogens (**A**), 4-OH-estrogens (**B**), or 16-OH-estrogens (**C**). Incubation was performed and radioactivity quantified, as described by Faucher et al.[12]

the formation of the semiquinone containing a one-electron system is responsible for the genotoxic effects and oxidative damage.[17,18] Although the quinone model could explain the activation of 4-hydroxy-estrogen, it could not apply to 16-hydroxy because the D ring is not aromatic. Moreover, our results show that estrogen sulfotransferase could metabolize 16-hydroxy-catecholestrogen as well as 4-hydroxy and 2-hydroxy catecholestrogen. The ability of the enzyme to metabolize 4- and 16-hydroxy-catecholestrogen, together with evidences suggesting that the metabolic by-products of estrogens can cause DNA damage,[19,20] and the potential of hEST to produce bioactive by-products strongly suggest that estrogen sulfotransferases could be involved in the activation of estrogen metabolites into mutagens. Following are additional observations that support the involvement of estrogen sulfotransferase in the formation of cancer promoters of estrogenic origin.

High Level of Estrogen Sulfate in Breast Cyst

Gross cystic disease of the breast is reportedly associated with a higher risk for the development of breast cancer.[21] Interestingly, it has been reported by Orlandi *et al.*[22] that E1S accumulated in breast cyst fluid. There was a difference in the concentrations of E1S between type 1 cysts (high K+, low Na+ concentrations) and type II cysts (low K+, high Na+ concentrations): it was fourfold higher in type 1 than in type 2. This is particularly interesting, because patients with type 1 cysts frequently have histological changes associated with an increased risk of cancer.[23] It is unlikely that E1S is responsible for the promotion of breast cancer, but a higher E1S level could indicate higher estrogen sulfotransferase activity and thus higher bioactive by-product formation.

Protective Effect of Oral Contraceptives

In a case-control study, Narod *et al.*[24] showed that the use of oral contraceptives was associated with a significant reduction in the risk of ovarian cancer among women with a mutation in the BRCA1 or BRCA2 gene. There was a 20% reduction in risk for up to 3 years of use, this reduction rising to 60% for 6 years or more. They recommended that administration of an oral contraceptive agent should be considered as part of a prevention program for women with BRCA1 or BRCA2 mutations who have not had ovarian cancer.

Protective Role of Phytoestrogens

It has been observed that Asians with high soy intake experience a lower cancer risk than do other populations.[25] However, when they migrate to the West, their risk of developing cancer increases, suggesting a causal role of environmental factors. The protective effect of soy intake seems to be stronger for breast, prostate, and colon cancers[26,27] and potentially also for endometrial cancer.[28] It has been suggested that the soy protective role is due to the presence of phytoestrogens. Indeed, isoflavones such as daidzein, genistein, and glycitein have been shown to prevent cancers.[29] The protective role of these compounds could be due to an ability to inhibit competitively the activation of promutagenic estrogen metabolites into carcinogens by estrogen sulfotransferases.

REFERENCES

1. RUDER, H.J., L. LORIAUX & M.B. LIPSETT. 1972. Estrone sulfate: production rate and metabolism in man. J. Clin. Invest. **51:** 1020–1033.
2. LABRIE, F. 1991. Intracrinology. Mol. Cell. Endocrinol. **78:** C113–118.
3. GLATT, H. et al. 1998. Sulfotransferase-mediated activation of mutagens studied using heterologous expression systems. Chem. Biol. Interact. **109:** 195–219.
4. LUU-THE, V. et al. 1989. Full length cDNA structure and deduced amino acid sequence of human 3β-hydroxy-5-ene steroid dehydrogenase. Mol. Endocrinol. **3:** 1310–1312.
5. LACHANCE, Y. et al. 1990. Characterization of human 3β-hydroxysteroid dehydrogenase/Δ^5-Δ^4 isomerase gene and its expression in mammalian cells. J. Biol. Chem. **265:** 20469–20475.
6. LUU-THE, V. et al. 1989. Characterization of cDNAs for human estradiol 17β-dehydrogenase and assignment of the gene to chromosome 17: evidence of two mRNA species with distinct 5′-termini in human placenta. Mol. Endocrinol. **3:** 1301–1309.
7. LUU-THE, V. et al. 1990. Structure of two in tandem human 17β-hydroxysteroid dehydrogenase genes. Mol. Endocrinol. **4:** 268–275.
8. YEN, P.H. et al. 1987. Cloning and expression of steroid sulfatase cDNA and the frequent occurrence of deletions in STS deficiency: implications for X-Y interchange. Cell **49:** 443–354.
9. JAMES, V.H. et al. 1987. Aromatase activity in normal breast and breast tumor tissues: in vivo and in vitro studies. Steroids **50:** 269–279.
10. SANTNER, S.J., P.D. FEIL & R.J. SANTEN. 1984. In situ estrogen production via the estrone sulfatase pathway in breast tumors: relative importance versus the aromatase pathway. J. Clin. Endocrinol. Metab. **59:** 29–33.
11. CHOU, H.C., N.P. LANG & F.F. KADLUBAR. 1995. Metabolic activation of the N-hydroxy derivative of the carcinogen 4-aminobiphenyl by human tissue sulfotransferases. Carcinogenesis **16:** 413–417.
12. FAUCHER, F. et al. 2001. High metabolization of catecholestrogens by type 1 estrogen sulfotransferase (hEST1). J. Steroid Biochem. Mol. Biol. **77:** 83–86.
13. BEATSON, G. 1898. On the treatment of inoperable cases of breast cancer by oophorectomy. Lancet **2:** 104–107.
14. KIRKMAN, H. 1974. Autonomous derivatives of estrogen-induced renal carcinomas and spontaneous renal tumors in the Syrian hamster. Cancer Res. **34:** 2728–2744.
15. OSBORNE, M.P. et al. 1993. Upregulation of estradiol C16 alpha-hydroxylation in human breast tissue: a potential biomarker of breast cancer risk. J. Natl Cancer Inst. **85:** 1917–1920.
16. SUTO, A. et al. 1992. Persistent estrogen responsiveness of ras oncogene-transformed mouse mammary epithelial cells. Steroids **57:** 262–268.
17. SUTO, A. et al. 1993. Experimental down-regulation of intermediate biomarkers of carcinogenesis in mouse mammary epithelial cells. Breast Cancer Res. Treat. **27:** 193–202.
18. ROY, D. & J.G. LIEHR. 1989. Changes in activities of free radical detoxifying enzymes in kidneys of male Syrian hamsters treated with estradiol. Cancer Res. **49:** 1475–1480.
19. SERVICE, R.F. 1998. New role for estrogen in cancer? Science **279:** 1631–1633.
20. FISHMAN, J., M.P. OSBORNE & N.T. TELANG. 1995. The role of estrogen in mammary carcinogenesis. Ann. N.Y. Acad. Sci. **768:** 91–100.
21. HAAGENSEN, C.D., C. BODIAN & D.E. HAAGENSEN, 1981. Breast Carcinoma: Risk and Detection. W.B. Saunders. Philadelphia, PA.
22. ORLANDI, F. et al. 1990. Estrone-3-sulfate in human breast cyst fluid. Ann. N.Y. Acad. Sci **595:** 464–466.
23. DIXON, J.M., A.B. LUMSDEN & W.R. MILLER. 1985. The relationship of cyst type to risk factors for breast cancer and the subsequent development of breast cancer in patients with breast cystic disease. Eur. J. Cancer Clin. Oncol. **21:** 1047–1050.
24. NAROD, S.A. et al. 1998. Oral contraceptives and the risk of hereditary ovarian cancer. Hereditary Ovarian Cancer Clinical Study Group. N. Engl. J. Med. **339:** 424–428.
25. BARNES, S. et al., 1994. Diet and Cancer: Markers, Prevention and Treatment. M. Jakobs, ed. :135–147. Plenum Press.

26. MESSINA, M.J. *et al.* 1994. Soy intake and cancer risk: a review of the *in vitro* and *in vivo* data. Nutr. Cancer **21:** 113–131.
27. KURZER, M.S. & X. XU. 1997. Dietary phytoestrogens. Annu. Rev. Nutr. **17:** 353–381.
28. GOODMAN, M.T., *et al.* 1997. Association of soy and fiber consumption with the risk of endometrial cancer. Am. J. Epidemiol. **146:** 294–306.
29. ZHENG, W. *et al.* 1999. Urinary excretion of isoflavonoids and the risk of breast cancer. Cancer Epidemiol. Biomarkers Prev. **8:** 35–40.

Prevention and Treatment of Breast Cancer by Suppressing Aromatase Activity and Expression

SHIUAN CHEN, DUJIN ZHOU, TOMOHARU OKUBO, YEH-CHIH KAO, ELIZABETH T. ENG, BAIBA GRUBE, ANNETTE KWON, CHUN YANG, AND BIN YU

Division of Immunology, Beckman Research Institute of the City of Hope, Duarte, California 91010, USA

ABSTRACT: Estrogen promotes the proliferation of breast cancer cells. Aromatase is the enzyme that converts androgen to estrogen. In tumors, expression of aromatase is upregulated compared to that of surrounding noncancerous tissue. Tumor aromatase is thought to stimulate breast cancer growth in both an autocrine and a paracrine manner. A treatment strategy for breast cancer is to abolish *in situ* estrogen formation with aromatase inhibitors. In addition, aromatase suppression in postmenapausal women is being evaluated as a potential chemopreventive modality against breast cancer. One area of aromatase research in this laboratory is the identification of foods and dietary compounds that can suppress aromatase activity. *In vitro* and *in vivo* studies have found that grapes and mushrooms contain chemicals that can inhibit aromatase. Therefore, a diet that includes grapes and mushrooms would be considered preventative against breast cancer. Another area of our aromatase research is the elucidation of the regulatory mechanism of aromatase expression in breast cancer tissue. Increased aromatase expression in breast tumors is attributed to changes in the transcriptional control of aromatase expression. Whereas promoter I.4 is the main promoter that controls aromatase expression in noncancerous breast tissue, promoters II and I.3 are the dominant promoters that drive aromatase expression in breast cancer tissue. Our recent gene regulation studies revealed that in cancerous versus normal tissue, several positive regulatory proteins (e.g., nuclear receptors and CREB1) are present at higher levels and several negative regulatory proteins (e.g., snail and slug proteins) are present at lower levels. This may explain why the activity of promoters II and I.3 is upregulated in cancerous tissue. In addition, our *in vitro* transcription/translation analysis using plasmids containing T7 promoter and the human snail gene as a reporter capped with different untranslated exon Is revealed that exon PII-containing transcripts were translated more effectively than were exon I.3-containing transcripts. An understanding of the molecular mechanisms of aromatase expression between noncancerous and cancerous breast tissue, at both transcriptional and translational levels, may help in the design of a therapy based on suppressing aromatase expression in breast cancer tissue.

KEYWORDS: breast cancer; aromatase; estrogen; enzyme; promoter; transcript

Address for correspondence: Dr. Shiuan Chen, Division of Immunology, Beckman Research Institute of the City of Hope, Duarte, CA. Voice: 626-359-8111, ext. 62601; fax. 626-301-8186.
schen@coh.org

INTRODUCTION

Estrogen can play a critical role in the development of breast cancer. Approximately 60% of premenopausal and 75% of postmenopausal patients have estrogen-dependent carcinoma. In estrogen-dependent breast tumors, by binding to the estrogen receptor protein, estrogen induces expression of peptide growth factors that are responsible for the proliferative responses of cancer cells. Aromatase is an enzyme that converts androgen to estrogen (FIG. 1). Because aromatase is the enzyme responsible for the synthesis of estrogen, and estrogen can have a major effect in the development of breast cancer, abnormal expression of aromatase in breast cancer cells and/or surrounding adipose stromal cells may have a significant influence on breast tumor development and growth in cancer patients. Aromatase is expressed at higher levels in human breast cancer tissue than in normal breast tissue, as measured by enzyme activity assay, immunocytochemistry, and reverse transcription-polymerase chain reaction (RT-PCR) analysis (e.g., Refs. 1–6). Furthermore, in postmenopausal patients, concentrations of estrogen in breast tumor tissues were several-fold higher than those in plasma.[7] These results support the hypothesis that estrogen is made and accumulates in the tumor. Cell culture,[8] animal experiments using aromatase-transfected breast cancer cells,[9] and transgenic mouse studies[10] demonstrated that *in situ* produced estrogen plays a more important role than circulating estrogens in breast tumor promotion. In addition, tumor aromatase stimulates breast cancer growth in both an autocrine and a paracrine manner.[11]

BREAST CANCER TREATMENT AND PREVENTION WITH AROMATASE INHIBITORS

A major treatment strategy for breast cancer is directed at abolishing the effects of estrogen. The stimulative effects of estrogen on tumor growth can be blocked by surgical ablation of hormonally active tissues, antiestrogens, and/or aromatase inhibitors.[12,13] Tamoxifen, an antiestrogen, is first-line therapy for estrogen-sensitive tumors in the postmenopausal woman.[14] Tamoxifen possesses both antiestrogenic and estrogenic properties.[15] Eventually, breast cancer cells develop resistance to tamoxifen and demonstrate tamoxifen-dependent proliferation.[15–19] Aromatase inhibitors have been used to treat tamoxifen-resistant tumors.[20,21] Newer aromatase inhibitors such as anatrozole, letrozole, and vorozole are very potent suppressors of serum estradiol (e.g., Ref. 22). Anatrozole and letrozole were recently approved by the US Food and Drug Adminstration for use as first-line agents against estrogen-responsive cancer. These compounds are different from tamoxifen in that they do not have estrogenic properties.

Hormonal blockade as a potential chemopreventive modality in breast cancer was investigated recently. Chemoprevention with tamoxifen reduced the incidence of invasive and noninvasive breast cancer in high-risk women.[23] An alternative strategy for hormonal modulation is the inhibition of aromatase.[24] The *in situ* reduction of estradiol synthesis by inhibition of aromatase could reduce estrogen-dependent cellular proliferation and estrogen conversion to genotoxic metabolites.[24] Phase I clinical trials have shown vorozole to be capable of reducing estradiol levels in premenopausal women with few side effects.[25] Similar reductions in serum estradiol

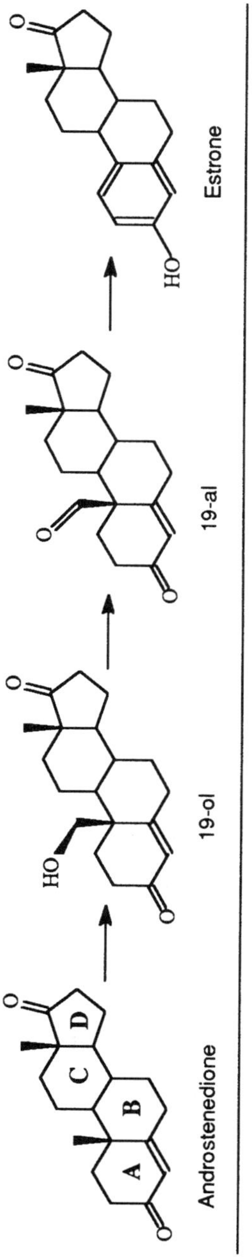

FIGURE 1. Aromatase converts androgens to estrogens.

levels in healthy postmenopausal female volunteers using Arimidex were demonstrated with no adverse effects on gonadotropins or adrenocorticoids.[22] In addition, both tamoxifen and aromatase inhibitors were evaluated for use in neoadjuvant endocrine therapy. It was found that a significant reduction in tumor volume was achieved by treating estrogen receptor-positive breast cancer with tamoxifen or aromatase inhibitors for 3 months.[26] This led to a conversion from mastectomy to breast conservation.

AROMATASE SUPPRESSION WITH PHYTOCHEMICALS IN FRUITS AND VEGETABLES

Whereas pharmaceutical agents have a therapeutic and preventative role in breast cancer, examination of foods and dietary compounds to prevent breast cancer is being vigorously explored. Cohort and case-controlled epidemiological studies have investigated the effect of certain vegetables and fruits on the incidence of cancer.[27,28] Among the intensely studied compounds are the phytoestrogens. Asian women have a four- to sixfold lower risk of breast cancer than do Western women.[29] One of the reported differences between these two populations is the increased consumption of soy protein.[30] Soy is high in phytoestrogens.[31] The best-known phytoestrogens are flavones, isoflavones, and lignans derived from whole grains, fruits, berries, and soy.[31,32] The phytoestrogens are plant compounds that may function as estrogens and/or antiestrogens by binding to the estrogen receptor.[32] Recent studies have also suggested that isoflavones[33] and flavones[34-39] suppress aromatase. Structure-function studies of aromatase in our laboratory have shown that phytoestrogens bind to aromatase in a different orientation than with the estrogen receptor.[40] Flavones bind to the active site of aromatase in an orientation in which their rings -A and -C mimic rings -D and -C of the androgen substrate, respectively. Phytoestrogens may therefore function as chemopreventive and/or chemotherapeutic agents by not only binding to the estrogen receptor, but also inhibiting aromatase.

During the last several years, our laboratory has initiated studies to address whether any fruits and vegetables contain phytochemicals that can suppress aromatase. We examined juices from eight kinds of fruit: orange, peach, grapefruit, plum, apple (Granny Smith), strawberry, and red seedless grape.[41] Our aromatase inhibition experiments revealed that red seedless grape juice contains chemicals that inhibit aromatase (FIG. 2). Furthermore, red seedless grape juice, green seedless grape juice, and black grape juice were equally effective in suppressing aromatase activity. Inhibition kinetic analysis indicates that the active components in grape juice inhibit aromatase by competing for the binding of the substrate androstenedione. Results from cell culture experiments suggest that chemicals in grape juice can act as weak agonists/antagonists of estrogen receptors and as aromatase inhibitors. Finally, the breast cancer-protective action of grape juice was demonstrated in a nude mouse model using MCF-7aro, an aromatase-transfected MCF-7 cell line (i.e., MCF-7aro).[11] It was found that tumor size in mice fed (by gavage) 0.5 ml of grape juice/day for 5 weeks is reduced 70% when compared to tumor size in animals not fed grape juice (FIG. 3).

We also examined heat stable extracts from seven kinds of vegetable: green onion, celery, carrot, bell pepper, broccoli, spinach, and white bottom mushroom for

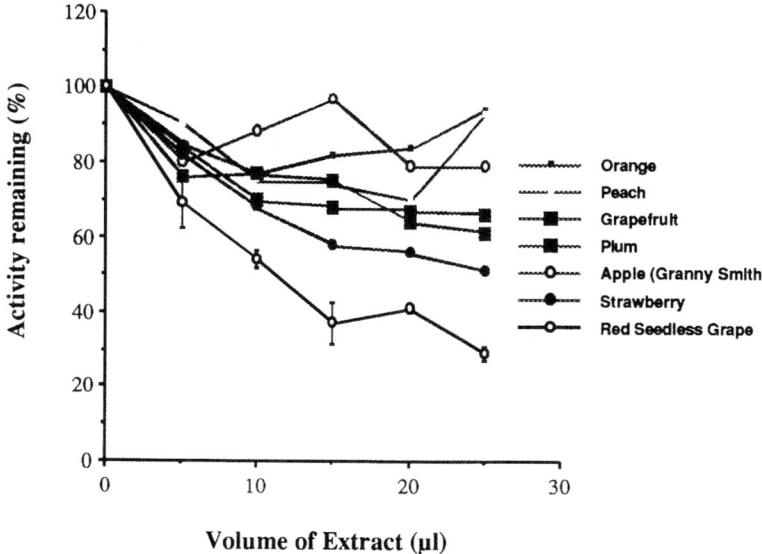

FIGURE 2. Inhibition of aromatase by fruit juices. Human aromatase activity was measured in the presence of various amounts of fruit juices. The activity of untreated samples was taken as 100%. The assay conditions are described in the publication by Chen et al.[41]

their abilities to suppress aromatase in a human placental microsomal assay. Among these vegetables, white bottom mushroom (species *Agaricus bisporus*) was the most effective inhibitor of aromatase. It suppressed aromatase activity in a dose-dependent fashion. Enzyme kinetics demonstrated mixed inhibition, suggesting the presence of multiple inhibitors or more than one inhibitory mechanism. "In cell" aromatase activity and cell proliferation was measured using MCF-7aro. In addition to inhibiting aromatase activity, the phytochemicals in mushrooms suppressed the androgen-induced proliferation of MCF-7aro cells.

A diet that includes grapes and mushrooms, therefore, would be considered preventative against breast cancer. Current efforts are being devoted towards the isolation and structural characterization of the active chemicals. In addition, we are evaluating their *in vivo* effects using animal experiments.

GENE REGULATION STUDIES

The human aromatase gene was mapped to chromosome 15, band q21.1 by *in situ* hybridization studies.[43] The gene contains nine translated exons. A complex mechanism is involved in the control of human aromatase expression. At least seven untranslated exons I (I.1, I.2, I.3, I.4, I.5, I.6, and PII) have been identified. Various exon I-containing RNA messages were found present at different levels in different aromatase-expressing tissues/cells. It is thought that aromatase expression in the tissues is driven by the promoters situated upstream from these exon Is, providing tis-

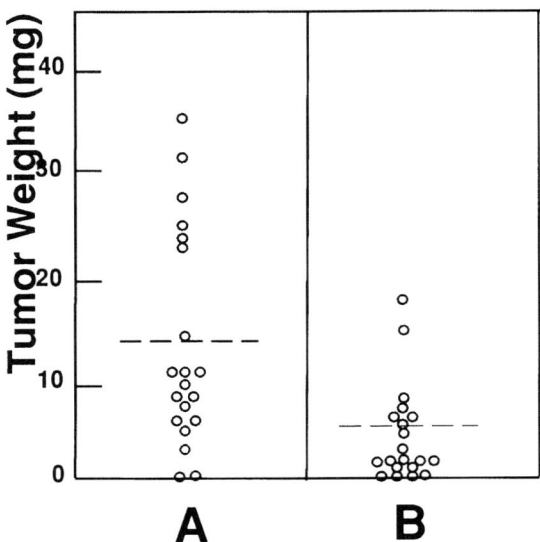

FIGURE 3. Suppression of MCF-7aro-induced tumor formation in nude mice by grape juice. The detailed procedure is described in the publication by Chen et al.[41] In this study, 10 mice were controls (**A**) and 10 mice were fed 0.5 ml green seedless grape juice/day for 5 weeks (**B**). Grape juice feeding started on the same day that MCF-7aro cells were injected. There were two injection sites per animal, and each site was injected with 4×10^6 cells. At the end of 5 weeks, mice were euthanized, and tumors were removed and weighted. The average weights of tumors from groups A and B were 14.6 and 4.5 mg, respectively (indicated by *dotted lines*). The differences between the control and the treated group are statistically significant ($p = 0.03$ using a Wilcoxon test).

sue-specific control of aromatase expression. In premenopausal women, the ovary (primarily in granulosa cells) is the major site of estrogen production. Aromatase expression in ovary is mainly driven by promoter II that is upregulated by cAMP. In pregnant women, the placenta produces a significant amount of estrogen. Aromatase expression in placenta is driven by promoter I.1 that is regulated through a protein kinase c-mediated mechanism. In postmenopausal women, estrogen is produced by skin cells and adipose tissue, including breast tissue. Aromatase expression in these tissues is driven by promoter I.4 that is regulated by glucocorticoids. Promoters I.2, I.5, and I.6 are less characterized than those promoters just described.

RT-PCR using exon 1-specific primers was performed to determine the exon I usage in aromatase mRNA in breast tumor specimens.[3] The results revealed that exon PII and I.3 are the major exons I present in aromatase mRNA isolated from breast tumors, suggesting that promoters II and I.3 are the major promoters driving aromatase expression in breast cancer and surrounding adipose stromal cells. Therefore, major promoter usage in breast tumors (both cancer cells and surrounding adipose stromal cells) (i.e., cAMP-stimulated promoters I.3 and II) is different from that in normal breast adipose tissue (i.e., glucocorticoid-stimulated promoter I.4). Aromatase was also found to be overexpressed in patients with gynecomastia or uterine disease.[44] Expression of aromatase in these patients was found to be driven mainly by promoters I.3 and II as well. Therefore, these two promoters are thought to be important promoters, driving abnormal aromatase expression/estrogen synthesis.

Promoters I.3 and II are approximately 200 bp apart from each other. Our laboratory has functionally characterized these promoters.[45,46] Furthermore, by DNA deletion and mutagenesis experiments, DNA mobility shift experiments, and DNAse I footprinting analyses, two regulatory regions have been identified near these promoters.[47,48] A regulatory element (S1) is situated between the two promoters, and the *trans*-factors that interact with the element are mainly nuclear receptors, as identified by the yeast one-hybrid screening of a human mammary gland cDNA expression library.[49] This element can function as an enhancer or a repressor element. S1 behaves as an enhancer when SF1 or ERRα-1 binds and as a repressor when COUP-TF or EAR-2 binds. The function of S1 depends on the expression levels of these nuclear receptors in cells. In addition, a CRE (i.e., CREaro) was identified near promoter I.3.[48] CREaro can be activated by CREB1, indicating that promoter I.3 is a cAMP-dependent promoter. However, our yeast one-hybrid screen has found that in noncancerous tissue, two zinc finger repressor proteins, snail and slug, bind to a site that overlaps with CREaro.[50] It is thought that snail and slug can quench CREaro activity. "Quenching" is a form of gene regulation whereby activators and repressors occupy neighboring sites in a target promoter, but the repressor blocks the ability of the activator to contact the transcription complex. Recent characterization of tran-

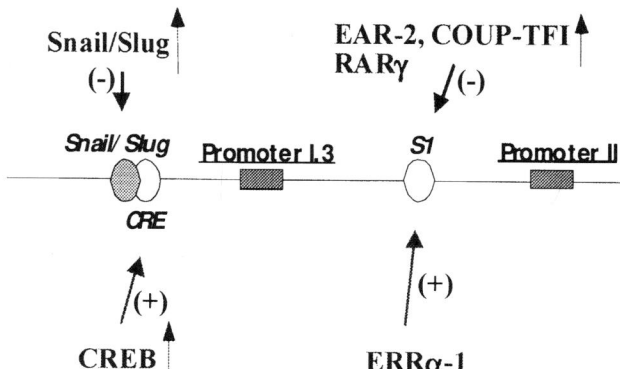

FIGURE 4. Modulation of the activity of promoters I.3 and II in normal breast tissue and cancer tissue.

scription factors that interact with these two important regulatory elements near promoters I.3 and II helps us better understand the mechanism of the switch of promoter usage between normal breast tissue and cancer tissue. By examining the results from RT-PCR analyses, it is thought that in normal breast tissue, the function of promoters I.3 and II is suppressed through the binding of EAR-2, COUP-TFI, and EARγ to S1 and through the binding of snail/slug proteins to their binding site that quenches the CREaro activity (FIG. 4). In cancer tissue, the expression levels of EAR-2, COUP-TF1, EARγ, snail, and slug decrease, and aromatase expression is then upregulated through the binding of ERRα-1 to S1 and the binding of CREB or related factors to CREaro.

Recently, we also investigated the effect of the 5′ untranslated regions (i.e., untranslated exon Is) on the translation of aromatase mRNA.[42] Our *in vitro* transcription/translation analysis using plasmids containing T7 promoter and the human snail gene as a reporter capped with different untranslated exon Is revealed that exon PII-containing transcripts were translated more effectively than exon I.3-containing transcripts. These results indicate that aromatase expression can also be regulated at the translational level.

This and several other laboratories have devoted significant efforts towards a clear understanding of the regulatory mechanism of aromatase expression in breast cancer tissue. Whereas the regulatory mechanism of aromatase expression in human breast tissue is complex, through a systematic approach, we begin to elucidate the molecular details of how aromatase expression is regulated in human breast cancer tissue. It is thought that through an understanding of the regulatory mechanism of aromatase expression in breast cancer tissue, a therapy based on suppressing aromatase expression can be developed.

ACKNOWLEDGMENTS

This research was supported in part by National Institutes of Health Grants ES 08258 and CA44735, UC Breast Cancer Research Grant 4PB-0115, and AICR Grant 99B054.

REFERENCES

1. JAMES, V.H.T., J.M. MCNEILL, L.C. LAI, *et al.* 1987. Aromatase activity in normal breast and breast tumor tissues: *in vivo* and *in vitro* studies. Steroids **50:** 269–279.
2. MILLER, W.R. & J. O'NEILL. 1987. The importance of local synthesis of estrogen within the breast. Steroids **50:** 537–548.
3. ZHOU, C., D. ZHOU, J. ESTEBAN, *et al.* 1996. Aromatase gene expression and its exon I usage in human breast tumors. Detection of aromatase messenger RNA by reverse transcription-polymerase chain reaction (RT-PCR). J. Steroid Biochem. Mol. Biol. **59:** 163–171.
4. ESTEBAN, J.M., Z. WARSI, H. HANIU, *et al.* 1992. Detection of intratumoral aromatase in breast carcinomas, an immunohistochemical study with clinico-pathologic correlation. J. Am. Pathol. **140:** 337–343.
5. SANTEN, R.J., J. MARTEL, M. HOAGLAND, *et al.* 1994. Stromal spindle cells contain aromatase in human breast tumors. J. Clin. Endocrinol. Metab. **79:** 627–632.
6. LU, Q., J. NAKAMURA, A. SAVINOV, *et al.* 1996. Expression of aromatase protein and messenger ribonucleic acid in tumor epithelial cells and evidence of functional sig-

nificance of locally produced estrogen in human breast cancers. Endocrinology **137**: 3061–3077.
7. PASQUALINI, J.R., G. CHETRITE, C. BLACKER, et al. 1996. Concentrations of estrone, estradiol, and estrone sulfate and evaluation of sulfatase and aromatase activities in pre- and postmenopausal breast cancer patients. J. Clin. Endocrinol. Metab. **81**: 1460–1464.
8. SANTNER, S.J., S. CHEN, D. ZHOU, et al. 1993. Effect of androstenedione on growth of untransfected and aromatase-transfected MCF-7 cells in culture. J. Steroid Biochem. Mol. Biol. **44**: 611–616.
9. YUE, W., D. ZHOU, S. CHEN & A. BRODIE. 1994. A new nude mouse model for postmenopausal breast cancer using MCF-7 cells transfected with the human aromatase gene. Cancer Res. **54**: 5092–5095.
10. TEKMAL, R.R., N. RAMACHANDRA, S. GUBBA, et al. 1996 Overexpression of int-5/aromatase in mammary glands of transgenic mice results in the induction of hyperplasia and nuclear abnormalities. Cancer Res. **56**: 3180–3185.
11. SUN, X.-Z., D. ZHOU & S. CHEN. 1997. Autocrine and paracrine actions of breast tumor aromatase. A three-dimensional cell culture study involving aromatase transfected MCF-7 andT-47D cells. J. Steroid Biochem. Mol. Biol. **63**: 29–36.
12. VOGEL, C. 1996. Hormonal approaches to breast cancer treatment and prevention: an overview. Semin. Oncol. **23**: 2–9.
13. BRODIE, A. 1996. Aromatase inhibitors and breast cancer. Semin. Oncol. **23**: 10–20.
14. EBCTCG. 1992. Systemic treatment of early breast cancer by hormonal, cytotoxic, or immune therapy. Lancet **Pt. 1**: 1–15; **Pt.12**: 71–85.
15. WIEBE, V., C.K. OSBORNE, W.L. MCGUIRE & M.W. DEGREGORIO. 1992. Identification of estrogenic tamoxifen metabolite(s) in tamoxifen-resistant human breast tumors. J. Clin. Oncol. **10**: 990–994.
16. OSBORNE, C. & S.A.W. FUQUA. 1994. Mechanisms of tamoxifen resistance. Breast Cancer Res. Treat. **32**: 49–55.
17. OSBORNE, C., E. CORONADO, D.C. ALLRED, et al. 1991. Acquired tamoxifen resistance: correlation with reduced breast tumor levels of tamoxifen and isomerization of trans-4-hyroxytamoxifen. J. Natl. Cancer Inst. **20**: 1477–1482.
18. GOTTARDIS M, S.-Y. JIANG, M.-H. JENG & V.C. JORDAN. 1989. Inhibition of tamoxifen-stimulated growth of an MCF-7 tumor variant in athymic mice by novel steroidal antiestrogens. Cancer Res. **49**: 4090–4093.
19. GOTTARDIS M. & V.C. JORDAN. 1988. Development of tamoxifen-stimulated growth of MCF-7 tumors in athymic mice after long-term antiestrogen administration. Cancer Res. **48**: 5183–5187.
20. GOSS, P., R.L. COOMBES, T.J. POWLES, et al. 1986. Treatment of advanced postmenopausal breast cancer using aromatase inhibitor, 4-hydroxyandrostenedione: phase 2 report. Cancer Res. **46**: 4823–4826.
21. SANTEN, R., T.J. WORGUL, A. LIPTON, et al. 1982. Aminoglutethimide as treatment of postmenopausal women with advanced breast carcinoma: correlation of clinical and hormonal responses. Ann. Int. Med. **96**: 94–101.
22. YATES, R., M. DOWSETT, G.V. FISHER, et al. 1996. Arimidex (ZD1033): a selective, potent inhibitor of aromatase in postmenopausal female volunteers. Br. J. Cancer **73**: 543–548.
23. FISHER, B., J.P. COSTANTINO, D.L. WICKERHAM, et al. 1998. National Surgical Adjuvant Breast and Bowel Project Investigators: tamoxifen for prevention of breast cancer: report of the National Surgical Adjuvant Breast and Bowel Project P-1 Study. J. Natl. Cancer Inst. **18**: 1371–1388.
24. SANTEN, R., W. YUE, F. NAFTOLIN, et al. 1999. The potential of aromatase inhibitors in breast cancer prevention. Endocr.-Related Cancer **6**: 235–243.
25. DECOSTER, R., W. WOUTERS, C.R. BOWDEN, et al. 1990. New non-steroidal aromatase inhibitors: focus on R76713. J. Steroid Biochem. Mol. Biol. **37**: 335–341.
26. DIXON, J.M. 2001. Neoadjuvant endocrine therapy. In Aromatase Inhibition and Breast Cancer. W.R. Miller & R.J. Santen, eds. :103–116. Marcel Dekker, Inc. New York. Basel.
27. POTTER, J. & K. STEINMETZ. 1996. Vegetables, fruit and phytoestrogens as preventive agents. IARC Sci. Publ. **139**: 61–90.

28. ZHANG, S.H., M.R. FORMAN, B.A. ROSNER, *et al.* 1999. Dietary carotenoids and vitamins A,C, and E and risk of breast cancer. J. Natl. Cancer Inst. **91:** 546–556.
29. KELSEY, J. & P.L. HORN-ROSS. 1993. Breast cancer: magnitude of the problem and descriptive epidemiology. Epidemiol. Rev. **15:** 7–16.
30. LEE, H., L. GOURLEY, S.W. DUFFY, *et al.* 1991. Dietary effects on breast-cancer risk in Singapore. Lancet **337:** 1197–1200.
31. BARNES, S., J. SFAKIANOS, L. COWARD & M. KIRK. 1996. Soy isoflavonoids and cancer prevention. Adv. Exp. Med. Biol. **401:** 87–100.
32. CLARKE, R., L. HILAKIVI-CLARKE, E. CHO, *et al.* 1996. Estrogens, phytoestrogens, and breast cancer. Adv. Exp. Med. Biol. **401:** 63–85.
33. ADLERCREUTZ, H., C. BANNWART, K. WAHALA, *et al.* 1993. Inhibition of human aromatase by mammalian lignans and isolavonoid phytoestrogens. J. Steroid Biochem. Mol. Biol. **44:** 147–153.
34. CAMPBELL, D. & M.S. KURZER. 1993. Flavonoid inhibition of aromatase enzyme activity in human preadipocytes. J. Steroid Biochem. Mol. Biol. **46:** 381–388.
35. IBRAHIM, A. & Y.J. ABUL-HAJJ. 1990. Aromatase inhibition by flavonoids. J. Steroid Biochem. Mol. Biol. **37:** 257–260.
36. KELLIS, J. & L.E. VICKERY. 1984. Inhibition of estrogen synthetase (aromatase) by flavones. Science **225:** 1032–1034.
37. PELISSERO, C.M. J.P. LENCZOWSKI, D. CHINZI, *et al.* 1996. Effects of flavonoids on aromatase activity: an *in vitro* study. J. Steroid Biochem. Mol. Biol. **57:** 215–223.
38. WANG, C., T. MAKELA, T. HASE, *et al.* 1994. Lignans and flavonoids inhibit aromatase enzyme in human preadipocytes. J. Steroid Biochem. Mol. Biol. **50:** 205–212.
39. CHEN, S., Y.-C. KAO & C.A. LAUGHTON. 1997. Binding characteristics of aromatase inhibitors and pytoestrogens to human aromatase. J. Steroid Biochem. Mol. Biol. **61:** 107–115.
40. KAO, Y.-C., C. ZHOU, M. SHERMAN, *et al.* 1998. Molecular basis of the inhibition of human aromatase by flavone and isoflavone phytoestrogens. A site-directed mutagenesis study. Environ. Health Perspect. **106:** 85–92.
41. CHEN, S., X.-Z. SUN, Y.-C. KAO, *et al.* 1998. Suppression of breast cancer cell growth with grape juice. Pharmaceut. Biol. **36:** 53–61.
42. OKUBO, T., S.C. MOK & S. CHEN. 2000. Regulation of aromatase expression in human ovarian surface epithelial cells. J. Clin. Endocrinol. Metab. **85:** 4889–4899.
43. CHEN, S., M.J. BESMAN, R.S. SPARKES, *et al.* 1988. Human aromatase: cDNA cloning, Southern blot analysis, and assignment of the gene to chromosome 15. DNA **7:** 27–38.
44. BULUN, S.E., L.S. NOBLE, K. TAKAYAMA, *et al.* 1997. Endocrine disorders associated with inappropriately high aromatase expression. J. Steroid Biochem. Mol. Biol. **61:** 133–139.
45. WANG, J. & S. CHEN. 1992. Identification of a promoter and a silencer at the 3′-end of the first intron of the human aromatase gene. Molec. Endocrinol. **6:** 1479–1488.
46. ZHOU, D., P. CLARKE, J. WANG & S. CHEN. 1996. Identification of a promoter that controls aromatase expression in human breast cancer and adipose stromal cells. J. Biol. Chem. **271:** 15194–15202.
47. ZHOU, D. & S. CHEN. 1998. Characterization of a silencer element in the human aromatase gene. Arch. Biochem. Biophys. **353:** 213–220.
48. ZHOU, D. & S. CHEN. 1999. Identification and characterization of a cAMP-responsive element in the region upstream from promoter I.3 of the human aromatase gene. Arch. Biochem. Biophys. **371:** 179–190.
49. YANG, C., D. ZHOU & S. CHEN. 1998. Modulation of aromatase expression in the breast tissue by ERRα-1 orphan receptor. Cancer Res. **58:** 5695–5700.
50. OKUBO, T., T.K. TRUONG, B. YU, *et al.* 2001. Down-regulation of promoter I.3 activity of the human aromatase gene in breast tissue by zinc-finger protein, snail (SnaH). Cancer Res. **61:** 1338–1346.

Anti-Aromatase Chemicals in Red Wine

E.T. ENG,[a] D. WILLIAMS,[a] U. MANDAVA,[b] N. KIRMA,[b]
R.R. TEKMAL,[b] AND S. CHEN[a]

[a]*Division of Immunology, Beckman Research Institute of the City of Hope,
Duarte, California 91010, USA*

[b]*Department of Gynecology & Obstetrics, Emory University,
Atlanta, Georgia 30322-4710, USA*

ABSTRACT: Estrogen synthesized *in situ* plays a more important role in breast cancer cell proliferation than does circulating estrogen. Aromatase is the enzyme that converts androgen to estrogen and is expressed at a higher level in breast cancer tissue than in surrounding noncancer tissue. A promising route of chemoprevention against breast cancer may be through the suppression of *in situ* estrogen formation using aromatase inhibitors. A diet high in fruits and vegetables may reduce the incidence of breast cancer, because they contain phytochemicals that can act as aromatase inhibitors. In our previous studies, we found that grapes and wine contain potent phytochemicals that can inhibit aromatase. We show that red wine was more effective than white wine in suppressing aromatase activity. Interestingly, our results from white wine studies suggest a weak inductive effect of alcohol on aromatase activity. On the other hand, the potent effect of anti-aromatase chemicals in red wine overcomes the weak inductive effect of alcohol in wine. Several purification procedures were performed on whole red wine to separate active aromatase inhibitors from nonactive compounds. These techniques included liquid-liquid extraction, silica gel chromatography, various solid phase extraction (SPE) columns, and high performance liquid chromatography. An active Pinot Noir red wine SPE C18 column fraction (20% acetonitrile:water) was more effective than complete Pinot Noir wine in suppressing aromatase assay. This red wine extract was further analyzed in a transgenic mouse model in which aromatase was over-expressed in mammary tissue. Our gavaged red wine extract completely abrogated aromatase-induced hyperplasia and other neoplastic changes in mammary tissue. These results suggest that red wine or red wine extract may be a chemopreventive diet supplement for postmenopausal women who have a high risk of breast cancer. Further research is underway to purify and characterize the active compounds in red wine that are responsible for the inhibition of aromatase.

KEYWORDS: aromatase; red wine; estrogen; breast cancer

Address for correspondence: Dr. S. Chen, Division of Immunology, Beckman Research Institute of the City of Hope, Duarte, CA 91010. Voice: 626-359-8111, ext. 62601; fax: 626-301-8186.
schen@coh.org

INTRODUCTION

Estrogen promotes the proliferation of breast cancer cells. Aromatase is the enzyme that converts androgen to estrogen. In tumors, expression of aromatase is upregulated compared to that of surrounding noncancerous tissue. Tumor aromatase is thought to stimulate breast cancer growth in both an autocrine and a paracrine manner. A treatment strategy for breast cancer is to abolish *in situ* estrogen formation with aromatase inhibitors. In addition, aromatase suppression in postmenopausal women is being evaluated as a potential chemopreventive modality against breast cancer.

Our laboratory reported that grape juice contains phytochemicals that can effectively suppress aromatase activity,[1] suggesting that drinking grape juice is a potential chemopreventive modality against breast cancer. However, without knowing the active chemicals and their levels, it is difficult to estimate the exact quantity of grape juice that is needed for chemoprevention. Considering the high sugar content in grape juice that hinders the isolation and characterization of the effective components, we initiated a study to determine whether wines contain similar chemicals that are capable of suppressing aromatase.

ANTI-AROMATASE ACTIVITY OF RED WINE

To determine if any components exist in red or white wines that may have any action on aromatase, we tested 11 red and 4 white wines (TABLE 1). Aromatase assay was performed using human placental microsomes as the source of the enzyme.[2] All red wines tested (50 μl in an assay volume of 1 ml), but not white wines, effectively suppressed aromatase. These results indicate that red wine contains active components that can suppress aromatase. Furthermore, it is thought that the inhibition does not result from alcohol in the wine, because both white and red wines contain similar levels of alcohol, but white wine was not able to suppress aromatase activity.

Alcohol has been indicated as a risk factor for breast cancer. Although the exact action of alcohol is not yet understood, alcohol ingestion has been shown to increase hepatic aromatase activity, to elevate plasma estradiol, and to decrease plasma testosterone levels.[3,4] To better understand the effect of alcohol in wine on aromatase activity, we performed a study that included de-alcoholized wine that was prepared by lyophilizing the wine and reconstituted in water to its original volume. For all dosages of red wine (Pinot Noir, Hacienda, 1996) studied, no differences were apparent in the complete wine versus the lyophilized wine reconstituted in an equal volume of water.[5] Therefore, by comparing it to the potent inhibitory effect of phytochemicals in red wine on aromatase, the effect of alcohol is insignificant. However, for all dosages of white wine (Fumé Blanc, Domaine Napa, 1996) studied, aromatase activity of the samples treated with the complete wine was slightly higher than that of the samples treated with the lyophilized wine. The stimulating effect of alcohol in white wine could be observed, because white wine does not contain any anti-aromatase chemicals. Estrogen is known to increase breast density,[6] and mammographic breast density is considered to be a significant risk factor for breast cancer. In an analysis of the association of breast density and dietary factors in 1,508 women in a historical cohort study of breast cancer families in Minnesota, Vachon *et al.*[7]

TABLE 1. Inhibitory effect on human placental aromatase activity with 50 µl of each of the complete red or white wines

Wine	Percent remaining aromatizer activity
Red wine	
Cabernet Sauvignon, Tanglewood, 1996	0.29
Cabernet Sauvignon, Glen Ellen Prp Reserve ,1997	7.7
Cabernet Sauvignon, San Andrés, 1998	0.36
Merlot, JW Morris, 1997	0.42
Merlot, Forest Ville, 1997	0.46
Merlot, Hacienda, 1997	3.29
Merlot, Hacienda, 1998	0.9
Zinfande, Black Mountain, 1996	0.39
Zinfandel, Sequoia Ridge ,1996	0.39
Pinot Noir, Cambiaso, 1996	0.34
Pinot Noir, Hacienda, 1996	2.16
White wine	
Chardonnay Woodbridge, 1998	99.1
Chardonnay, Santa Rita Reserve, 1999	80
Fumé Blanc, Domaine Napa, 1996	112.5
Sauvignon Blanc, Turning Leaf, 1998	106.5

found that wine intake among postmenopausal women was significant in that white wine showed a positive association and red wine an inverse association with percentage of breast density. The findings from this and other laboratories support the hypothesis that red wine, but not white wine, contains chemicals that suppress aromatase.

CHARACTERIZATION OF ANTI-AROMATASE CHEMICALS IN RED WINE

Red wine, compared to white wine, is a rich source of polyphenolic compounds, because skins and seeds are not removed during the grape-crushing process for red wine. Quercetin, resveratrol, and rutin are well-characterized chemicals in grape and red wine. Among them, resveratrol was shown to be an agonist for the estrogen receptor in different test systems.[8] More recent studies indicate that the binding affinity of resveratrol to estrogen receptor is relatively weak.[9,10] Freyberger et al.[11] revealed that in an animal study, resveratrol mildly decreased uterine weight, whereas histology did not reveal differences between controls and resveratrol-treated rats. This recent finding is considered important in that the estrogenic activity of resveratrol as determined by *in vitro* studies cannot be substantiated in an *in vivo* study. Our aromatase assay has revealed that up to 100 µM, quercetin, resveratrol, and rutin are ineffective in suppressing aromatase (FIG. 1). These results indicate that these

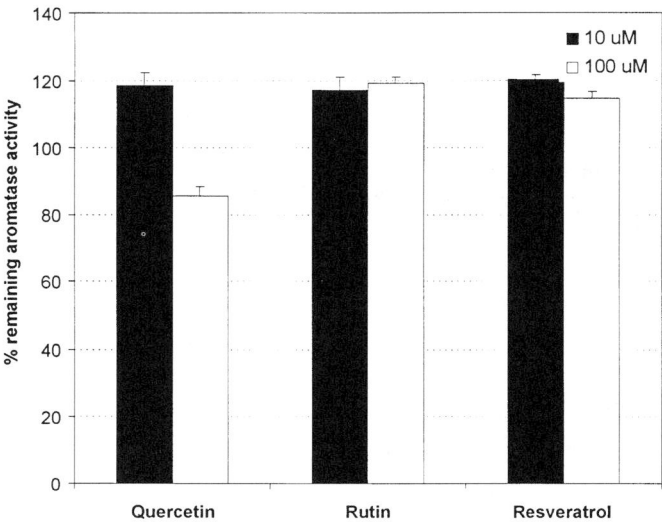

FIGURE 1. Quercetin, rutin, and trans-resveratrol known compounds found in grapes and wine were analyzed for their ability to inhibit aromatase in a human placental microsome assay.

three compounds are not the chemicals in grape or red wine that inhibit aromatase. The concentrations of these chemicals in 50 µl of red wine should be much lower than 100 µM.

A major part of our efforts has been dedicated towards optimizing the purification of this complex wine mixture into more refined crude fractions and in large quantities that are required for structure characterization. Our strategy was to simplify the wine mixture by first removing some of the inactive compounds. Complete wine was processed in a liquid-liquid extractor containing 750 mls of a whole bottle of wine and about 1.5 liters of ethyl acetate. Each extraction took about 16 hours for boiling ethyl acetate to adequately and sufficiently evaporate, condense, and diffuse through the wine. This procedure extracted any wine compounds that were soluble in ethyl acetate. Strong polar compounds remained in the aqueous phase of the wine extract. Six separate extractions using one bottle each of Pinot Noir (Hacienda, 1996) were carried out and later combined. Upon separation of the aqueous and organic phases, the total organic phase was rotovapped down to a 20-ml volume and then loaded on the top of the silica column. Our initial separation procedure used silica gel chromatography for a crude separation of the red wine extract. A silica preparative column was prepared to 11-cm diameter × 30-cm length with silica mesh 70–230 (Sigma-Aldrich, Milwaukee, WI) and preconditioned with ethyl acetate (Burdick and Jackson, AlliedSignal, Muskegon, MI). The 20 mls of the wine organic phase was applied to the top of the silica column. A glass bulb was attached to the top of the silica column serving as a solvent reservoir to provide a constant flow of ethyl acetate over the column. The chemicals were eluted off the column based on their binding affinity to the silica gel. Five-milliliter fractions were collected until all colored chemicals were eluted. One milliliter of each 5-ml silica fraction was dried to completion by vacufuge and rehydrated with water to a 1-ml volume. Each of these silica fractions was tested in the human placental microsome assay to determine where the active aromatase inhibitors are distributed. A clearly evident region of wine aromatase inhibitors was located in the front end of the column eluting after about 100 mls at the start of when colored compounds began to elute off the silica column.

A secondary phase of semipreparative purification was separation of the active chemicals using pre-packed solid phase extraction (SPE) resin columns. The method development kits containing a variety of SPE columns (AccuBond, J&W Scientific, Folsom, CA) were used to determine the best column to de-convolute our complex wine samples. Amino, cyano, diol, methyl, phenyl, and octadecyl (C18) resin columns were used. One of the most active silica fractions was taken, dried, and rehydrated in equal volume with water, and then a 100-µl aliquot was loaded on top of the pre-equilibrated column. A stepwise gradient of acetonitrile (Burdick and Jackson, AlliedSignal, Muskegon, MI) and water was loaded into each column and pulled through by gravity flow without ever letting the column go to dryness. For each eluted acetonitrile:water fraction, a 1-ml sample was dried by lyophilization and reconstituted to a 1-ml volume of water or water and ethyl alcohol (Aaper Alcohol and Chemical Co., Shelbyville, KY) for the more nonpolar fractions. The reconstituted fractions were checked for their ability to inhibit aromatase in the human placental microsome assay. We found that amino, cyano, and diol columns did not provide a good separation of compounds, because the active chemicals do not bind to the resins (example shown in FIG. 2A). The separational column was good when the different acetonitrile:water fractions showed a distribution of aromatase inhibitory activity. Two promising separatory columns are the methyl and phenyl columns. Methyl columns are useful to isolate polar multifunctional compounds, whereas phenyl columns are helpful to separate aromatic compounds. Both the methyl and phenyl columns both provided an adequate distribution of aromatase suppression (FIG. 2B and 2C). These results suggest that the active chemicals are aromatic compounds. Among the columns that best separated the aromatase inhibitory activity across a range of increasing organic solvent, we selected the most active fractions and analyzed them by another stage of chromatography using high performance liquid chromatography (HPLC) with a reverse-phase C18 column (Vydac, Western Analytical Products, Hesperia, CA). Several active fractions from reverse-phase HPLC separation have been identified. Currently, we are performing large-scale isolation and chemical structural analyses using mass spectrometry and NMR.

We tested the 20% MeCN fraction (Pinot Noir, Hacienda, 1996) from a C18 SPE separation in a hybrid *in vitro* aromatase assay using CHO cells transfected with human wild-type aromatase. Similar to whole wine, the wine extract was able to inhibit CHO cell aromatase in a dose-dependent fashion (FIG. 3). Our active wine compounds appear to be midpolar in nature and cannot easily penetrate the cell membrane to interact with aromatase. In the hybrid assay, the CHO cells were briefly treated with trypsin.

We also examined the efficacy of the Pinot Noir (Hacienda, 1996) 20% MeCN fraction in an *in vivo* model using a transgenic mouse model containing a mouse mammary tumor virus promoter attached to the human aromatase gene. Control mice develop hyperplastic lesions in the mammary glands. This is a good model to test the validity of our red wine extract as a potential chemopreventive agent against

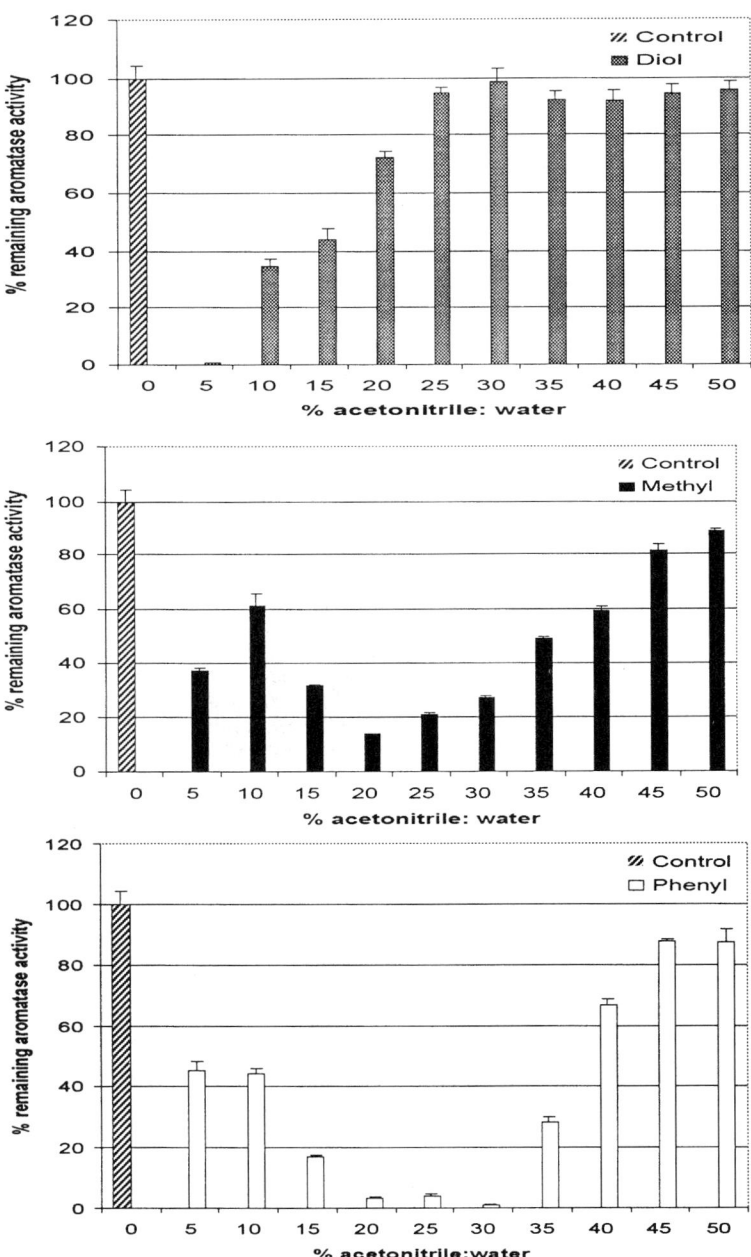

FIGURE 2. Chemical separation of complete red wine, Pinot Noir, to generate crude pre-purification fractions using diol (FIG. 2A), methyl (FIG. 2B), or phenyl (FIG. 2C) solid phase extraction (SPE) columns.

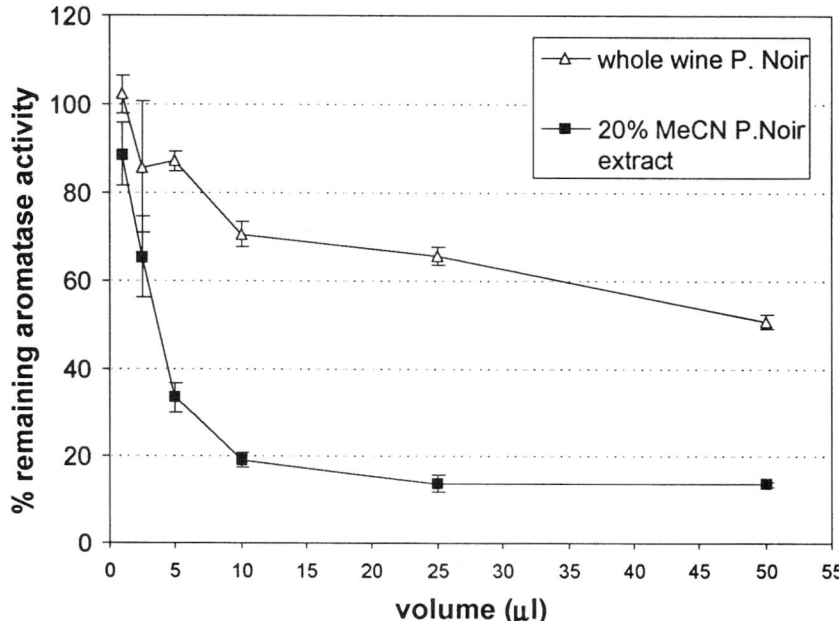

FIGURE 3. Hybrid microsome assay using CHO cell line transfected with human wild-type aromatase (pHβ) challenged with a water control, complete Pinot Noir (Hacienda, 1996) red wine, and a 10× concentrated 20% acetonitrile:water fraction of Pinot Noir (Hacienda, 1996). All samples are compared to a water control (taken as 100%).

breast cancer. The Pinot Noir 20% MeCN fraction was gavage fed to mice at 100 μl per day per mouse for 3 weeks. Two control groups were maintained: one was gavage fed water and the other received 5 μg/mouse/daily Letrozole, a clinically approved aromatase inhibitor. After 3 weeks of treatment, all mice were euthanized and the mammary glands, uteri, and ovaries were removed, weighed, and histologically evaluated. We found that the wine extract was able to completely inhibit the development of hyperplastic lesions in the mammary glands and was as effective as the Letrozole treatment. These results indicate that although the active chemicals are midpolar, they can be processed and absorbed by the mammary gland *in vivo*. In addition, the wine extract generated an estrogen-deprived environment that affected other endocrine organs. Atrophy of endothelial cells lining the lumen of the uterus and the appearance of large hyperchromatic nucleated cells in the uterus lumen and multiple ovarian cysts, impaired follicle growth, and ovum release were observed in the red wine extract and Letrozole-treated mice.

In summary, our wine studies reveal that red wine contains chemicals that can suppress aromatase activity *in vitro* and more importantly *in vivo*. Moderate red wine consumption may help postmenopausal women from developing breast cancer by suppressing estrogen formation in breast tissue. Our current efforts are to purify and to structurally characterize the active chemicals. This information is critical for us to better understand the molecular basis of the aromatase inhibitory effect of red wine.

ACKNOWLEDGMENT

This research was supported in part by National Institutes of Health Grants ES 08258 and CA44735, UC Breast Cancer Research Grant 4PB-0115, and a National Institutes of Health predoctoral fellowship (F31AT00059) to E.T. Eng.

REFERENCES

1. CHEN, S., X.-Z. SUN, Y.-C. KAO, et al. 1998 Suppression of breast cancer cell growth with grape juice. Pharm. Biol. **36** (Suppl): 53–61.
2. THOMPSON, E.A., JR. & P.K. SIITERI. 1974. Utilization of oxygen and reduced nicotinamide adenine dinucleotide phosphate by human placental microsomes during aromatization of androstenedione. J. Biol. Chem. **249:** 5364–5372.
3. GORDON, G.G., A.L. SOUTHREN, J. VITTEK & C.S. LIEBER. 1979. The effect of alcohol ingestion on hepatic aromatase activity and plasma steroid hormones in the rat. Metabolism **28:** 20–24.
4. VAN THIEL, D.H., J.S. GAVALER, P.K. EAGON, et al. 1981 Hypogonadism and feminization in alcoholic men: the past, present and future. Curr. Alcohol **8:** 29–40.
5. ENG, E.T., D. WILLIAMS, U. MANDAVA, et al. 2001. Suppression of aromatase (estrogen synthetase) by red wine phytochemicals. Breast Cancer Res. Treat. In press.
6. RUTTER, C.M, M.T. MANDELSON, M.B. LAYA, et al. 2001. Changes in breast density associated with initiation, discontinuation, and continuing use of hormone replacement therapy. JAMA **285:** 171–176.
7. VACHON, C.M., R.A. KING, L.D. ATWOOD, et al. 2000. Association of diet and mammographic breast density in the Minnesota breast cancer family cohort. Cancer Epidemiol. Biomarkers Prev. **9:** 151–160.
8. GEHM, B.D., J.M. MCANDREWS, P.Y. CHIEN & J.L. JAMESON. 1997. Resveratrol, a polyphenolic compound found in grapes and wine, is an agonist for the estrogen receptor. Proc. Natl. Acad. Sci. USA **94:** 14138–14143.
9. ASHBY, J., K. TINWELL, W. PENNIE, et al. 1999. Partial and weak oestrogenicity of the red wine constituent resveratrol: consideration of its superagonist activity in MCF-7 cells and its suggested cardiovascular protective effects. J. Appl. Toxicol. **19:** 39–45.
10. BOWERS, J.L., V.V. TYULMENKOV, S.C. JERNIGAN & C.M. KLINGE. 2000. Resveratrol acts as a mixed agonist/antagonist for estrogen receptors alpha and beta. Endocrinology **141:** 3657–3667.
11. FREYBERGER, A., E. HARTMANN, H. HILDEBRAND & F. KROTLINGER. 2001. Differential response of immature rat uterine tissue to ethinylestradiol and the red wine constituent resveratrol. Arch. Toxicol. **74:** 709–715.

Diet and Breast Cancer

H. LEON BRADLOW AND DANIEL W. SEPKOVIC

David and Alice Jurist Institute for Research, Hackensack University Medical Center, Hackensack, New Jersey 07601, USA

> ABSTRACT: The preponderance of evidence suggests a role for fat and alcohol as risk factors for breast cancer. The role of milk is more controversial with some studies suggesting that milk is a risk factor and others that consumption of milk is protective against breast cancer. No other major nutrient appears to play a significant role in increasing breast cancer risk. On the other hand, there is increasing evidence that a variety of micronutrients and hormones appear to have significant anticancer activity. These range from steroids such as dehydroepiandrosterone (DHEA) and its analysis to indoles, isothiocyanates, and isoflavone derivatives. These compounds act directly by interfering with cyclins and promoting apoptosis as well as indirectly by altering estrogen metabolism in a favorable direction. These effects are not merely theoretical actions in cell culture and tissue explants; they have been demonstrated in human patients as a range of studies have demonstrated.
>
> KEYWORDS: diet; breast cancer; micronutrients; indoles; isothiocyanates; alcohol; milk; obesity

INTRODUCTION

The interaction of diet and breast cancer risk needs to be divided into two distinct roles: (1) the effects of major dietary components, particularly dietary fat intake; and (2) the role of micronutrients acting as antitumor agents. The role of dietary fat has had a long and convoluted history. When epidemiologists looked at the striking variations in breast cancer incidence in different countries and how the incidence changed as people migrated from one country to another, diet became the object of intense investigation. Early on, attention focused on fat, as illustrated in the famous plot correlating fat consumption by countries versus breast cancer incidence (FIG. 1).[1] Secondary to the investigation of total consumption of fat was the question of which fatty acids (saturated, unsaturated, w-6 polyunsaturated fatty acids, or w-3 fatty acids) might be risk promoting and which might be protective. There is good animal data that saturated and w-6 fatty acids are risk promoting, whereas w-3 fatty acids are not.[2,3] However, contrary to epidemiologic studies, which clearly indicate a risk from dietary fat, case control studies, most notably the Nurses Health Study, found no correlation between dietary fat consumption and breast cancer risk.[4,5]

Address for correspondence: Dr. H. Leon Bradlow, David and Alice Jurist Institute for Research, Hackensack University Medical Center, Hackensack, NJ 07601. Voice: 201-336-8104; fax: 201-487-1882.

leon@bradlow.net

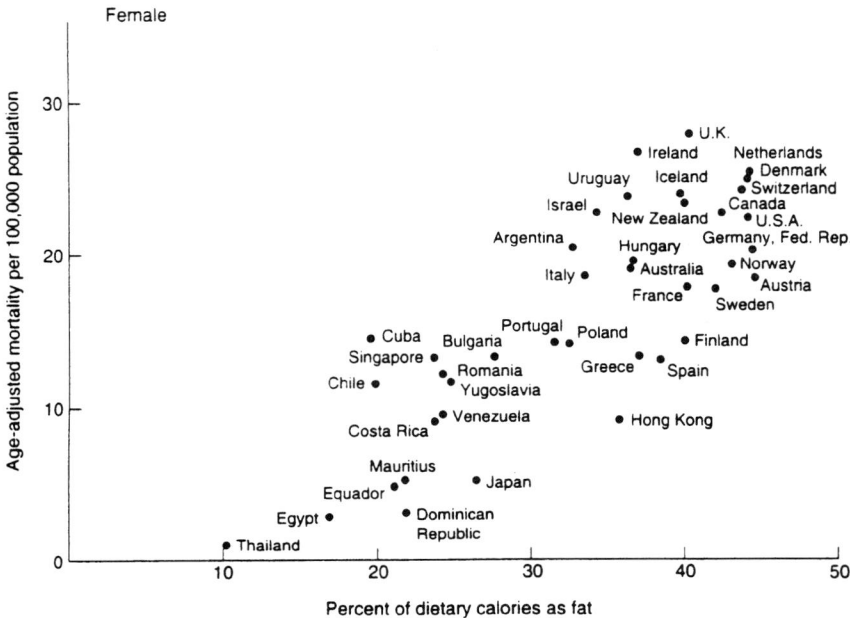

FIGURE 1. Correlation between % calories as fat and breast cancer mortality (Carroll[1]).

These studies were based on recall of current diets at the time of entry into the study and do not necessarily reflect dietary fat intake in earlier years. In a prospective study over a 20-year period, Knekt et al.[6] reported a weakly positive correlation between dietary fat and breast cancer incidence, which was increased when fat intake was adjusted for total energy consumption. In a meta-analysis of dietary fat and breast cancer risk, Boyd et al.[7] reported that European studies were more likely to show an increased relative risk associated with breast cancer and dietary fat than were studies done in other countries,[7] although no mechanism was offered. The failure to connect fat intake with breast cancer risk led investigators to the next step, which was to look at a possible role for stored fat in the body. Whether one consumes excess calories as fat or carbohydrates, it ultimately ends up being deposited as fat in adipocytes. It has been established that obese postmenopausal women show a greater risk of breast cancer.[8,9] Obesity, premenopausally, appears to decrease breast cancer incidence, presumably because it decreases the number of ovulatory cycles, so that there is less exposure to estrogen between menarche and menopause. Because fat is not likely to act merely by being consumed, but only after it is taken up into adipocytes, a possible explanation is the effect of fat-laden adipocytes on estrogen metabolism. Previous studies from this laboratory showed that 2-hydroxylation, yielding the biologically weakly estrogenic 2-OHE1, was greatly reduced in obese subjects.[10] Conversely, in anorectic girls and female athletes with minimal fat depots, 2-OHE1 levels were significantly elevated.[11,12] We recently demonstrated that

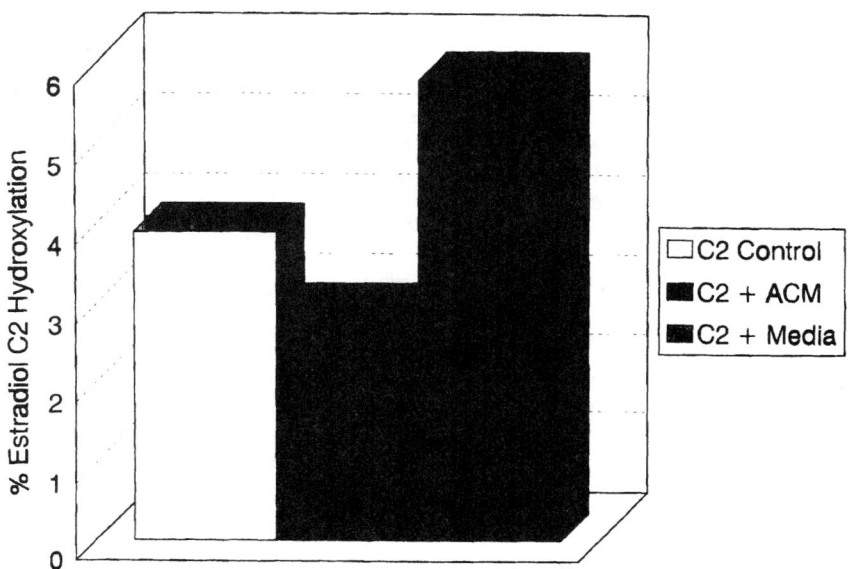

FIGURE 2. Estradiol C2 hydroxylation in MCF7 cells. ACM, adipocyte conditioned media.

human adipocytes in culture secrete a 30-kD protein that inhibits 2-hydroxylation of estradiol in cell culture studies (FIG. 2).[13]

Obesity plays yet another role in increasing breast cancer risk. As Frisch[14] pointed out, body fat is critical in the early initiation of menarche, expanding the period between menarche and menopause, thereby increasing total exposure to estrogen.

Animal studies have shown that exposure to increased body fat *in utero* increased subsequent susceptibility to breast cancer.[15] This raises the possibility that a similar risk may arise in the children of women who gain much more weight during pregnancy than they did in the past. This is a problem that remains to be investigated.

Another disputed diet item in terms of breast cancer risk is the consumption of milk. In 1975, Armstrong and Doll[16] reported an association between the intake of milk products and increased breast cancer mortality. Subsequently, Rose *et al,.*[17] in an international comparison, also concluded that a strong positive correlation existed between breast cancer rates and milk consumption. Conversely, in 1990, Stock and Karn[18] concluded that there was an inverse relation between milk consumption and breast cancer incidence. A subsequent 11-year study in Norway by Ursin *et al.*[19] of a population of 16,000 patients found only a weak positive risk for breast and other cancers except for lymphatic cancer for which a significantly increased risk was observed. In 1995 Knekt *et al.,*[20] following up on an earlier Finnish study, concluded that there was "a protective effect of milk consumption that overwhelms the associations between other factors and the risk of breast cancer." A recent follow-up study by Hjartaker *et al.*[21] of 50,000 patients in the Nowac study concluded that women drinking three glasses of milk or more per day had less than 50% of the risk of women who did not drink milk at all. The protective effect was present whether one drank whole, reduced-fat, or skim milk. The increased consumption of the calcium and vitamin D found in milk was suggested as part of the protective response, although no experimental evidence was offered. Recent data from the Nurses Health Study summarized by Willett et al.[22] have raised doubts about the value of milk in the diet. With all of these conflicting data, the role of milk in breast cancer risk must be considered an unresolved issue, requiring further study.

Another dietary component, reputed to play a role in breast cancer risk, is alcohol consumption. A positive correlation between alcohol consumption and breast cancer risk was observed in premenopausal but not in postmenopausal women.[23–28] This has raised a possible dietary conflict, because there are increasing data that modest alcohol consumption has cardioprotective effects.[29] No correlation has been reported for the consumption of protein or carbohydrate and breast cancer risk.

A particularly active field of study in recent years has been that of micronutrients as protective agents against a wide variety of cancers including the various hormonally related cancers. Micronutrients comprise a diverse collection of compounds, ranging from steroids such as dehydroepiandrosterone to indole derivatives such as indole-3-carbinol and diindolylmethane, isothiocyanates such as sulforaphane, isoflavonoids from soy, catechins such as epigallocatechin gallate found in green tea, and some vitamins and vitamin precursors.

DEHYDROEPIANDROSTERONE

Work by Schwartz[30] has shown that DHEA and some of its synthetic analogs are potent anticancer agents. The mechanism by which DHEA acts as an antitumor agent has not been established. The use of these synthetic analogs as antitumor agents is under active investigation.[31] Clinical trials on the 16-F analog of DHEA as an antitumor agent are underway (FIG. 3).

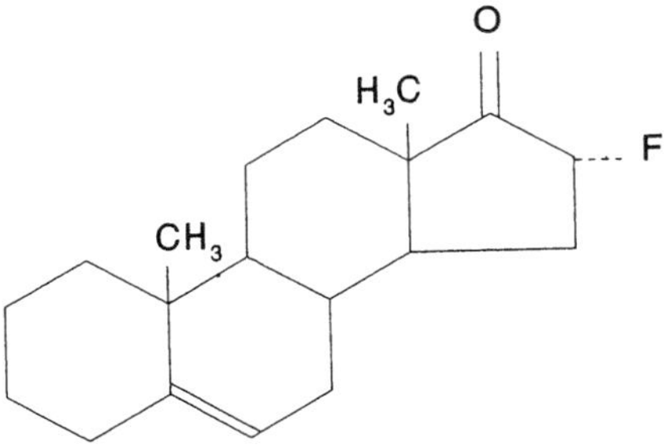

FIGURE 3. 16-fluoro-androst-5-en-17-one.

ISOTHIOCYANATES

A great deal of work has been done on isothiocyanates occurring naturally as glucosinolates, primarily in cruciferous vegetables. Enzymatic action by the enzyme

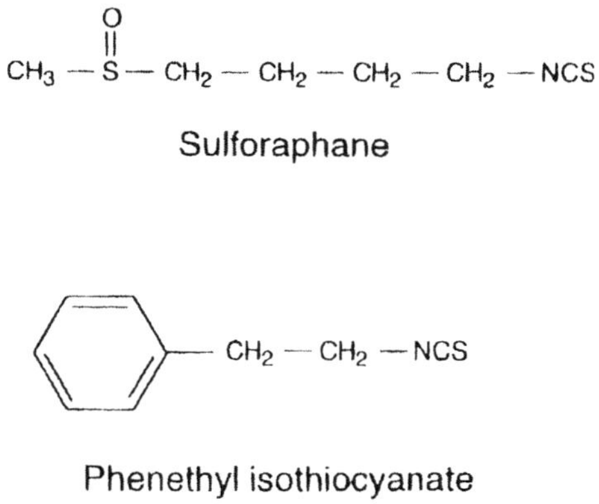

$$CH_3 - \underset{\underset{O}{\|}}{S} - CH_2 - CH_2 - CH_2 - CH_2 - NCS$$

Sulforaphane

Phenethyl isothiocyanate

FIGURE 4. Structure of sulforaphane.

myrosinase also present in these plants cleaves these compounds to yield the isothiocyanates. The greatest interest has been in sulforaphane, which is most abundant in broccoli,[32] and in phenethylisothiocyanate,[33] which is most abundant in watercress (FIG. 4). Both of these compounds were found to have potent antitumor activity in cell culture and in animal models. Both compounds act primarily as phase II inducers. increasing the clearance of carcinogens by conjugation with a variety of conjugating agents including glucosiduronic acid, sulfate, and glutathione, which render the carcinogens inactive and make them watersoluble, facilitating their clearance through the kidney. In animal models given carcinogens, the simultaneous administration of these compounds decreased the incidence of mammary tumors[34] and lung tumors.[35] Activity of sulforaphane against LNCAP prostate cancer cells was recently reported.[36] The level of these compounds in cruciferous vegetables has proved to be highly variable, ranging 15-fold, depending on seed stock, sunshine, moisture, and soil.[37] Recently, a strain of broccoli was bred in which the level of sulforaphane is elevated in 3- to 5-day-old sprouts. Attempts have been made to commercialize their use as a chemopreventive agent.[38] Although extensive cell culture and animal studies have been carried out with both compounds, proving their activity as antitumor agents, no human studies have been reported on their use.

A number of analogs of sulforaphane have been prepared, some of which show substantial activity. Isobornylisothiocyanate has been shown to possess significant activity in cell culture.[39] Recently, Gerhauser et al.[40] described sulforamate {4-methylsulfinyl-1-{S-methyldithiocarbamyl} butane} with activity comparable to that of sulforaphane, but with one third the toxicity of the latter compound. Both acted to block preneoplastic lesions in carcinogen-treated mouse mammary glands in organ culture. Bonnesen reported that the combination of indolylcarbazole and sulforathane acted synergistically to protect against benz-α-pyrene than did either compound alone. The same was true for H_2O_2 as the genotoxic agent. This was true for both LS-174 and CaCO2 cells. The combination acts to increase both apoptosis and intracellular defenses.[41]

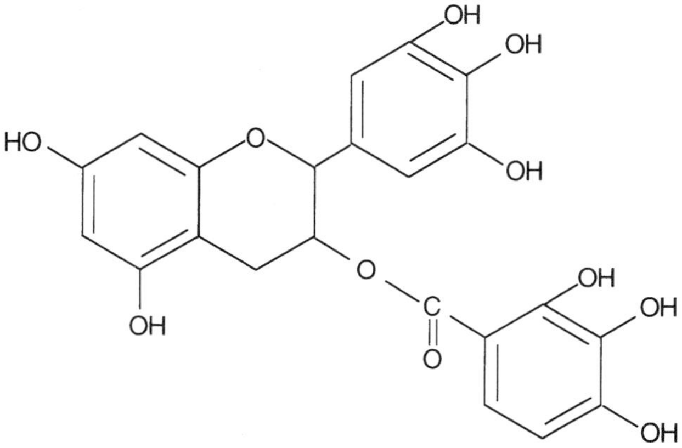

FIGURE 5. Epigallocatechin-3-gallate (EGCG).

Studies by Brooks et al.[42] suggest that protection by sulforaphane is related to the GSTM1 phenotype, with protection being achieved when the null phenotype was present. Protection was not achieved in the presence of wild-type GSTM1.

The isothiocyanates are metabolized first to thiocarbamates, which in turn are converted to watersoluble mercapturic acids.[43]

EPIGALLOCATECHIN GALLATE

Epigallocatechin gallate (ECGC) (FIG. 5), a compound found in green tea and, to a lesser extent, in black tea, has been extensively studied for its activity as an antitumor agent in a remarkably diverse variety of tumors.[44] It was shown to be active as a topical agent against skin tumors induced by carcinogens and promoted by TPA.[45] It also exhibited dramatic activity in various lung tumor models including NNK tumor induction.[46] When tested against various gastrointestinal carcinogens including N-ethyl-N1-nitro-N-nitrosoguanidine, N-methyl-N1-nitro-N-nitrosoguanidine, azoxymethane, etc., it showed substantial inhibitory activity. It has also been shown to be active *in vivo* against prostate cancer and breast cancer and *in vitro* against the corresponding cell lines.[47,48] Recent studies by Menegazzi et al.[49] have shown that EGCG acts to block gamma interferon by specific inhibition of STAT-1 by interfering with tyrosine phosphorylation.

When studied in breast cancer cell lines, EGCG showed significant ability to alter estrogen metabolism in a protective direction, increasing the ratio of C-2/C16a metabolites.[50] However, it is primarily considered to be active as an antioxidative agent. Despite extensive literature from China and Japan where green tea is consumed in large amounts, EGCG as the compound or as green tea has failed to be considered as an antitumor agent in Europe and America despite its substantial potency and absence of toxicity. The lack of a corporate champion may well be one of the problems. When compared with I3C and genistein for its ability to block proliferation and in-

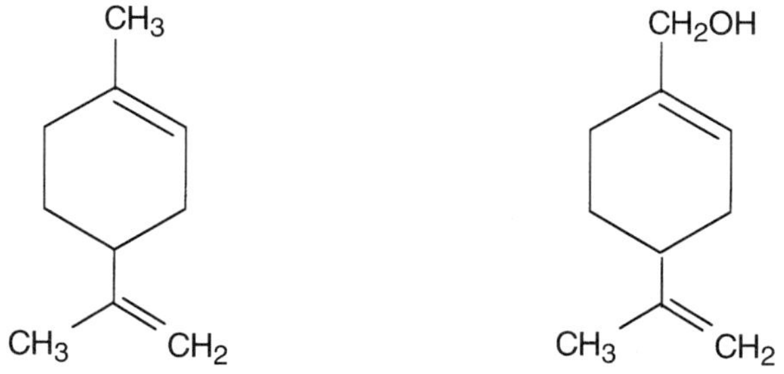

FIGURE 6. (*Left*) limonene; (*right*) perillyl alcohol.

duce apoptosis, EGCG was intermediate in potency, more potent than I3C but less potent than genistein.[51]

LIMONENE

This compound is a monoterpene found in citrus peel along with its monooxygenated derivative, perillyl alcohol. It has been extensively studied for its antitumor activity by Gould and colleagues[52] (FIG. 6). On a molar basis, limonene is less potent than some of the other phytochemicals under study. In animal studies, limonene must be used at doses up to 5% of the diet. Limonene is believed to act as an inhibitor of farnesylation of the RAS oncogene.[53,54] In addition, it is thought to interfere with the first steps in isoprenylation from hydroxymethylglutarate. Phase I clinical trials of a perilyl alcohol extract have been reported.[53]

GENISTEIN

This compound is a weak phytoestrogen found at relatively high concentrations in soy products such as tofu, soymilk, and various high-protein soy concentrates (FIG. 7). It was thought to be one reason that Asian women go through menopause with fewer symptoms than Western women.[56] Although genistein is a weak estrogen relative to estrogen receptor α (ER-α), because it is present in high concentrations in women who consume large amounts of soy products, it can compete for estradiol for receptor binding sites. Newer studies on estradiol receptor β showed that genistein competes very effectively with estradiol for this receptor.[57] Because the β receptor is present in high concentration in certain tissues, genistein may be more of an agonist than was previously thought. Recent studies by Kurzer and colleagues[58,59] have shown that consumption of soy concentrates alters estrogen metabolism in the direction of increased 2-hydroxylation and decreased 16α-hydroxylation. These results are in conflict with other studies. Slavin et al.[60] reported the response to be much less, though still positive. Similar findings have been reported by Kishida et al.[61] and Lu et al.[62] A soy diet containing isoflavones increased the 2/

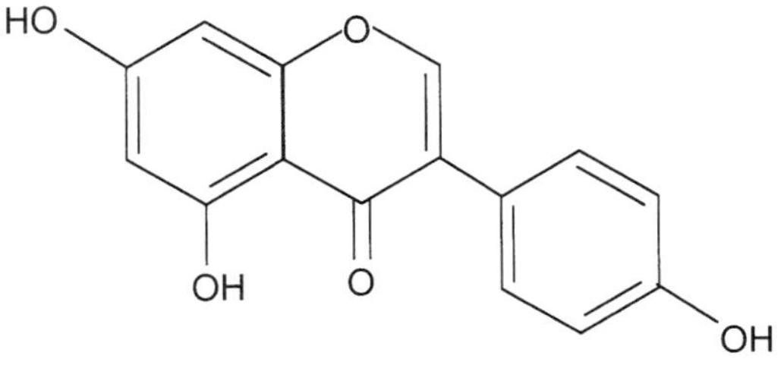

Genistein

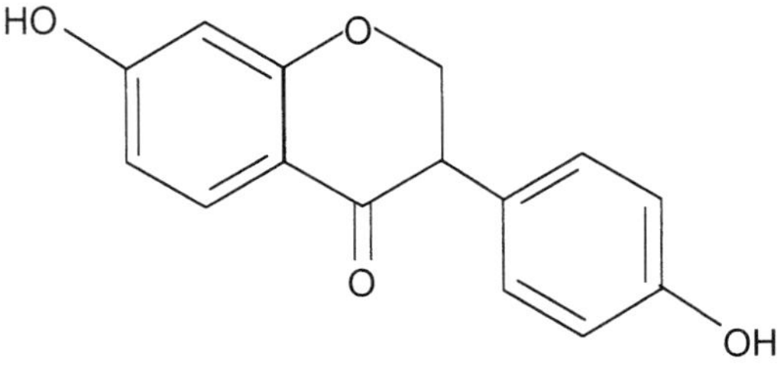

Daidzein

FIGURE 7.

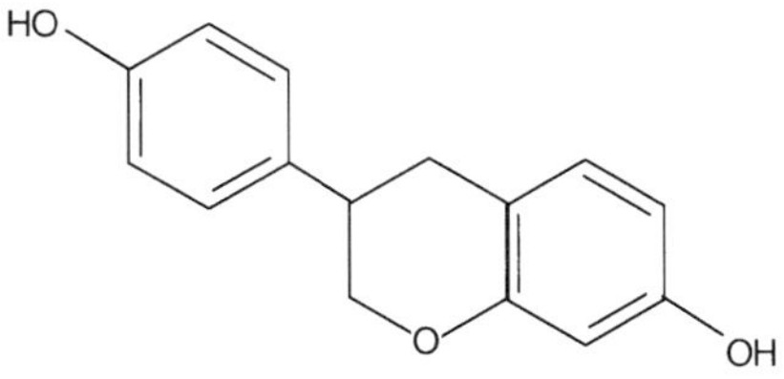

Equol

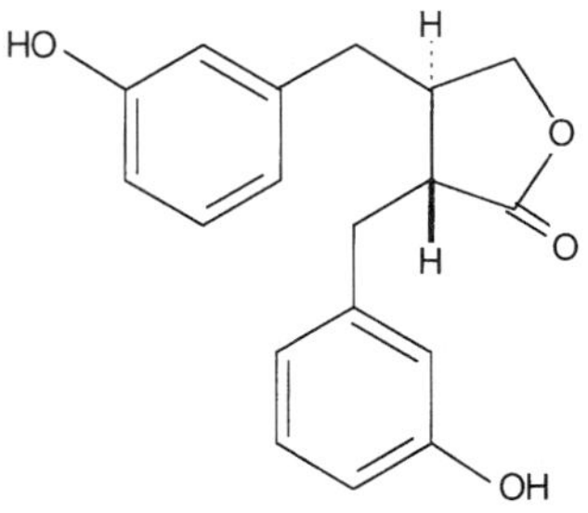

Enterolactone

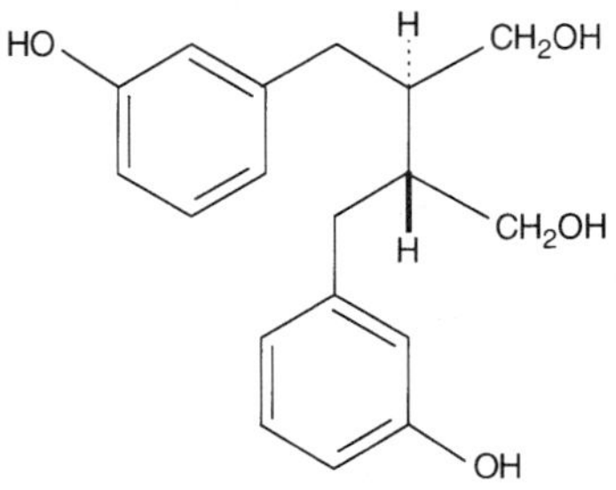

Enterodiol

FIGURE 8.

16 metabolite ratio more than did an isoflavone-free soy diet. The primary effect was exerted on 2-hydroxylation with little or no change in 16-OHE1 formation.[63]

Recently, both Maskarinec et al.[64] and Persky et al.[65] reported finding no effect of soy products on the estrogen metabolite ratio. Cell cycle kinetic studies by Telang et al.[66] showed that genistein at the maximum tolerated dose was more potent than I3C or EGCG in blocking proliferation by holding the cells at a given point in the cell cycle. On the other hand, a recent study by Tonkelaar et al.[67] on a Dutch population found no protective effect from soy consumption on breast cancer incidence in a case control study. The suitability of genistein as a preventive chemotherapeutic agent is still not clear, because in large doses Setchell et al.[68] reported that it produced major alterations in the menstrual cycle. Further studies on this compound are in progress. Berrino[69] recently reported that administration of soy products to patients with breast cancer increased the rate of recurrence compared to that with a non-soy diet. The final story on these compounds remains to be settled. Similar caveats apply to related compounds such as daidzein and the lignan derivatives (FIG. 8). Further studies by Setchell et al.[70] have suggested that bacterial conversion of daidzein to equol is important, because equol appears to be more potent as a protective agent. Not all people carry the bacterial flora effecting this reduction.

HYDROXYCINNAMIC ACID DERIVATIVES

This group of polyhydroxycinnamic acid derivatives has been studied with varying levels of interest for the different members of this class of antitumor agents. These include caffeic acid and its phenylethyl ester (CAPE), ferulic acid, and its dimer, curcumin III. These compounds are potent cyclooxygenase and lipoxygenase inhibitors[1] (FIG. 9).

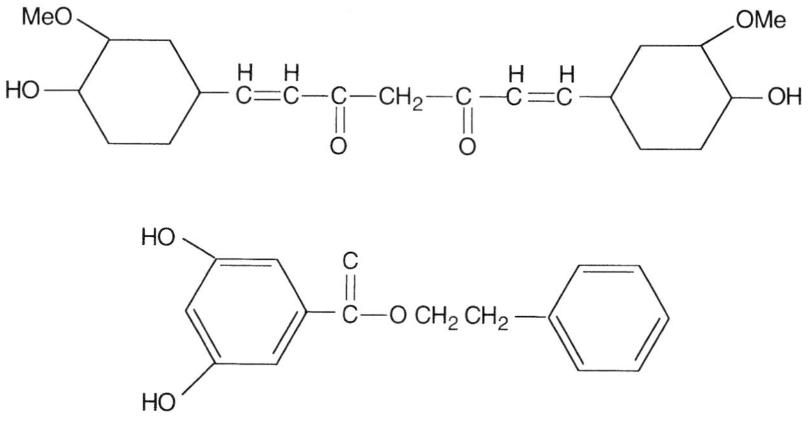

FIGURE 9. (**Top**) Curcumin; (**Bottom**) caffeic acid phenethyl ester.

Curcumin, a constituent of the traditional Indian spice, turmeric, has been regarded as an anticancer agent dating back to Indian folk medicine. Curcumin has been shown to be a mixture of curcumin I, the desmethoxy compound, curcumin II, the monomethoxy compound, and curcumin III, the dimethoxy compound and the most potent of the group. Recent studies have shown that it is active against DMBA-induced mammary tumors and DMBA-DNA adduct formation in female rats,[72] although other studies have reported a lesser response. Curcumin also inhibited azoxymethane-induced colon tumors in Fischer rats from a 47% incidence down to 19% at a low dose (8 g/kg) and 0.06% at a high dose (16 g/kg).[73] It was also shown that curcumin partially reverses the metabolic abnormalities in experimentally induced diabetes.[74] Curcumin III causes 74% inhibition of Ehrlich ascites tumors.[75] It also induces apoptosis in human leukemia cells with a response that was dose and time dependent. In part, it acts by modulating CyP450 formation.[76,77] It substantially blocks croton oil-induced skin tumors. Despite this promise in animal models, extrapolating the effective dose of 16 g/kg in rats to persons suggests that enormous and clearly impractical doses might be necessary in people. In addition, pharmacokinetic studies indicate that it is rapidly cleared from the body in people, making its use as an effective human anticancer agent impractical. In a recent phase I study, doses up to 12 g per day were required.[79]

Studies on CAPE in the minmouse as well as cell culture studies suggested antitumor activity for this compound originally isolated from propopolis.[71,79,80]

INDOLES

Indole-3-Carbinol

Structure and Initial Metabolism (FIG. 10). Indole-3-carbinol is present as a glucosinolate complex (glucobrasicanin) in cruciferous vegetables. When the vegetables are crushed or eaten, the enzyme myrosinase is liberated, cleaving the glucosinolate to yield indole-3-carbinol, unlike the sulfur-containing glucosinolates, which yield isothiocyanates under the same conditions. Indole-3-carbinol is an unstable prodrug, which is not active when administered intraperitoneally or intravenously.[81] When added to cell culture media or even in distilled water, it is specifically converted to diindolylmethane (DIM).[82] When fed to animals or people, the acid in the stomach converts it to DIM as well as to a series of linear and cyclic trimers (FIG. 10). The relative proportions of the various compounds formed depend on the acidity of the stomach. At lower pH levels the extent of trimer formation is greater, whereas as the pH level increases towards pH 5, the proportion of DIM formed is increased. In neutral solutions in water or tissue culture media, only DIM is formed.

Cytochrome Induction. All of these compounds bind in varying degree to the AH receptor binding site upstream from the 5′ end of the DNA sequence for Cyp 1A1/2 and to a lesser extent to 3A4.[83] Induction of CyP1A1 produces a hydroxylase that converts estradiol to yield 2-OHE1 and simultaneously inhibits 4-hydroxylation of estradiol to yield 4-OHE1, a known carcinogen.[84] Although it has been a concern that this enzyme induction would activate carcinogens such as DMBA, in practice

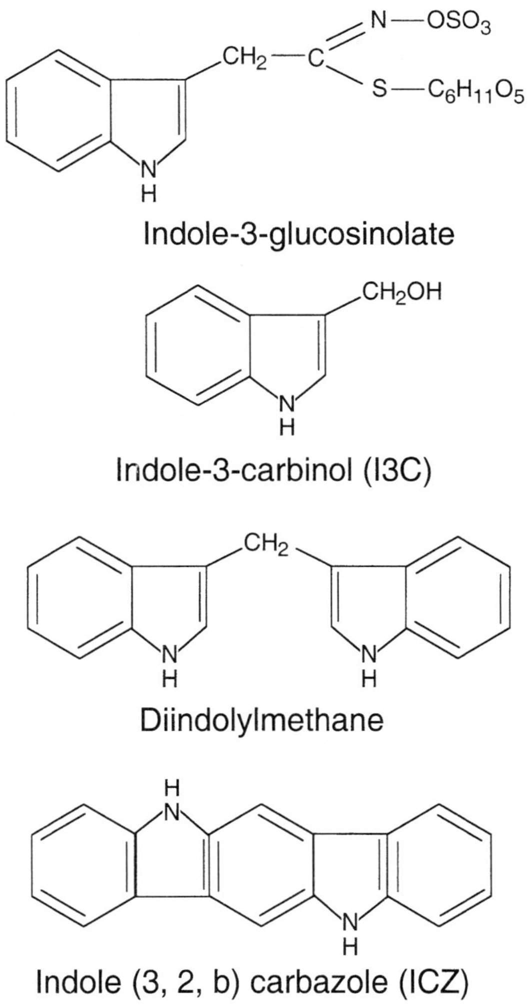

FIGURE 10.

this has not happened. The addition of I3C blocks the action of DMBA on estrogen metabolism and on cell proliferation.[85] Administration of I3C prior to B-α-P decreased the incidence of single-strand DNA breaks.[41] DIM is relatively specific in inducing only P4501A1 but not P4503A4, the enzyme responsible for 16α-hydroxylation, whereas the trimers derived from I3C also induce 3A4 to some extent.

Cyclin Action. Several studies by Bjeldanes *et al.*[86] and Safe *et al.*[87] have shown that DIM and related compounds can act directly on cyclin D to inhibit the cell cycle and block proliferation. Recent reports have indicated that indoles can also promote apoptosis by altering the Bax/Bcl2 ratio.[88,89]

Indirectly by promotion of 2-hydroxylation, proliferation of HPV is also blocked by turning off the E6 and E7 exons, key elements in cell growth.[90] Direct addition of 2-OHE1 has been shown to be equally potent in effecting this blockade of HPV proliferation.

Enzyme Inhibition and Activation. Studies by Manson et al.[91] have shown that I3C inhibits ornithine decarboxylase and several other enzymes in a dose-dependent manner and also acts to inhibit cell growth and proliferation. In addition to the induction of cytochromes, I3C has also been shown to induce phase II enzymes, which increase conjugation and elimination of carcinogens.

Synergistic Response. Cell culture studies by Firestone and Bjeldanes[92] have shown a synergistic response between tamoxifen and I3C. In preliminary data from human studies in breast cancer patients receiving tamoxifen, the addition of DIM results in a substantial increase in 2-OHE1/16OHE1.[93] This increase was the result of a specific enzyme induction in cell cultures. Further studies on this effect are underway. Because this metabolite ratio is related to breast cancer survival, studies affecting this metabolite ratio are of considerable importance. Preliminary studies also indicate synergism between ICZ and sulforaphane.[41]

Animal Studies. Treatment of mice carrying MMTV showed that feeding I3C in the diet resulted in substantial inhibition of mammary tumor formation and multiplicity.[94,95] Additional studies by Grubbs et al.[96] showed that feeding I3C virtually eliminated mammary tumors in mice given DMBA as a specific tumor inducer. A substantial decrease in NMU-induced mammary tumors was also observed.[96] Kojima et al.[97] also reported that I3C decreased tumor formation in the Donryku rat. Other studies have shown that I3C acts to block both tumor initiation and, in most cases, tumor promotion. Under certain circumstances, particularly with aflatoxin as the carcinogen, I3C can act as a tumor promoter when given after initiation has already occurred.[98] Human studies show no evidence of tumor promotion by I3C.

The I3C trimer ICZ binds to the Ah receptor and induces P4501A1 expression both *in vivo* and *in vitro*. A broad spectrum of antiestrogenic responses, including inhibition of cell proliferation, thymidine uptake, PR binding, and CAT activity, is observed. ICZ can also bind directly to the estrogen receptor with weak affinity and exhibits weak estrogen-like activity. ICZ antiestrogenic responses can also be observed in circumstances in which EROD activity is unchanged. ICZ is less desirable, because it can exhibit both estrogenic and antiestrogenic activities.[99] Because of the mixed character of the response to ICZ, the use of DIM, which is stable and not converted to ICZ, is preferable. Increased formation of 2-OHE1 is also of interest, because its further metabolite, 2-methoxyestradiol, has been reported to be an antiantigenic agent.[100]

I3C has also been shown to accelerate the metabolism of 4-(methylnitrosamino)-1-3-pyridyl)-1-butanone and its clearance in smokers. The formation of the corresponding alcohol and its glucuronide was decreased, alhtough the ratio of the conjugate to the free compound was increased.[101] Studies in A/J mice treated with NNK showed that I3C inhibited tumor formation by 40%. The mechanism appeared to be decreased availability of NNK, because of I3C induced further metabolism of NNK and a decrease in DNA methylation.[102]

2,3,7,8-Tetrachlorodibenzo-*p*-dioxin and DIM differentially induce CyP450 1A1, 1B1, and 19 in H295R human adrenocortical carcinoma cells. DIM alters estrogen metabolism and blocks the effect of estrogens via inhibition of AhR:ER cross-talk. TCDD and DIM reduced EROD metabolism. DIM, but not TCDD, increased aromatase activity, TCDD increased CyP 1A1 and 1B1 but not CyP 19, and DIM increased all three. Multiple pathways are involved.[103] AhR, CyP 1A1, and its mRNA were measured in DMBA-induced mammary tumors. Higher AhR amd high AhR mRNA levels were found in tumor tissue. Whereas initially AhR induces 1A1 and 1B1 levels, only 1B1 nRNA activity remained elevated in tumors. This is a partial explanation for the mechanism. 1B1 may be a key marker.[104]

DIM at 10–50 mM results in rapid AhR complex formation and induction of 1A1 such as TCDD. DIM at these doses inhibits DMBA tumor proliferation by E2. At low doses (5 mg/kg) DIM inhibits DMBA-induced tumors in SD rats without CyP-1A1 induction.[105]

Carcinogenesis by aflatoxin B1 is promoted by I3C when given after initiation has occurred. The influence of dose level, duration, and intermittent dosing were explored. I3C fed before and during aflatoxin B dosing inhibited tumor promotion, whereas I3C given afterwards acts as a promoter. In trout, I3C was as good at blocking tumors when given before as it was potent as a promoter when given afterwards.[106]

In a review, Zhu and Conney[107] proposed that 2-OHE1 and 2-MeOE2 may be protective against tumors, although no mechanism was offered. DIM at 50 mM induces apoptosis. It acts by a pathway that is independent of the P53 pathway.[108]

The effect of broccoli consumption on human *in vivo* drug-metabolizing enzymes was studied by Vang. Broccoli increased the 2/16 metabolite ratio, but CyP 2E1 was less affected.[109]

I3C was studied in CaSKI cervical cells. E2 enhanced transcription of HPY16 E6 and E7 exons. Both I3C and 2-OHE1 inhibited viral E6/E7 expression. 1B1 expression was also decreased. I3C appears to be act via increased 2-OHE1.[110] I3C prevents cervical cancer in KMHPY15 transgenic mice. E2 promotes tumor formation, whereas I3C inhibits initiation of HPV16 cervical cancer in mice.[111] Evidence for I3C as scavenger of free radicals *in vitro*. I3C and indole-3-acetic acid are both good scavengers, but I3C is better. Indole-3-aldehyde is the product of the scavenging reaction. Adducts from scavenging have also been detected.[112]

Cytostatic and antiestrogenic effects of 2(indol-3-methyl)-3,3′-diindolylmethane (LTR_ (a major metabolite of I3C) were studied. LTR inhibited the growth of estrogen-dependent MCF-7 and MDA MB 231 cells. At 25 mM, LTR only works in the presence of E2. LTR-1 inhibits E2-induced binding of ER to the DNA response element and increased 1A1.[113]

Human Studies

These studies have focused on two distinct responses: (1) inhibition of HPV-induced tumors; and (2) breast cancer, in which a number of studies have shown that breast cancer risk is associated with a decrease in the 2/16 hydroxyestrone metabolite ratio.

Laryngeal Papillomatosis. Based on animal studies showing that administration of I3C prevents the formation of papillomatous cysts in nude mice,[114] a treatment regimen was developed for children with laryngeal papillomas.[115–117] Following clearing of any papillomas present in the throat, treatment with I3C (~200 mg) was started. Its efficacy was monitored by measuring the urinary 2/16-metabolite ratio. Approximately two thirds of the children showed an increase in the metabolite ratio, which corresponded with the absence of further papilloma development. In some cases, children who failed to respond to I3C responded when DIM was substituted for I3C.

Cervical Dysplasia. Because the same virus is present in cervical dysplasia, a double-blind study in which I3C or a placebo was administered to groups of women for 12 weeks was carried out. Approximately 50% of the women showed a favorable response. A larger trial using DIM is currently underway.[118]

A series of case control and prospective studies on newly diagnosed cases of breast cancer carried out in different countries has shown that the 2/16 metabolite ratio is lower in cases than in controls.[119–124] The ratio was lowest in severe cases.[124,126] Studies by Kuller and others[126–129] have shown two interlinking findings: (1) that high bone

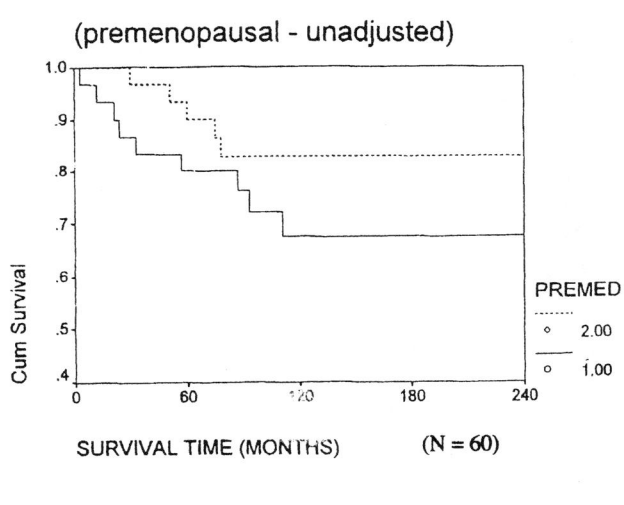

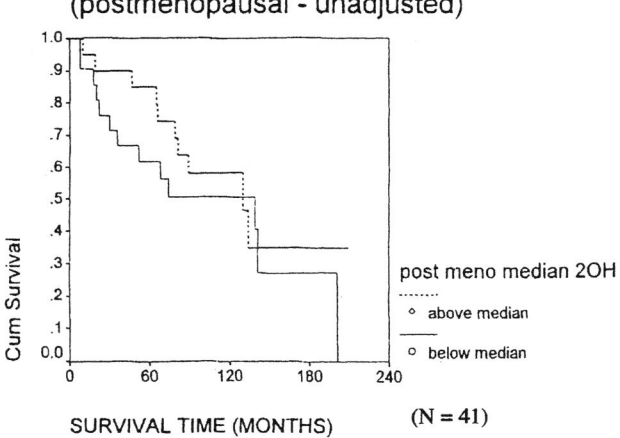

FIGURE 11. Survival by median 20HE. (**Top**) Premenopausal, unadjusted. (**Bottom**) Postmenopausal, unadjusted.

density is associated with both increased breast cancer risk and increased 16-hydroxylation; and (2) conversely, that women with low bone density show decreased breast cancer risk and an increase in 2-hydroxylation. These findings are among the strongest evidence for the role of the metabolite ratio in breast cancer.

When the metabolite ratios in cases in the prospective study, carried out on Guernsey, were ranked from high to low, those patients with ratios above the median level lived longer than did those patients with ratios below the median level (FIG. 11).

Recent results in women from remote areas of China, Japan, and the Philippines showed higher metabolite ratios than those in women from the same countries living in cities or migrants to the west.[130] The migrants consistently showed lower metabolite ratios. Studies to see if the metabolite ratio in women with breast cancer can be elevated by treatment with DIM are being performed. Timing of the studies is critical. If one selects a subset of patients who survived for many years free of disease, these women have metabolite ratios comparable to those of control subjects.[131,132] These results are similar to our findings on Guernsey.

SUMMARY

As just outlined, a promising role for a variety of micronutrients, both in chemoprevention and in chemotherapy of hormone-related tumors, is clear. Both cell cultures and animal studies have shown successful responses against tumors with a variety of promising agents. Successful results have been obtained in human patients against HPV-induced tumors including laryngeal papillomas, cervical dysplasia, and warts. Exploratory work is underway at expanding this progress to human breast cancer. Initial results show that the combination of micronutrients such as Dim or sulforathane together with chemotherapeutic agents such as tamoxifen produces better responses than does either agent alone. In early studies the combination of tamoxifen and DIM resulted in a higher 2/16a-metabolite ratio than did either compound alone. The same is true for mixtures of DIM and isothiocyanates. It seems clear that the future is the use of combinations of micronutrients acting in different ways to produce an enhanced response. The role of obesity, milk, or alcohol consumption as major nutrients is still somewhat controversial, but they may play an important role as risk factors.

REFERENCES

1. CARROLL, K.K. 1991. Nutrition and Cancer: Fat, Nutrition, Toxicity and Cancer. :439–453.CRC Press. Boca Raton, FL.
2. CARROLL, K.K. 1975. Experimental evidence of dietary factors and hormone dependent cancers Cancer Res. **35:** 3374–3383.
3. CARROLL, K.K. & L.M. BRADEN. 1985. Dietary fat and mammary carcinogenesis. Nutr. Cancer **6:** 254–259.
4. COLDITZ, G.A. 1993. Epidemiology of breast cancer. Cancer **71:** 1480–1489.
5. HOLMES, M.D., D.J. HUNTER, G.A. COLDITZ, et al. Association of dietary intake of fat and fatty acids with risk of breast cancer J. Am. Med. Assoc. **281:** 914–920.
6. KNEKT, P., D. ALBANES, R. SEPPANEN, et al. 1990. Dietary fat and risk of breast cancer. J. Clin. Nutr. **52:** 903–908.

7. BOYD, N.F., L.J. MARTIN, M. NOFFEL, *et al.* 1993. A meta-analysis of studies of dietary fat and breast cancer risk. Br. J. Cancer **68:** 627–636.
8. PAFFENBERGER, R.S., J.B. KAMPERT & H.G. CHANG. 1980. Characteristics that predict risk of breast cancer before and after the menopause. Am. J. Epidemiol. **112:** 258–268.
9. KIRSCHNER, M.A., G. SCHNEIDER, N.H. ERTEL, *et al.* 1982. Obesity, androgens, estrogens and cancer risk. Cancer Res. **85:** 578–583.
10. SCHNEIDER, J., H.L. BRADLOW, G. STRAIN, *et al.* 1983. Effects of obesity on estradiol metabolism: decreased formation of non-nutero-tropic metabolites. J. Clin. Endocrinol. Metab. **56:** 973–978.
11. SNOW, R., R. BARBIERI & R. FRISCH. 1991. Estrogen 2-hydroxylase oxidation and menstrual function among elite oarswomen. J. Clin. Endocrinol. Metab. **69:** 369–376.
12. FISHMAN, J. & H.L. BRADLOW. 1977. Effect of mallnutrition on the metabolism of sex hormones in man. Clin. Pharmacol. Ther. **22:** 721–723.
13. BRADLOW, H.L., R. TIWARI, D.W. SEPKOVIC, *et al.* 2002. The role of adipocytes as a breast cancer risk factor. Anticancer Res. In press.
14. FRISCH, R.E. & R. REVELLE. 1971. Height and weight at menarche and a hypothesis of menarche. Arch. Dis. Child. **46:** 695–701.
15. HILAKIVI-CLARKE, L.R., I. ONOJAFE, M. RAYGADA, *et al.* 1997. A maternal diet high in n-6 polyunsaturated fats alters human breast gland development, puberty onset, and breast cancer risk among female rat offspring. Proc. Soc. Acad. Sci. USA **94:** 9372–9377.
16. ARMSTRONG, B. & R. DOLL. 1975. Environmental factors and cancer incidence and mortality in different countries, with special refrence to dietary practices. Int. J. Cancer **15:** 617–631.
17. ROSE, D.P., A.P. BOYAR & E.L. WYNDER. 1986. International comparisons of mortality rates for cancer of the breast, ovary, prostate, and colon and per capita food consumption. Cancer **58:** 2363–2371.
18. STOCKS, P. & M.N. KARN. 1933. A coooperative study of home life, dietary and family hostories of 430 cancer paatients and an equal number of control patients. Ann. Eugenics **5:** 237–242.
19. URSIN, G., E. BJELKE, I. HEUCH & S.E. VOLLSET. 1990. Milk consumption and cancer incidence: a Norwegian prospective study. Br. J. Cancer **61:** 454–459.
20. KNEKT, P., R. JARVINEN, R. SEPPANEN, *et al.* 1996. Intake of dairy products and the risk of breast cancer. Br. J. Cancer **73:** 687–691.
21. HJARTAKER, A., P. LAAKE & E. LUND. 2001. Childhood and adult milk consumption and risk of premenopausal breast cancer in a cohort of 48,844 women: the Norwegian women and cancer study. Int. J. Cancer **93:** 888–893.
22. WILLETT, W.C. 2001. Eat, Drink and Be Healthy. Simon & Schuster. New York.
23. HOWE, G., T. ROHAN, A. DECARLLI, *et al.* 1991. The association between alcohol and breast cancer risk: evidence from the combined analysis of six dietary case-control studies. Int. J. Cancer **47:** 707–710.
24. LONGNECKER, M.P. 1994. Alcoholic beverage consumption in relation to risk of breast cancer: meta-analysis and review. Cancer Causes Control **5:** 73–82.
25. LONGNECKER, M.P., J.A. BERLIN, M.J. ORZA, *et al.* 1988. A meta-analysis of alcohol consumption in relation to risk of breast cancer. J. Am. Med. Assoc. 260: 652–656.
26. MUTI, P., M. TREVISON, A. MICHELI, *et al.* 1998. Alcohol consumption and total estradiol in premenopausal women. Cancer Epidemiol. Biomarkers Prev. **7:** 1890–1893.
27. PUROHIT, V. 1998. Moderate alcohol consumption and estrogen levels in postmenopausal women. Alcoholism: Clin. Exp. Res. **22:** 994–997.
28. COLDITZ, G.A., E. GIOVANNUCCI, E.B. RIMM, *et al.* 1991. Alcohol intake in relation to diet and obesity in women and men. Am. J. Clin. Nutr. **54:** 49–55.
29. RIMM, E.B. 1996. Alcohol consumption and coronary heart disease: good habits may be more important than just good wine. Am. J. Epidemiol. **143:** 1094–1098.
30. SCHWARTZ, A.G. 1979. Inhibition of spontaneous breast cancer formation in female C3H (A vy/a) mice by long-term treatment with dehydroepiandrosterone. Cancer Res. Colditz **39:** 1129–1132.
31. SCHWARTZ, A.G., J.M. WHITCOMB, J.W. NYCE, *et al.* 1988. Dehydroepiandrosterone and structural analogs: a new class of cancer chemopreventive agents. Adv. Cancer Res. **51:** 391–424.

32. ZHANG, Y., P. TALALAY, C.G. CHO, et al. 1992. A major inducer of anticarcinogenic protective enzymes from broccoli: isolation and elucidation of structure. Proc. Natl. Acad. Sci. USA **89:** 2399–2403.
33. TACHE, S., G. PEIFFER, A.-S. MILLET & D.E. CORPET. 2000. Inhibition of methyl-*n*-amylnitrosamine hydroxylation by diallyl sulfide and phenethylisothiocyanate in the rat. Nutr. & Cancer **37:** 299–305.
34. ZHANG, Y., K.L. WADE, T. PRESTERA & P. TALALAY. 1996. Quantitative determination of isothiocyanates, dithiocarbamates, carbon disulfide, and related thiocarbonyl compounds by cyclocondensation with 1,2-benzenedithiol. Anal. Biochem. **239:** 160–167.
35. ZHANG, Y., R.H. KOLM, B. MANNERVIK & P. TALALAY. 1995. Reversible conjugation of isothiocyanates with glutathione catalyzed by human glutathione transferases. Biochem. Biophys. Res. Commun. **206:** 748–755.
36. DEPRIMO, S.E. & J.D. BROOKS. 2000. Microarray analysis and prostate cancer research. CTCL.Comsult.com
37. ROSA, E., R.K. HEANEY, R. FENWICK & C.A.M. PORTAS. 1996. Changes in glucosinolate concentrations in Brassica crops (*Brassica oleracea* and *B. napus*) throughout growing seasons. J. Sci. Food Agric. **71:** 237–244.
38. FAHEY, J.W., Y. ZHANG & P. TALALAY. 1997. Broccoli sprouts: an exceptionally rich source of inducers of enzymes that protect against chemical carcinogens. Proc. Natl. Acad. Sci.USA **94:** 10367–10371.
39. POSNER, G.H., C.G. CHO, J.V. GREEN, et al. 1994. Design of bifunctional isothiocyanate analogs of sulforaphane: correlation between structure and potency as inducers of anti-carcinogenic detoxification enzymes. J. Med. Chem. **37:** 170–176.
40. GERHAUSER, C. et al. 1997. Cancer chemopreventive potential of sulforamate, a novel analogue of sulforaphane that induces phase 2 drug-metabolizing enzymes. Cancer Res. **57:** 272–277.
41. BONNESEN, C., I.M. EGGLESTON & I.D. HAYES. 2001. Dietary indoles and isothiocyanates that are generated from cruciferous vegetables can both stimulate apoptosis and confer protection against DNA damage in human colon cell lines. J. Cancer Res. **61:** 6120–6130.
42. BROOKS, J.D., V.G. PATON & G. VIDANES. 2001. Potent induction of phase 2 enzymes in human prostate cells by sulforaphane. Cancer Epidemiol. Biomarkers Prev. **10:** 949–954.
43. ZHANG, Y., R.H. KOLM, B. MANNERVIK & P. TALALAY. 1994. Reversible conjugation of isothiocyanates with glutathione catalyzed by human glutathione transferases. J. Med. Chem. **37:** 170–176.
44. JUNSHI, C. 1992. The antimutagenic and anticarcinogenic effects of tea, garlic and other natural foods in China: a review. Biomed. Environ. Sci. **5:** 1–17.
45. HUANG, M.T., C.T. HO, Z.Y. WANG, et al. 1992. Inhibitory effect of topical application of a green tea polyphenol fraction on tumor initiation and promotion in mouse skin. Carcinogenesis **13:** 947–954.
46. SAKAGAMI, H., K. ASANO, Y. HARA & T. SHIMAMURA. 1992. Stimulation of human monocyte and polymorphonuclear cell iodination and interleukin-1 production by epigallocatechin gallate. J. Leukocyte Biol. **51:** 478–483.
47. GAO, Y.T., J.K. MCLAUGHLIN, W.J. BLOT, et al. 1994. Reduced risk of esophageal cancer associated with green tea consumption. J. Natl. Cancer Inst. **86:** 855–858.
48. JAIN, A.K., K. SHIMOI, Y. NAKAMURA, et al. 1989. Crude tea extracts decrease the mutagenic activity of *N*-methyl-*N*1-nitro-*N*-nitrosoguanidine *in vitro* and in intragastric tract of rats. Mutat. Res. **210:** 1–8.
49. MENAGAZZI, M., E. TEDESCHI, D. DUSSIN, et al. 2001. Anti-interferon g action of epigallocatechin-3-gallate mediated by specific inhibition of STAT1 activation. Faseb J. **15:** 1309–1311.
50. MICHNOVICZ, J.J. & H.L. BRADLOW. 1994. Dietary cytochrome P450 modifiers in the control of estrogen metabolism. *In* Food Phytochemicals for Cancer Prevention. I. M.T. Huang, T. Osawa, C.T. Ho & R.T. Rosen, eds. :282–293. American Chemical Society. Washington, DC.
51. FUJIKI, H., M. SUGANUMA, H. SUGURI, et al. 1990. New antitumour promoters: (1)-epigallocatecin gallate and sarcophytols A and B. *In* Basic Life Sciences: Antimutagen-

esis and Anticarcinogenesis Mechanisms II. Vol. 52. Y. Kuroda, D.M. Shankel, & M.D. Waters, eds. :205–212. Plenum Press. New York.
52. CROWELL, P.L., W.S. KENNAN, J.D. HAAG, *et al.* 1992. Chemoprevention of mammary carcinogenesis by hydroxylated derivatives of d-limonene. Carcinogenesis **13:** 1261–1264.
53. CROWELL, P.L., R.R. CHANG, Z. REN, *et al.* 1991. Selective inhibition of isoprenylation of 21-26-kDa proteins by the anticarcinogen d-Limonene and its metabolites. J. Biol. Chem. **266:** 17679–17685.
54. CROWELL, P.L., Z. REN, S. LIN, *et al.* 1994. Structure-activity relationships among monoterpene inhibitors of protein isoprenylation and cell proliferation. Biochem. Pharmacol. **47:** 1405–1415.
55. RIPPLE, G.H., M.N. GOULD, J.A. STEWART, *et al.* 1998. Phase I clinical trial of perillyl alcohol administered daily. Clin. Cancer Res. **4:** 1159–1164.
56. BAIRD, D.D., D.M. UMBACH, L. LANSDELL, *et al.* 1990. Dietary intervention study to assess estrogenicity of dietary soy among postmenopausal women. J. Clin. Endocrinol. Metab. **80:** 1685–1690.
57. KUIPER, G.G.J.M., B. CARLSSON, K. GRANDIEN, *et al.* 1997. Comparison of the ligand binding specificity and transcript tissue distribution of estrogen receptors alpha and beta. Endocrinology **138:** 863–870.
58. XU, X., A.M. DUNCAN, B.E. MERX & M.S. KURZER. 1998. Effects of soy isoflavones on estrogen and Phytoestrogen metabolism in premenopausal women Cancer Epidemiol. Biomarkers Prev. **7:** 1101–1108.
59. XU, X., A.M. DUNCAN, K.E. WANEN & M.S. KURZER. 2000. Soy consumption alters endogenous estrogen metabolism in postmenopausal women. Cancer Epidemiol. Biomarkers Prev. **9:** 781–786.
60. MARTINI, M.C., B.B. DANCISAK, C.J. HAGGANS, *et al.* 1999. Effects of soy intake on sex hormone metabolism in premenopausal women. Nutr. Cancer **34:** 133–139.
61. KISHIDA, T., M. BEPPU, K. NASHIKI, *et al.* 2000. Effect of dietary soy isoflavone aglycones on the urinary 16alpha-to-2-hydroxyestrone ratio in C3H/HeJ mice. Nutr. Cancer **38:** 209–214.
62. LU, J.W., M. CREE, S. JOSYULA *et al.* 2000. Increased urinary excretion of 2-hydroxyestrone but not 16a-hydroxyestrone in menopausal women during a soya diet containing isoflavones. Cancer Res. **60:** 1299–1305.
63. CREE, M., S. JOSYULA, K.E. ANDERSON, *et al.* 1999. Altered urinary excretion of 2-OH-estrone to 16-OH-estrone in women after soya isoflavone consumption (Abstr 2007). Proc. Am. Assoc. Cancer Res. **40:** 302.
64. MASKARINEC, G., A. FRANKE, J.S. INOUYE, *et al.* 2000. Estrogen metabolism in an isoflavone intervention among premenopausal women. Proc. Am. Assoc. Cancer Res. **42:** 311.
65. PERSKY, V.W., M.E. TURYK, L. WANG, *et al.* 2002. The effect of soy protein on endogenous hormones in postmenopausal women. Am. J. Clin. Nutr. **75:** 145–153.
66. TELANG, N.T., R. NARAYANAN, H.L. BRADLOW & M.P. OSBORNE. 1991. Coordinated expression of intermediate biomarkers for tumorigenic transformation in RAS transfected mouse mammary epithelial cells. Cancer Res. Treat. **13:** 155–163.
67. TONKELAAR, I. DEN, L. KEINAN-BOKER, P. VAN'T VEER, *et al.* 2001. Urinary phytoestrogens and postmenopausal breast cancer risk. Cancer Epidemiol. Biomarkers Prev. **10:** 223–228.
68. MURKIES, A.L., C. LOMBARD, B.J.G. STRAUSS, *et al.* 1995. Dietary flour supplementation decreases postmenopausal hot flushes: effect of soy and wheat. Maturitas **21:** 189–195.
69. BERRINO, F. 2001. Private communication.
70. SETCHELL, K.D.R., A.M. LAWSON, S.P. BORRIELLO, *et al.* 1981. Lignan formation in man: microbial involvement and possible roles in relation to cancer. Lancet **ii**(8236): 4–7.
71. MICHALUART, P. & J.L. MASFERRER, A.M. CAROTHERS, *et al.* 1999. Inhibitory effects of caffeic acid phenethyl ester (CAPE) on the activity and expression of cyclooxygenase-2 in human oral epithelial cells and in a rat model of inflammation. Cancer Res. **59:** 2347–2352.
72. CHANG, S.E., M.L. KU, C.H. HSU, *et al.* 2000. Curcumin-containing diet inhibits diethylnitrosoamine-induced mouse hepatocarcinogenesis. Carcinogenesis **21:** 331–335.

73. RAO, C.V., A. RIVENSON, B. SIMI & B.S. REDDY. 1995. Chemoprevention of colon carcinogenesis by dietary curcumin, a naturally occurring plant phenolic compound. Cancer Res. **59:** 259–266.
74. BABU, P.S. & K. SRINIVASAI. 1995. Influence of dietary curcumin and cholesterol on the progression of experimentally induced diabetes in albino rats. Molec. Cell. Biochem. **152:** 13–21.
75. RUBY, A., G. KUTTEN, K.D. BABU, et al. 1995. Anti-tumor and anti-oxidant activity of natural curcuminoids. Cancer Lett. **94:** 79–83.
76. ANTO, R.J., J. GEORGE, K.V.D. BABU & K.N. RAJASIKHARER. 1996. Anti-mutagenic and anti-carcinogenic activity of natural and synthetic curcuminoids. Mutat. Res. **370:** 127–131.
77. FIROZI, P.F., D.S. ABOOBKER, R.Y. BHATTACHARNJA, et al. 1996. Action of curcumin on the cytochrome-P450 system catalyzing the activation of aflatoxin B1. Chem. Biol. Interact. **100:** 41–51.
78. CHENG, A.L., C.-H. HSU, J.-K. LIN, et al. 2001. Phase I clinical trial for curcumin, a chemopreventive agent, in patients with high-risk or pre-malignant lesions. Anti-Cancer Res. **21:** 2895–2900.
79. GUARINI, L., X.X. SU, S. XUCJER, et al. 1992. Growth Inhibition and antigenic phenotype in human melanoma and glioblastoma multiforme cells by caffeic acid phenylethyl ester. Cell. Molec. Biol. **38:** 513–527.
80. HUANG, M.T., Y.R. LOU, W. MA, et al. 1994. Inhibitory effects of dietary curcumin on forstomach, duodenal, and colon carcinogenesis in mice. Cancer Res. **58:** 5841–5847.
81. JELLINCK, P.H., P.G. FORKERT, D.S. RIDDICK, et al. 1992. Ah receptor binding properties of indole carbinols and induction of hepatic estradiol hydroxylation. Biochem. Pharmacol. **45:** 1139–1152.
82. BRADLOW, H.L., J.J. MICHNOVICZ, N.T. TELANG & M.P. OSBORNE. 1991. Effect of dietary indole-3 carbinol on estradiol metabolism and spontaneous mammary tumors in mice. Carcinogenesis **12:** 1571–1574.
83. BJELDANES, L.J., J.Y. KIM, K.R. GROSS, et al. 1991. Aromatic hydrocarbon responsiveness-receptor agonists generated from indole-3-carbinol *in vitro* and *in vivo*: comparisons with 2,3,7,8-tetrachlorodibenzo-*p*-dioxin. Proc. Natl. Acad. Sci. **88:** 9543–9547.
84. YUAN, F., D. CHEN, K. LIU, et al. 1999. Anti-estrogenic effect of indole-3-carbinol in cervical cancer cells: implications for estrogen-related carcinogenesis. Anticancer Res. **19:** 673–680.
85. TELANG, N.T., M. BRADLOW & M.P. OSBORNE. 1997. Estradiol metabolism: an endocrine biomarker for modulation of human mammary carcinogenesis. Environ. Health Perspect. **109:** 559–562.
86. HONG, C., G.F. FIRESTONE & L.F. BELDANES. 2000. 3,3'-Diindolylmethane (DIM), a dietary indole, has multiple cell suppressive effects on MCF-7 human breast cancer cells. Am. Soc. Cell Biol. 40th annual meeting.
87. CHEN, I., A. MCDOUGAL, F. WONG & S. SAFE. 1998. Carcinogenesis **19:** 1631–1639.
88. HONG, C., G.F. FIRESTONE & L.F. BJELDANES. 2000. BCL-2 family mediated apoptotic effects of 3,3'-diindolylmethane (DIM) in human breast cancer cells. Biochem. Pharmacol. **63:** 1085–1097.
89. COVER, C.M., S.J. HSIEH, S.H. TRAN, et al. 1998. Indole-3-carbinol inhibits the expression of cyclin-dependent kinase-6 and induces a G1 cell cycle arrest of human breast cancer cells independent of estrogen receptor signaling. J. Biol. Chem. **273:** 3838–3847.
90. LIANG, J., Q. MEI, C. DA-ZHI, et al. 1999. Indole-3-carbinol prevents cervical cancer in human papilloma virus type 16 (HPV16) transgenic mice. Cancer Res. **59:** 3991–3997.
91. MANSON, M.M., E.A. HUDSON, H.W. BALL, et al. 1998. Chemoprevention of aflatoxin B1-induced carcinogenesis by indole-3-carbinol in rat liver-predicting the outcome using early biomarkers. Carcinogenesis **19:** 1829–1836.
92. COVER, C.M., S.J. HSIEH, E.J. CRAM, et al. 1999. Indole-3-carbinol and tamoxifen cooperate to arrest the cell cycle of MCF-7 human breast cancer cells. Cancer Res. **59:** 1244–1251.

93. ZELIGS, M. Private communication.
94. BRADLOW, H.L., R.J. HERSHCOPF, C.P. MARTUCCI & J. FISHMAN. 1985. Estradiol 16α-hydroxylation in the mouse correlates with mammary tumor incidence and presence of murine mammary tumor virus: a possible model for the hormonal etiology of breast cancer in humans. Proc. Natl. Acad. Sci. USA **82:** 6295–6299.
95. MALLOY, V., H.L. BRADLOW, J. MATIAS & N. ORENTREICH. 1998. Interaction between a semisynthetic diet and indole-3-carbinol on mammary tumor incidence in Balb/cfC3H mice. Anticancer Res. **17:** 4333–4338.
96. GRUBBS, C., V.E. STEELE, T. CASEBOLT, *et al.* 1995. Chemoprevention of chemically induced mammary carcinogenesis by indole-3-carbinol. Anticancer Res. **15:** 709–716.
97. KOJIMA, T., T. TANAKA & M. MORI. 1994. Chemoprevention of spontaneous endometrial cancer in female Donryku rats by dietary indole-3-carbinol. Cancer Res. **54:** 1446–1449.
98. DASHWOOD, R.H., A.T. FONG, D.E. WILLIAMS, *et al.* 1991. Promotion of afiotoxin B1 carcinogenesis by the natural tumor modulator indole-3-carbinol: influence of dose, duration, and intermittent exposure on indole-3-carbinol promotional potency. Cancer Res. **51:** 2362–2365.
99. LIU, H., M. WORMKE, S.H. SAFE & L.F. BJELDANES. 1994. Indolo[3,2-b]carbazole: a dietary-derived factor that inhibits both antiestrogenic and estrogenic activity. J. Natl. Cancer Inst. **86:** 1758–1765.
100. FOTSIS, T., Y. ZHANG, M.S. PEPPER, *et al.* 1994. The endogenous estrogen metabolite 2-methoxuestradiol inhibits angiogenesis and suppresses tumor growth. Nature **368:** 237–239.
101. TAIOLI, E., S. GARBERS, H.L. BRADLOW, *et al.* 1997. Effect of indole-3-carbinol on the mechanism of 4-(methylnitrosoamino)-1-(pyridyl)-1-butanone in smokers. Cancer Epidemiol. Biomarkers Prevent. **6:** 517–522.
102. MORSE, M.A., S.D. LAGRECA, S.G. AMIN & F.-L. CHUNG. 1990. Effects of indole-3-carbinol on lung tumorigenesis and dna methylation induced by 4-(methylnitrosoamino)-1-(3-pyridyl)-1-butanone (NNK) and on the metabolism and disposition of NNK in A/J mice. Cancer Res. **50:** 2613–2617.
103. SANDERSON, J.T., L. SLOBBE, W.A. LANSVERGEN, *et al.* 2001. 2,3,7,8-Tetrachlorodibenzo-*p*-dioxin and diindolylmethanes differentially induce cytochrome P450 1A1, 1B1, and 19 in H295R human adrenocortical carcinoma cells. Toxicol. Sci. **61:** 40–48.
104. TROMBINO, A.F., R.I. NEAR, R.A. MATULKA, *et al.* 2000. Expression of the aryl hydrocarbon receptor/transcription factor (AhR) and AhR-regulated CYP1 gene transcripts in a rat model of mammary tumorigenesis. Breast Cancer Res. & Treatment **63:** 117–131.
105. CHEN, I., A. MCDOUGAL, F. WONG & S. SAFE. 1998. Aryl hydrocarbon receptor-mediated antiestrogenic and antitumorigenic activity of diindolylmethane. Carcinogenesis **19:** 1631–1639.
106. TAKAHASHI, N., R.H. DASHWOOD, L.F. BJELDANES, *et al.* 1995. Mechanisms of indole-3-carbinol (I3C) anticarcinogenesis: inhibition of aflatoxin B1-DNA adduction and mutagenesis by I3C acid condensation products. Food Chem.Toxicol. **33:** 851–857.
107. ZHU, B.T. & A.H. CONNEY. 1998. Is 2-methoxyestradiol an endogenous estrogen metabolite that inhibits mammary carcinogenesis. Cancer Res. **58:** 2269–2277.
108. CHEN, I., A. MCDOUGAL, F. WONG & S. SAFE. 1998. Aryl hydrocarbon receptor-mediated antiestrogenic and antitumorigenic activity of diindolylmethane. Carcinogenesis **19:** 1631–1639.
109. KALL, M.A., O. VANG & J. CLAUSEN. 1996. Effects of dietary broccoli on human *in vivo* drug metabolizing enzymes: evaluation of caffeine, estrone and chlorzoxazone. Carcinogenesis **30:** 793–799.
110. NEWFIELD, L., A. GOLDSMITH, H.L. BRADLOW & K. AUBORN. 1993. Estrogen metabolism and human papillomavirus-induced tumors of the larynx: chemoprophylaxis with indole-3-carbinol. Anticancer Res. **13:** 337–341.

111. AUBORN, K., A. ABRAMSON, H.L. BRADLOW, et al. 1995. Cruciferous vegetables as adjunct therapy for laryngeal papillomatosis, a pilot study workshop on respiratory papillomatosis. Quebec, Canada, July 1995.
112. JIN, L., M. QI, D.Z. CHEN, et al. 1999. Indole-3-carbinol prevents cervical cancer in human papilloma virus type 16 (HPV16) transgenic mice. Cancer Res. **59:** 3991–3997.
113. ARNAO, M.B., J. SANCHEZ-BRAVO & M. ACOSTA. 1996. Indole-3-carbinol as a scavenger of free radicals. Biochem. Molec. Biol. Int. **39:** 1125–1134.
114. CHANG, Y.C., J. RIBY, G.H.F. CHANG, et al. 1999. Cytostatic and antiestrogenic effects of 2-(indol-3-ylmethyl-3, 3′-diindolylmethane, a major *in vivo* product of dietary indole-3-carbinol. Biochem. Pharmacol. **58:** 825–834.
115. AUBORN, K., A. ABRAMSON, H.L. BRADLOW, et al. 1998. Estrogen metabolism and laryngeal papillomatosis: a pilot study. Anticancer Res. **18:** 4569–4573.
116. COLL, D.A., C.A. ROSEN, K. AUBORN, et al. 1997. Treatment of recurrent respiratory papillomatosis with indole-3-carbinol. Am. J. Otolaryngol. **18:** 283–285.
117. ROSEN, C.A., G.E. WOODSON, J.W. THOMPSON, et al. 1998. Preliminary results of the use of indole-3-carbinol for recurrent respiratory papillomatosis. Otolaryngol. Head Neck **118:** 810–815.
118. BELL, M.C., P. CROWLEY-NOWICK, H.L. BRADLOW, et al. 2000. Placebo-controlled trial of indole-3-carbinol in the treatment of CIN. Gynecol. Oncol. **78:** 123–129.
119. MEILAHN, E.N., B. DE STAVOLA, D.S. ALLEN, et al. 1998. Do urinary estrogen metabolites predict breast cancer? Follow up of the Guernsey III cohort. Br. J. Cancer **78:** 1250–1255.
120. KABAT, G.C., C.J. CHANG, J.A. SPARANO, et al. 1997. Urinary estrogen metabolites and breast cancer: a case-control study. Cancer Epidemiol. Biomarkers Prevent. **6:** 505–509.
121. HO, G.H., X.W. LUO, C.Y. JI, et al. 1998. Using 2/16 alpha-hydroxyestrone ratio: correlation with serum insulin-like growth factor binding protein-3 and a potential biomarker of breast cancer risk. Ann. Acad. Med. Singapore **27:** 294–299.
122. MUTI, P., H.L. BRADLOW, A. MICHELI, et al. 2000. Estrogen metabolism and risk of breast cancer: a prospective study of the 2:16 alpha-hydroxyestrone ratio in premenopausal and postmenopausal women. Epidemiology **11:** 635–640.
123. FOWKE, J.H., D. QI, H.L. BRADLOW, et al. 2002. Modification of the estrogen metabolite and breast cancer association by urine collection protocol in the Shanghai Breast Cancer Study. Cancer Epidemiol. Biomarkers Prevent. In press.
124. DUPONT, E., T. KLUG, C. MCCANN, et al. 2000. The prognostic value of altered estrogen metabolism in breast cancer. Ann. Surg. Oncol. 7(suppl): Abstr 24.
125. FLEISHER, M., D. SEPKOVIC, H.L. BRADLOW & M.K. SCHWARTZ. 1996. Estrogen metabolite ratios as biomarkers of hormonally related breast cancer risk. Clin. Chem. **42:** Abstr 5361.
126. KULLER, L.H., J.A. CAULEY, L. LUCAS, et al. 1997. Sex steroid hormones, bone mineral density and risk of breast cancer. Environ. Health Perspect. **105:** (suppl. 3) 593–599.
127. KULLER, L.H., K.A. MATTHEWS & E.N. MEILHAN. 2000. Estrogens and women's health: interrelation of coronary heart disease, breast cancer, and osteoporosis. J. Steroid. Biochem. **74:** 297–309.
128. LEELAWATTANA, R., Z. ZIAMBARAS, J. ROODMAN-WEISS, et al. 2000. The oxidative metabolism of estradiol conditions post-menopausal bone density and bone loss. J. Bone Miner Res. **15:** 2513–2520.
129. ZMUDA, J.M., J.A. CAULEY, B.M. LJUNG, et al. 2001. Bone mass and breast cancer risk in older women: differences by stage at diagnosis. J. Natl. Cancer Inst. **93:** 930–936.
130. FALK, K. 2002. Private communication.
131. URSIN, G., S. LONDON, F.Z. STANCZYK, et al. 1999. Urinary 2-hydroxyestrone/16alpha-hydroxyestrone ratio and risk of breast cancer in postmenopausal women. J. Natl. Cancer Inst. **91:** 1967–1972.
132. SENIE, R. 2002. Private communication.

Effects of Weight Control and Physical Activity in Cancer Prevention

Role of Endogenous Hormone Metabolism

RUDOLF KAAKS AND ANNEKATRIN LUKANOVA

International Agency for Research on Cancer, 69372 Lyon Cedex 08, France

> ABSTRACT: Excess body weight and/or lack of physical activity are increasingly recognized as major risk factors for cancer of the colon, breast, endometrium, and prostate. This paper reviews the effects of excess body weight and physical inactivity on endogenous hormone metabolism (insulin, the IGF-I/IGFBP system, and sex steroids) and of endocrine alterations with risk of cancer of the endometrium, breast, prostate, and colon.
>
> KEYWORDS: weight control; physical activity; cancer prevention; endogenous hormone metabolism

INTRODUCTION

The cancer-preventive potential of chronically restricted dietary energy intake has long been known from animal studies.[1] Although there is little direct evidence for a similar protective effect of chronic energy restriction in humans, substantial epidemiologic evidence indicates that a relative excess of energy intake relative to the average daily expenditure is associated with an increased risk of several forms of cancer that are frequent in affluent societies. An international working group at the International Agency for Research on Cancer[2] recently judged that there was sufficient evidence that being overweight (as indicated by body mass index [BMI]; BMI = weight/height^2 greater than 25 kg/m^2) or obese (BMI >30 kg/m^2) is associated with increased risks of cancers of the endometrium, colon, kidney (renal cell tumors), as well as esophageal adenomas. In addition, excess body weight was associated with an increased risk of breast cancer diagnosed several years after menopause, whereas before menopause, paradoxically, obesity appears to confer mild protection against breast cancer. However, excess body weight appears to be unrelated to the risk of cancer of the rectum or prostate.

In addition to the risks of excess body weight, many epidemiologic studies have shown that regular physical activity may protect against cancers of the colon and breast and possibly other tumors such as those of the endometrium and prostate.[2] Globally, it was estimated that between one quarter and one third of the incidence of

---

Address for correspondence: Dr. Rudolf Kaaks, International Agency for Research on Cancer, 150 cours Albert Thomas, 69372 Lyon Cedex 08, France. Voice: 00 33 4 72 73 8553; fax: 00 33 4 72 73 8361.

kaaks@iarc.fr/lukanova@iarc.fr

cancers of the endometrium, colon, breast, kidney, and esophagus could be attributed to the combination of excess body weight and lack of physical activity.[2]

Physiologic mechanisms that have been proposed to explain the foregoing relationships of cancer risk with excess weight and lack of physical activity include increased gastric reflux and harmful effects of gastric acids on the esophageal mucosa, increased intestinal transit times and hence prolonged mucosal exposures to intraluminal cancer-initiating or cancer-promoting agents, alterations in endogenous free radical formation and oxidative damage, reduced DNA repair capacity, or altered activities of carcinogen-metabolizing enzymes. The present paper discusses some major effects of excess weight and physical inactivity on endogenous hormone metabolism and the possible relationships of these hormonal alterations with cancer risk. Emphasis is placed on the endogenous metabolism of insulin, the IGF-I/IGFBP system, and sex steroids in relation to cancers of the endometrium, breast, and prostate and colon.

EFFECTS OF OBESITY AND PHYSICAL INACTIVITY ON ENDOGENOUS HORMONE METABOLISM

Insulin Resistance

One major effect of both excess body weight and physical inactivity is the development of insulin resistance, that is, a reduced response of skeletal muscle, liver, and other tissue to the physiologic effects of insulin. Insulin resistance causes an increase in insulin secretion and in fasting and nonfasting (postprandial) plasma levels of insulin, so as to compensate for the reduction in tissue response and to maintain blood glucose concentrations within narrow, acceptable limits. There is generally a linear, continuous rise in fasting insulin with increasing body mass index (BMI), even within the range of BMI (of 20–25 kg/m^2) generally defined as "normal" or "healthy." Associated metabolic phenomena are increases in fasting plasma glucose, increased plasma levels of glucose and insulin after a standard oral glucose dose, rises in triglycerides and very-low-density lipoproteins (VLDLs), and a decrease in HDL cholesterol. Together, this constellation of metabolic changes, often also associated with a rise in blood pressure, is also referred to as the insulin resistance syndrome, or "syndrome X."[3]

Nutritionally induced insulin resistance (as opposed to some rare, genetically determined forms) is largely a consequence of increased muscular and hepatic uptake and oxidation of plasma free fatty acid for energy metabolism. Through complex intracellular regulatory mechanisms, this increase in uptake and oxidation of free fatty acids affects the tissues' capacity to absorb glucose and store glucose in the form of glycogen.[4] An increase particularly in intraabdominal fat stores (visceral adipose tissue), from which free fatty acids are easily mobilized and released into the circulation, is associated with reduced insulin sensitivity. Weight reduction and especially a loss of visceral adipose tissue has consistently been found to improve insulin sensitivity,[2,5] whereas weight regain usually is followed by a relative loss of insulin sensitivity.

Physical activity is generally associated with better insulin sensitivity and lower fasting plasma insulin levels in both cross-sectional studies and human intervention studies.[6,7] Even a single session of sustained submaximal exercise can improve insulin sensitivity acutely, although only for a limited duration of several days, through mechanisms unrelated to body weight or weight change. In the long term, regular physical activity may also improve insulin sensitivity by limiting weight gain or reducing excess weight.

IGF-I and IGF Binding Proteins

Insulin-like growth factors (IGFs) I and II are both central to the regulation of anabolic (growth) processes. The IGFs stimulate the proliferation and inhibit the programmed death (apoptosis) of cells. The bioactivity of IGF-I and IGF-II is modulated by at least six IGF-binding proteins (IGFBPs) that bind the IGFs with an affinity. The IGFs and IGFBPs are synthesized in all human tissues; however, most (over 80%) of the two IGFs and of IGFBPs in blood plasma originate in the liver. Major physiologic functions of the IGFBPs are to form a pool of IGF-I and IGF-II in the circulation, to regulate the efflux of IGFs from blood plasma towards target tissues, and to regulate the binding of IGFs to its cellular receptors. Several of the binding proteins (e.g., IGFBP-3 and IGFBP-5) have also been shown to exert physiologic effects through their own specific binding sites on cellular membranes. The biologic function of the IGFBPs themselves is further modulated by enzymatic phosphorylation or by cleavage of the IGFBPs by specific proteases. In the circulation, more than 90% of IGF-I and IGF-II is bound in a ternary complex of IGF-I, IGFBP-3, and another glycoprotein called "acid-labile subunit." Much smaller fractions of IGF-I in blood are bound to IGFBP-5, which also forms a complex with the acid-labile subunit, and to IGFBPs-1, -2, -4, and -6. Globally, IGF bioactivity is the overall result of endocrine, paracrine, and autocrine effects of IGFs and the various IGFBPs.

Plasma levels of IGF-I and IGFBP-1, -2, and -3, but not IGF-II and the other IGFBPs (-4, -5, and -6), depend on the amount of energy available from diet or body fat stores as well as the availability of essential nutrients, especially the essential amino acids.[8,9] The remainder of this text will therefore focus uniquely on IGF-I. The nutritional regulation of IGF-I and these three binding proteins is regulated largely along two physiologic axes, one for growth hormone and one for insulin.[8] Growth hormone provides the key stimulus for the synthesis of IGF-I in both the liver and other tissues and directly or indirectly also stimulates the synthesis of IGFBP-3. This stimulatory effect of growth hormone, however, is modulated by insulin, which increases cellular growth hormone-receptor levels[10,11] and which in general stimulates the cellular uptake of amino acids for protein synthesis.[8,12] In addition, insulin directlly inhibits the synthesis of IGFBP-1 and, possibly through less direct mechanisms, also appears to reduce the synthesis of IGFBP-2.[8] Plasma levels of IGFBP-1 and IGFBP-2 are generally inversely correlated with levels of insulin[13–15] and positively with plasma-free IGF-I.[15,16] Due to these mechanisms, conditions of low endogenous insulin production, such as chronic fasting, but also insulin-dependent diabetes mellitus, cause resistance of tissues to the effects of growth hormone and hence a dramatic decrease in plasma IGF-I levels. In addition, plasma levels of IGFBP-1 and IGFBP-2 rise. As an overall result, the bioavailability of IGF-I to tissue receptors is strongly reduced.[9] By contrast, conditions of comparatively elevated endogenous insulin production, such as obesity, but also non-insulin-dependent diabetes mellitus, are associated with decreased IGFBPs-1 and -2 and increased free plasma IGF-I. Paradoxically, however, obesity (BMI >30 kg/m^2) has not generally been found to increase, but rather to mildly reduce circulating IGF-I levels, probably because increased plasma-free IGF-I inhibits the pituitary secretion of growth hormone and hence reduces the primary stimulus of IGF-I synthesis.[9] There is some evidence that IGF-I levels correlate directly with BMI in lean subjects (BMI up to 25), whereas at higher BMI levels this relation is inversed.[17,18]

Human intervention studies have shown that physical activity causes an acute but transient, moderate increase in circulating growth hormone and IGF-I levels and a strong (up to 20-fold) increase in levels of IGFBP-1.[9] The increase in IGFBP-1 during exercise as well as during fasting may be explained not only by a decrease in pancreatic insulin secretion, but also by the rise in plasma cortisol, which stimulates IGFBP-1 synthesis.[19,20] The longer term effects of physical activity on the IGF-I system have not been studied much so far.

TOTAL AND BIOAVAILABLE PLASMA SEX STEROIDS

Both overall adiposity and intraabdominal body fat have been associated with differences in plasma levels of sex-hormone-binding globulin (SHBG) and plasma total and bioavailable androgens and estrogens. These relationships can be explained by a number of mechanisms: (1) Obesity increases levels of insulin and reduces IGFBP-1 and IGFBP-2; increases in insulin and bioactive IGF-I, in turn, inhibit the hepatic production of SHBG[21,22] and thus increase levels of plasma estradiol and testosterone unbound to SHBG; (2) Insulin and bioavailable IGF-I may stimulate the gonadal and adrenal synthesis of androgens, which are the direct precursors for estrogen synthesis;[22–24] (3) Within adipose tissue, androgens (Δ4-androstenedione and testosterone) are converted into estrogens (estrone and estradiol, respectively) by the enzyme aromatase; increased adiposity augments total aromatase capacity[25] and increases plasma levels of androgens unbound to SHBG, available for conversion into estrogens.

Obesity thus reduces plasma SHBG levels in both men and women of all ages.[21,22] The associations of obesity with total and bioavailable plasma sex steroids, however, depend on gender and menopausal status. Furthermore, among premenopausal women the associations depend on the presence or absence of polycystic ovary syndrome, an endocrine disorder that affects 4–8% of premenopausal women and that is characterized by ovarian androgen excess, frequent anovulation, and oligomenorrhea.

In normoandrogenic premenopausal women, BMI or fasting plasma insulin levels are not associated with levels of bioavailable estradiol unbound to SHBG and are either uncorrelated or weakly inversely correlated with total plasma estradiol levels.[26–29] This relative stability of total and bioavailable estrogen levels with respect to BMI is most likely due to a physiologic regulation of estradiol levels through feedback mechanisms, such as circulating estrogens on pituitary gonadotropin secretion. BMI and plasma fasting insulin do correlate directly with levels of bioavailable testosterone unbound to SHBG, [30–34] although there is no correlation with absolute levels of testosterone.

In premenopausal women with polycystic ovary syndrome, obesity and chronic hyperinsulinemia markedly increase the ovarian (and in many women also adrenal) production and total plasma levels of androstenedione and testosterone.[35–39] Hyperinsulinemia clearly is central to the development of androgen excess in women with polycystic ovary syndrome.[23] (1) Insulin increases the expression and activity of key enzymes involved in synthesis of sex steroids and stimulates the production of androstenedione and testosterone by ovarian stroma *in vitro;* (2) Women with polycystic ovary syndrome are generally insulin resistant and hyperinsulinemic; and (3) Treatment with insulin-lowering drugs diminishes excess androgen.[40] In women with polycystic ovary syndrome, BMI and fasting insulin levels both correlate directly with the frequency of anovulation and amenorrheic cycles and thus are a negative determinant of progesterone production. Plasma estradiol levels are usually within the normal range, but do not show the cyclic variation observed in normally menstruating women.

In postmenopausal women, BMI correlates directly with both plasma estrone and estradiol,[26,41,42] but there are no clear associations with either total or free testosterone.[42–45]

In men versus women, BMI and fasting plasma insulin correlate inversely with plasma total testosterone (reviewed in Refs. 46 and 47). This inverse correlation can be explained by feedback inhibition by free plasma testosterone of the pituitary secretion of luteinizing hormone, which provides the primary stimulus for testicular testosterone synthesis. Plasma total testosterone levels and SHBG are thus coregulated, so that when SHBG levels decrease (e.g., due to excess body weight), so does the testicular production of testosterone. In men with a BMI above 30 kg/m^2, however, not only plasma levels of total testosterone, but also bioavailable testosterone levels are reduced due to additional mechanisms that are less well understood. In men, plasma estrogens correlate directly with the degree of adiposity, because adipose tissue is the major site of estrogen synthesis.

In both men and women, weight reduction is generally associated with a rise in SHBG levels.[2] The effects of weight loss on total or bioavailable plasma sex steroids, however, are variable and again depend on gender, menopausal status, and presence or absence of ovarian hyperandrogenism. In overweight or obese women with polycystic ovary syndrome, weight loss has consistently been shown to reduce levels of both total and bioavailable androgens.[48–50] However, in normoandrogenic premenopausal women as well as postmenopausal women, these effects are less clear as reviewed in Ref. 2. Physical activity causes an acute, but transient, and relatively minor increase in plasma SHBG.[51–53] The long-term effects of moderate-intensity, regular physical activity on total or bioavailable sex steroids have not been studied enough to draw definite conclusions.

RELATION OF ENDOGENOUS HORMONES WITH CANCER RISK

Risk of cancers of the endometrium and breast is related to factors such as age at menarche and menopause, age at first full-term pregnancy, and parity. In addition, the rise in the incidence of these two forms of cancer with increasing age is less rapid after menopause. Together, these observations suggest a role of ovarian activity and sex steroids as risk factors for these cancers, and this is confirmed by studies showing associations of risk with the use of exogenous hormones for contraception of postmenopausal replacement therapy. Strong indications for the implication of sex steroids in prostate cancer development are that androgen ablation therapy often dramatically improves the clinical course of disease and that administration of testosterone to Noble rats enhances prostate tumor development.

The association of obesity with increased risks of cancers of the colon, endometrium, and breast (in postmenopausal women) suggests that chronic hyperinsulinemia might be a direct cause of disease. Insulin, like the IGFs, stimulates cell proliferation and inhibits apoptosis either through its cognate receptor or because of cross-binding to the receptors for IGF-I and IGF-II. In addition, insulin reduces levels of IGFBP1 and IGFBP-2 and thus may increase the bioactivity of the IGFs.

Endometrial Cancer

A number of case-control studies have shown an increase in risk among women who have comparatively low plasma SHBG and elevated plasma total androgen levels (androstenedione and testosterone). Among postmenopausal women, patients with endometrial cancer had elevated levels of estrone and total and bioavailable estradiol.[54–56]

The predominant theory concerning endometrial cancer is that risk is increased in women who have normal or elevated bioavailable estrogens, but low levels of progesterone (unopposed estrogen hypothesis).[55] This theory is supported by observations that postmenopausal estrogen replacement alone increases the risk of endometrial cancer, whereas combined estrogen plus progestogen replacement reduces the risk.[57] Furthermore, progesterone specifically increases IGFBP-1 levels in endometrial tissue. In endometrial tissue, IGFBP-1 is the most abundantly expressed IGF binding protein, and strongly inhibits the mitogenic action of IGF-I.[58]

The unopposed estrogen hypothesis would predict that women with polycystic ovary syndrome who have chronic anovulation, and hence a progesterone deficit, would have an increased risk of endometrial cancer. This hypothesis is supported by a large number of case reports of polycystic ovary syndrome among premenopausal endometrial cancer patients[54] and by several case-control and cohort studies that have shown an increased endometrial cancer risk in women with polycystic ovary syndrome.[59–62] The unopposed estrogen hypothesis also fits the observation of an increased risk in obese premenopausal women, because obesity and hyperinsulinemia increase the frequency of anovulation (at least in hyperandrogenic women) and thus inhibit progesterone production.

The hypothesis that chronic hyperinsulinemia may enhance endometrial cancer risk finds indirect support in observations that the risk of cancers of the endometrium is increased in diabetics.[63,64] Many of these studies lacked details as to whether diabetes was of early onset (type I) and insulin dependent or of adult onset (type II) and non-insulin dependent. Nevertheless, it seems reasonable to assume that the "diabetes" risk factor addressed in these studies was of type II, because in the general population the vast majority of diabetics have type II and are non-insulin dependent (NIDDM). NIDDM is usually associated with elevated pancreatic insulin secretion as well as glucose intolerance. One large case-control study showed an increase in endometrial cancer risk in postmenopausal women with elevated serum C-peptide levels.[65] Two additional, small case-control studies showed that, compared to disease-free controls, endometrial cancer patients had increased fasting plasma insulin levels,[65] decreased plasma levels of IGFBP-1,[66] and decreased expression of the IGFBP-1 gene in endometrial tissue samples.[67] Chronic hyperinsulinemia may increase endometrial cancer risk by aggravating ovarian hyperandrogenism in women with polycystic ovary syndrome, thus increasing the frequency of anovulatory menstrual cycles and progesterone deficiency. In addition, insulin decreases IGFBP-1 levels in the circulation and in endometrial tissue.

Breast Cancer

Several prospective cohort studies (reviewed in Ref. 68), but also traditional case-control studies (reviewed in Ref. 69), have shown an increased risk among postmenopausal women who have comparatively elevated plasma levels of both androgens (androstenedione and testosterone) and estrogens (estrone, total estradiol, and non-SHBG-bound estradiol). The common interpretation of these results is that the increase in risk is due mainly to higher concentrations of bioavailable estrogens, which strongly stimulate breast cell proliferation (estrogen excess hypothesis). These findings may also explain the increase in postmenopausal breast cancer risk among obese women, because in postmenopausal women obesity increases total and bioavailable estrogen levels. An interesting hypothesis is that risk is increased in women with comparatively elevated combined exposure to both estradiol and progesterone (estrogen-plus-progestogen hypothesis). This hypothesis is supported by observations that the use of estrogens combined with progestogens for postmenopausal hormone replacement increases breast cancer risk more than does the use of estrogens alone.[57,70–72] In premenopausal women, the hypothesis might explain the mildly inverse relation of breast cancer risk with obesity, because obesity in some women may lead to ovarian androgen excess, chronic anovulation, and impaired progesterone production.

Two case-control studies showed an association of insulin or C-peptide levels with both premenopausal[73,74] and postmenopausal[74] breast cancer risk, but this was not confirmed by one prospective study with measurements of (nonfasting) C-peptide.[75] Another prospective study also showed no association of breast cancer risk with fasting glucose levels or glucose levels 2 hours after a standard oral glucose dose.[76] Many studies have not globally shown any clear association of breast cancer risk with preexisting diabetes.[22]

Regarding IGF-I and IGFBP-3, case control studies[77,78] and prospective cohort studies[75,79] have shown an increased risk of breast cancer among women with comparatively elevated plasma IGF-I measured either as absolute levels or relative to levels of IGF's major binding protein, IGFBP-3. In most studies, this association was confined to younger, premenopausal women. Other case-control studies[73,80] and a cohort study[81] did not show any association between IGF-I and breast cancer risk, although one study indicated a possible increase in risk for postmenopausal women, but only in a subcohort.

Prostate Cancer

Prospective cohort studies globally did not provide consistent evidence that prostate cancer risk is related to prediagnostic plasma levels of either total or bioavailable testosterone,[46,82] although one study[83] did show this relation. Besides circulating androgens, estrogens have also been proposed to either enhance or inhibit prostate cancer development,[84,85] but the lack of association of prostate cancer risk with plasma estrogens supports neither of these hypotheses. Despite these globally negative results, some genetic association studies have shown an increase in prostate cancer risk in men who carry specific polymorphisms in the androgen receptor gene that are related to increased receptor transactivation.[86] Furthermore, risk has also been associated with polymorphisms in the 5α-reductase gene that increase the enzyme's activity.[86] The 5α-reductase enzyme converts testosterone into dihydrotestosterone, which binds and activates the androgen receptor with a more than fourfold higher efficacy than does testosterone. It is possible that elevated intraprostatic dihydrotestosterone provides the principal androgenic stimulus to prostate tumor development. It is unknown, however, whether and how increased prostatic dihydrotestosterone formation is related to nutritional life style factors and energy balance.

In line with the absence of a relation between obesity and prostate cancer risk, one prospective cohort study showed no association of prostate cancer risk with plasma levels of fasting insulin, IGFBP-1, and IGFBP-2.[87] Prostate cancer risk also appears to be unrelated to NIDDM.[46] By contrast, several case-control[88,89] and prospective cohort studies[87,90,91] have shown a direct association of risk with circulating IGF-I levels or with elevated levels of IGF-I for a given concentration of IGFBP-3 (i.e., in a multivariate model adjusting for IGFBP-3 levels).

Colorectal Cancer

A number of studies have shown an increase in colon cancer risk among NIDDM patients.[92,93] Furthermore, a recent cohort study showed an increase in colorectal cancer risk in men and women who had comparatively elevated fasting plasma glucose levels and higher plasma levels of glucose and insulin 2 hours after a standard dose of oral glucose.[94] The association of colorectal cancer with fasting glucose levels confirmed results from previous studies reviewed in detail elsewhere.[92,93] Another study in New York showed an approximately fourfold increase in colorectal cancer risk comparing subjects in the highest and lowest quartiles of (nonfasting) serum C-peptide.[95] This association with C-peptide remained unaltered after adjustment for BMI. Furthermore, this study showed inverse associations of colorectal cancer risk with levels of IGFBP-1 and IGFBP-2.[95]

Relatively independent of obesity-related metabolic dysregulations, prospective studies have shown mild, statistically nonsignificant increases in risk with increasing IGF-I.[95–97] In two of these studies, this association became stronger and statistically significant when the statistical analyses were adjusted for levels of IGFBP-3.[96,97] In a further prospective study,[98] absolute IGF-I levels showed a significantly direct association with the risk of colon cancer, but an inverse association with the risk of rectal cancer. Traditional case-control studies also showed a significant direct association of colorectal cancer risk with IGF-I before or after adjustment for IGFBP-3.[99]

CONCLUSIONS

Taken together, evidence indicates that endometrial cancer risk is increased in women who are obese and have hyperinsulinemia, increased plasma androgen levels, and elevated plasma estrogen levels after menopause. Endometrial cancer risk may be increased particularly in women with polycystic ovary syndrome. This increase in risk might be due to elevated IGF-I activity within the endometrium, because of reduced IGFBP-1 (as a consequence of elevated insulin and low progesterone) and because estrogens induce IGF-I synthesis in endometrial stroma. Globally, these various observations are all in line with the unopposed estrogen hypothesis.

For breast cancer in postmenopausal women, evidence clearly indicates an increased risk in relation to excess body weight and lack of physical activity, and this may be explained by increases in bioavailable estrogens. For premenopausal women, obesity is mildly inversely related to risk of breast cancer, possibly because of reduced progesterone levels (especially in women with a tendency towards ovarian hyperandrogenism). However, there is lack of data on relationships with circulating sex steroids. Data relating breast cancer risk to insulin levels are inconsistent.

Data suggest an absence of a relation between prostate cancer risk and obesity, fasting plasma insulin, and plasma levels of IGFBP-1 and IGFBP-2. Furthermore, there are no clear associations of risk with total or bioavailable plasma testosterone levels, although some results indicate a mildly inverse relation with SHBG levels. Interestingly, the data do suggest an inverse relation between prostate cancer risk and physical activity levels.

Colon cancer risk is clearly associated with obesity and physical inactivity and has also been associated with increased plasma glucose and insulin and decreased plasma IGFBP-1 and IGFBP-2.

Elevated plasma IGF-I, either as absolute concentrations or adjusted for levels of IGFBP-3, appears to increase the risk of cancer of the prostate, colorectum, and breast. However, although plasma levels of IGF-I and IGFBP-3 are strongly reduced in conditions of chronic energy restriction, relations with body composition (BMI) and physical activity levels remain unclear.

Further prospective cohort studies are needed to examine the relations of circulating sex steroids, insulin, IGF-I, and IGFBPs with the risk of these various cancers. These should include prospective studies on endometrial cancer and on breast cancer in premenopausal women. Further research is also needed to understand the relation of circulating IGF-I levels with diet, levels of physical activity, energy balance, and body composition.

REFERENCES

1. KRITCHEVSKY, D. 1999. Caloric restriction and experimental carcinogenesis. Toxicol. Sci. **52:** 13–16.
2. IARC WORKING GROUP. 2002. IARC Handbook of Cancer Prevention: Weight Control and Physical Activity. IARC Press. Lyon.
3. REAVEN, G.M. 1993. Role of insulin resistance in human disease (syndrome X): an expanded definition. Annu. Rev. Med. **44:** 121–131.
4. EBELING, P. & V.A. KOIVISTO. 1994. Non-esterified fatty acids regulate lipid and glucose oxidation and glycogen synthesis in healthy men. Diabetologia **37:** 202–209.
5. GOODPLASTER, B.H., D.E. KELLEY, R.R. WING, et al. 1999. Effects of weight loss on regional fat distribution and insulin sensitivity in obesity. Diabetes **48:** 839–847.
6. KELLEY, D.E. & B.H. GOODPASTER. 1999. Effects of physical activity on insulin action and glucose tolerance in obesity. Med. Sci. Sports Exercise **31:** S619–S623.
7. BORGHOUTS, L.B. & H.A. KEIZER. 2000. Exercise and insulin sensitivity: a review. Int. J. Sports Med. **21:** 1–12.

8. THISSEN, J.P., J.M. KETELSLEGERS & L.E. UNDERWOOD. 1994. Nutritional regulation of the insulin-like growth factors. Endocr. Rev. **15:** 80–101.
9. KAAKS, R. & A. LUKANOVA. 2001. Energy balance and cancer: the role of insulin and insulin-like growth factor-I. Proc. Nutr. Soc. **60:** 91–106.
10. BAXTER, R.C. & J.R. TURTLE. 1978. Regulation of hepatic growth hormone receptors by insulin. Biochem. Biophys. Res. Commun. **84:** 350–357.
11. TOLLET, P., B. ENBERG & A. MODE. 1990. Growth hormone (GH) regulation of cytochrome P-450IIC12, insulin-like growth factor-I (IGF-I), and GH receptor messenger RNA expression in primary rat hepatocytes: a hormonal interplay with insulin, IGF-I, and thyroid hormone. Mol. Endocrinol. **4:** 1934–1942.
12. STRAUS, D.S. 1994. Nutritional regulation of hormones and growth factors that control mammalian growth. FASEB J. **8:** 6–12.
13. WABITSCH, M., W.F. BLUM, R. MUCHE, et al. 1996. Insulin-like growth factors and their binding proteins before and after weight loss and their associations with hormonal and metabolic parameters in obese adolescent girls. Int. J. Obes. Relat. Metab Disord. **20:** 1073–1080.
14. ARGENTE, J., N. CABALLO, V. BARRIOS, et al. 1997. Multiple endocrine abnormalities of the growth hormone and insulin-like growth factor axis in patients with anorexia nervosa: effect of short- and long-term weight recuperation. J. Clin. Endocrinol. Metab. **82:** 2084–2092.
15. NAM, S.Y., E.J. LEE, K.R. KIM, et al. 1997. Effect of obesity on total and free insulin-like growth factor (IGF)-1, and their relationship to IGF-binding protein (BP)-1, IGFBP-2, IGFBP-3, insulin, and growth hormone. Int. J. Obes. Relat. Metab. Disorders **21:** 355–359.
16. FRYSTYK, J., E. VESTBO, C. SKJAERBAEK, et al. 1995. Free insulin-like growth factors in human obesity. Metabolism **44:** 37–44.
17. LUKANOVA, A., S. SODERBERG, P. STATTIN, et al. 2001. Non-linear relationship of insulin-like growth factor (IGF-I) and IGF-I/IGF-binding protein-3 ratio with indices of adiposity and plasma insulin concentrations. Cancer Causes & Control. In press.
18. KAAKS, R., S. SODERBERG, T. OLSSON, et al. 2001. Response: re: plasma insulin-like growth factor-i, insulin-like growth factor-binding proteins, and prostate cancer risk: a prospective study. J. Natl. Cancer Inst. **93:** 650–651.
19. UNTERMAN, T.G. 1993. Insulin-like growth factor binding protein-1: identification, purification, and regulation in fetal and adult life. Adv. Exp. Med. Biol. **343:** 215–226.
20. LEE, P.D., L.C. GIUDICE, C.A. CONOVER & D.R. POWELL. 1997. Insulin-like growth factor binding protein-1: recent findings and new directions. Proc. Soc. Exp. Biol. Med. **216:** 319–357.
21. PUGEAT, M., J.C. CRAVE, M. ELMIDANI, et al. 1991. Pathophysiology of sex hormone binding globulin (SHBG): relation to insulin. J. Steroid Biochem. Mol. Biol. **40:** 841–849.
22. KAAKS, R. 1996. Nutrition, hormones, and breast cancer: is insulin the missing link? Cancer Causes Control **7:** 605–625.
23. PORETSKY, L., N.A. CATALDO, Z. ROSENWAKS & L.C. GIUDICE. 1999. The insulin-related ovarian regulatory system in health and disease. Endocrinol. Rev. **20:** 535–582.
24. CARA, J.F. 1994. Insulin-like growth factors, insulin-like growth factor binding proteins and ovarian androgen production. Horm. Res. **42:** 49–54.
25. SIITERI, P.K. 1987. Adipose tissue as a source of hormones. Am. J. Clin. Nutr. **45:** 277–282.
26. VERKASALO, P.K., H.V. THOMAS, P.N. APPLEBY, et al. 2001. Circulating levels of sex hormones and their relation to risk factors for breast cancer: a cross-sectional study in 1092 pre- and postmenopausal women (United Kingdom). Cancer Causes & Control **12:** 47–59.
27. DORGAN, J.F., M.E. REICHMAN, J.T. JUDD, et al. 1995. The relation of body size to plasma levels of estrogens and androgens in premenopausal women (Maryland, United States). Cancer Causes & Control **6:** 3–8.
28. NAGATA, C., N. KANEDA, M. KABUTO & H. SHIMIZU. 1997. Factors associated with serum levels of estradiol and sex hormone-binding globulin among premenopausal Japanese women. Environ. Health Perspect. **105:** 994–997.

29. THOMAS, H.V., T.J. KEY, D.S. ALLEN, et al. 1997. Re: reversal of relation between body mass and endogenous estrogen concentrations with menopausal status. J. Natl. Cancer Inst. **89:** 396–398.
30. DE RIDDER, C.M., P.F. BRUNING, M.L. ZONDERLAND, et al. 1990. Body fat mass, body fat distribution, and plasma hormones in early puberty in females. J. Clin. Endocrinol. Metab. **70:** 888–893.
31. KIRSCHNER, M.A., E. SAMOJLIK, M. DREJKA, et al. 1990. Androgen-estrogen metabolism in women with upper body versus lower body obesity. J. Clin. Endocrinol. Metab. **70:** 473–479.
32. LEENEN, R. VAN DER, K. KOOY, J.C. SEIDELL, et al. 1994. Visceral fat accumulation in relation to sex hormones in obese men and women undergoing weight loss therapy. J. Clin. Endocrinol. Metab. **78:** 1515–1520.
33. BERNASCONI, D., P. DEL MONTE, M. MEOZZI, et al. 1996. The impact of obesity on hormonal parameters in hirsute and nonhirsute women. Metabolism **45:** 72–75.
34. PENTTILA, T.L., P. KOSKINEN, T.A. PENTTILA, et al. 1999. Obesity regulates bioavailable testosterone levels in women with or without polycystic ovary syndrome. Fertil. Steril. **71:** 457–461.
35. BURGHEN, G.A., J.R. GIVENS & A.E. KITABCHI. 1980. Correlation of hyperandrogenism with hyperinsulinism in polycystic ovarian disease. J. Clin. Endocrinol. Metab. **50:** 113–116.
36. SHOUPE, D., D.D. KUMAR & R.A. LOBO. 1983. Insulin resistance in polycystic ovary syndrome. Am. J. Obstet. Gynecol. **147:** 588–592.
37. EVANS, D.J., J.H. BARTH & C.W. BURKE. 1988. Body fat topography in women with androgen excess. Int. J. Obes. **12:** 157–162.
38. LANZONE, A., A.M. FULGHESU, S. PAPPALARDO, et al. 1990. Growth hormone and somatomedin-C secretion in patients with polycystic ovarian disease. Their relationships with hyperinsulinism and hyperandrogenism. Gynecol. Obstet. Invest. **29:** 149–153.
39. HOLTE, J., T. BERGH, G. GENNARELLI & L. WIDE. 1994. The independent effects of polycystic ovary syndrome and obesity on serum concentrations of gonadotrophins and sex steroids in premenopausal women. Clin. Endocrinol. (Oxf.) **41:** 473–481.
40. EHRMANN, D.A. 1999. Insulin-lowering therapeutic modalities for polycystic ovary syndrome. Endocrinol. Metab. Clin. North Am. **28:** 423–438.
41. AUSTIN, H., J.M. AUSTIN, JR., E.E. PARTRIDGE, et al. 1991. Endometrial cancer, obesity, and body fat distribution. Cancer Res. **51:** 568–572.
42. KAYE, S.A., A.R. FOLSOM, J.T. SOLER, et al. 1991. Associations of body mass and fat distribution with sex hormone concentrations in postmenopausal women. Int. J. Epidemiol. **20:** 151–156.
43. CAULEY, J.A., J.P. GUTAI, L.H. KULLER, et al. 1989. The epidemiology of serum sex hormones in postmenopausal women. Am. J. Epidemiol. **129:** 1120–1131.
44. NEWCOMB, P.A., R. KLEIN, B.E. KLEIN, et al. 1995. Association of dietary and life-style factors with sex hormones in postmenopausal women. Epidemiology **6:** 318–321.
45. TURCATO, E., M. ZAMBONI, G. DE PERGOLA, et al. 1997. Interrelationships between weight loss, body fat distribution and sex hormones in pre- and postmenopausal obese women. J. Intern. Med. **241:** 363–372.
46. KAAKS, R., A. LUKANOVA & B. SOMMERSBERG. 2000. Plasma androgens, IGF-I, body size, and prostate cancer risk: a synthetic review. Prostate Cancer Prostatic Dis. **3:** 157–172.
47. GIAGULLI, V.A., J.A. KAUFMAN & A. VERMEULEN. 1994. Pathogenesis of the decreased androgen levels in obese men. J. Clin. Endocrinol. Metab. **79:** 997–1000.
48. CRAVE, J.C., S. FIMBEL, H. LEJEUNE, et al. 1995. Effects of diet and metformin administration on sex hormone-binding globulin, androgens, and insulin in hirsute and obese women. J. Clin. Endocrinol. Metab. **80:** 2057–2062.
49. BATES, G.W. & N.S. WHITWORTH. 1982. Effect of body weight reduction on plasma androgens in obese, infertile women. Fertil. Steril. **38:** 406–409.
50. KIDDY, D.S., D. HAMILTON-FAIRLEY, A. BUSH, et al. 1992. Improvement in endocrine and ovarian function during dietary treatment of obese women with polycystic ovary syndrome. Clin. Endocrinol. (Oxf.) **36:** 105–111.

51. GRAY, A.B., R.D. TELFORD & M.J. WEIDEMANN. 1993. Endocrine response to intense interval exercise. Eur. J. Appl. Physiol. Occup. Physiol. **66:** 366–371.
52. KRAEMER, W.J., J.S. VOLEK, J.A. BUSH, et al. 1998. Hormonal responses to consecutive days of heavy-resistance exercise with or without nutritional supplementation. J. Appl. Physiol. **85:** 1544–1555.
53. ZMUDA, J.M., P.D. THOMPSON & S.J. WINTERS. 1996. Exercise increases serum testosterone and sex hormone-binding globulin levels in older men. Metabolism **45:** 935–939.
54. GRADY, D. & V.L. ERNSTER. 1996. Endometrial cancer. In Cancer Epidemiology and Prevention. D. Schottenfeld & F.J. Fraumeni, eds. :1058–1089. Oxford University Press. Cambridge.
55. KEY, T.J. & M.C. PIKE. 1988. The dose-effect relationship between 'unopposed' oestrogens and endometrial mitotic rate: its central role in explaining and predicting endometrial cancer risk. Br. J. Cancer **57:** 205–212.
56. POTISCHMAN, N., R.N. HOOVER, L.A. BRINTON, et al. 1996. Case-control study of endogenous steroid hormones and endometrial cancer. J. Natl. Cancer Inst. **88:** 1127–1135.
57. IARC MONOGRAPHS ON THE EVALUATION OF CARCINOGENIC RISKS TO HUMAN. 1998. Hormonal contraception and post-menopausal hormonal therapy. In 1-660. IARC Press. Lyon, France.
58. RUTANEN, E.M. 1998. Insulin-like growth factors in endometrial function. Gynecol. Endocrinol. **12:** 399–406.
59. DAHLGREN, E., L.G. FRIBERG, S. JOHANSSON, et al. 1991. Endometrial carcinoma; ovarian dysfunction--a risk factor in young women. Eur. J. Obstet. Gynecol. Reprod. Biol. **41:** 143–150.
60. SHU, X.O., L.A. BRINTON, W. ZHENG, et al. 1991. A population-based case-control study of endometrial cancer in Shanghai, China. Int. J. Cancer **49:** 38–43.
61. NIWA, K., A. IMAI, M. HASHIMOTO, et al. 2000. A case-control study of uterine endometrial cancer of pre- and post-menopausal women. Oncol. Rep. **7:** 89–93.
62. COULAM, C.B., J.F. ANNEGERS & J.S. KRANZ. 1983. Chronic anovulation syndrome and associated neoplasia. Obstet. Gynecol. **61:** 403–407.
63. WEIDERPASS, E., G. GRIDLEY, I. PERSSON, et al. 1997. Risk of endometrial and breast cancer in patients with diabetes mellitus. Int. J. Cancer **71:** 360–363.
64. WEIDERPASS, E., I. PERSSON, H.O. ADAMI, et al. 2000. Body size in different periods of life, diabetes mellitus, hypertension, and risk of postmenopausal endometrial cancer (Sweden). Cancer Causes & Control **11:** 185–192.
65. TROISI, R., N. POTISCHMAN, R.N. HOOVER, et al. 1997. Insulin and endometrial cancer. Am. J. Epidemiol. **146:** 476–482.
66. AYABE, T., O. TSUTSUMI, H. SAKAI, et al. 1997. Increased circulating levels of insulin-like growth factor-I and decreased circulating levels of insulin-like growth factor binding protein-1 in postmenopausal women with endometrial cancer. Endocr. J. **44:** 419–424.
67. RUTANEN, E.M., T. NYMAN, P. LEHTOVIRTA, et al. 1994. Suppressed expression of insulin-like growth factor binding protein-1 mRNA in the endometrium: a molecular mechanism associating endometrial cancer with its risk factors. Int. J. Cancer **59:** 307–312.
68. KEY, T.J. 1999. Serum oestradiol and breast cancer risk. Endocr. Relat. Cancer **6:** 175–180.
69. BERNSTEIN, L. & R.K. ROSS. 1993. Endogenous hormones and breast cancer risk. Epidemiol. Rev. **15:** 48–65.
70. ROSS, R.K., A. PAGANINI-HILL, P.C. WAN & M.C. PIKE. 2000. Effect of hormone replacement therapy on breast cancer risk: estrogen versus estrogen plus progestin. J. Natl. Cancer Inst. **92:** 328–332.
71. SCHAIRER, C., J. LUBIN, R. TROISI, et al. 2000. Menopausal estrogen and estrogen-progestin replacement therapy and breast cancer risk. JAMA **283:** 485–491.
72. MAGNUSSON, C., J.A. BARON, N. CORREIA, et al. 1999. Breast-cancer risk following long-term oestrogen- and oestrogen-progestin-replacement therapy. Int. J. Cancer **81:** 339–344.

73. DEL GIUDICE, M.E., I.G. FANTUS, S. EZZAT, et al. 1998. Insulin and related factors in premenopausal breast cancer risk. Breast Cancer Res. Treat. **47:** 111–120.
74. BRUNING, P.F., J.M. BONFRER, P.A. VAN NOORD, et al. 1992. Insulin resistance and breast-cancer risk. Int. J. Cancer **52:** 511–516.
75. TONIOLO, P., P.F. BRUNING, A. AKHMEDKHANOV, et al. 2000. Serum insulin-like growth factor-I and breast cancer. Int. J. Cancer **88:** 828–832.
76. MANJER, J., R. KAAKS, E. RIBOLI & G. BERGLUND. 2001. Risk of breast cancer in relation to anthropometry, blood pressure, blood lipids and glucose metabolism: a prospective study within the Malmo Preventive Project. Eur. J. Cancer Prev. **10:** 33–42.
77. PEYRAT, J.P., J. BONNETERRE, B. HECQUET, et al. 1993. Plasma insulin-like growth factor-1 (IGF-1) concentrations in human breast cancer. Eur. J. Cancer **29A:** 492–497.
78. BRUNING, P.F., J. VAN DOORN, J.M. BONFRER, et al. 1995. Insulin-like growth-factor-binding protein 3 is decreased in early-stage operable pre-menopausal breast cancer. Int. J. Cancer **62:** 266–270.
79. HANKINSON, S.E., W.C. WILLETT, J.E. MANSON, et al. 1998. Plasma sex steroid hormone levels and risk of breast cancer in postmenopausal women. J. Natl. Cancer Inst. **90:** 1292–1299.
80. NG, E.H., C.Y. JI, P.H. TAN, et al. 1998. Altered serum levels of insulin-like growth-factor binding proteins in breast cancer patients. Ann. Surg. Oncol. **5:** 194–201.
81. KAAKS, R., E. LUNDIN, J. MANJER, et al. 2001. Prospective study of IGF-I, IGF-binding proteins and breast cancer risk, in Northern and Southern Sweden. Cancer Causes & Control. In press.
82. EATON, N.E., G.K. REEVES, P.N. APPLEBY & T.J. KEY. 1999. Endogenous sex hormones and prostate cancer: a quantitative review of prospective studies. Br. J. Cancer **80:** 930–934.
83. GANN, P.H., C.H. HENNEKENS, J. MA, et al. 1996. Prospective study of sex hormone levels and risk of prostate cancer. J. Natl. Cancer Inst. **88:** 1118–1126.
84. BOSLAND, M.C. 2000. The role of steroid hormones in prostate carcinogenesis. J. Natl. Cancer Inst. Monogr. 39–66.
85. FARNSWORTH, W.E. 1996. Roles of estrogen and SHBG in prostate physiology. Prostate **28:** 17–23.
86. ROSS, R.K., M.C. PIKE, G.A. COETZEE, et al. 1998. Androgen metabolism and prostate cancer: establishing a model of genetic susceptibility. Cancer Res. **58:** 4497–4504.
87. STATTIN, P., A. BYLUND, S. RINALDI, et al. 2000. Plasma insulin-like growth factor-I, insulin-like growth factor-binding proteins, and prostate cancer risk: a prospective study. J. Natl. Cancer Inst. **92:** 1910–1917.
88. MANTZOROS, C.S., A. TZONOU, L.B. SIGNORELLO, et al. 1997. Insulin-like growth factor 1 in relation to prostate cancer and benign prostatic hyperplasia. Br. J. Cancer **76:** 1115–1118.
89. WOLK, A., C.S. MANTZOROS, S.O. ANDERSSON, et al. 1998. Insulin-like growth factor 1 and prostate cancer risk: a population-based, case-control study. J. Natl. Cancer Inst. **90:** 911–915.
90. CHAN, J.M., M.J. STAMPFER, E. GIOVANNUCCI, et al. 1998. Plasma insulin-like growth factor-I and prostate cancer risk: a prospective study. Science **279:** 563–566.
91. HARMAN, S.M., E.J. METTER, M.R. BLACKMAN, et al. 2000. Serum levels of insulin-like growth factor I (IGF-I), IGF-II, IGF-binding protein-3, and prostate-specific antigen as predictors of clinical prostate cancer. J. Clin. Endocrinol. Metab. **85:** 4258–4265.
92. MCKEOWN, E.G. 1994. Epidemiology of colorectal cancer revisited: are serum triglycerides and/or plasma glucose associated with risk? Cancer Epidemiol. Biomarkers Prev. **3:** 687–695.
93. GIOVANNUCCI, E. 1995. Insulin and colon cancer. Cancer Causes Control **6:** 164–179.
94. SCHOEN, R.E., C.M. TANGEN, L.H. KULLER, et al. 1999. Increased blood glucose and insulin, body size, and incident colorectal cancer. J. Natl. Cancer Inst. **91:** 1147–1154.
95. KAAKS, R., P. TONIOLO, A. AKHMEDKHANOV, et al. 2000. Serum C-Peptide, Insulin-Like Growth Factor (IGF)-I, IGF-Binding Proteins, and Colorectal Cancer Risk in Women. J. Natl. Cancer Inst. **92:** 1592–1600.

96. MA, J., M.N. POLLAK, E. GIOVANNUCCI, *et al.* 1999. Prospective study of colorectal cancer risk in men and plasma levels of insulin-like growth factor (IGF)-I and IGF-binding protein-3. J. Natl. Cancer Inst. **91:** 620–625.
97. GIOVANNUCCI, E., M.N. POLLAK, E.A. PLATZ, *et al.* 2000. A prospective study of plasma insulin-like growth factor-1 and binding protein-3 and risk of colorectal neoplasia in women. Cancer Epidemiol. Biomarkers Prev. **9:** 345–349.
98. PALMQVIST, R, G. HALLMANS, S. RINALDI, *et al.* 2002. Plasma, IGF-I, IGF-binding proteins and risk of colorectal cancer: A prospective study in Northern Sweden. Gut **50:** 642–646.
99. MANOUSOS, O., J. SOUGLAKOS, C. BOSETTI, *et al.* 1999. IGF-I and IGF-II in relation to colorectal cancer. Int. J. Cancer **83:** 15–17.

The Mediet Project

L. CASTAGNETTA,[a,b] O.M. GRANATA,[a] R. CUSIMANO,[c] B. RAVAZZOLO,[d] M. LIQUORI,[d] L. POLITO,[a] M. MIELE,[a] A. DI CRISTINA,[a] P. HAMEL,[e] AND A. TRAINA[d]

[a]*Unit of Experimental Oncology & Palermo Branch of IST-GE, and* [d]*Cancer Registry, Department of Clinical Oncology, "M. Ascoli" Cancer Hospital Centre, A.R.N.A.S., Civico, Palermo, Italy*

[b]*Department of Experimental Oncology and Clinical Application, University Medical School, Palermo, Italy*

[c]*Department of Epidemiology, A.L.S.L. 6, Palermo, Italy*

[e]*Department of Internal Medicine, A.R.N.A.S., Civico, Palermo, Italy*

ABSTRACT: Preliminary evidence from a case control study of healthy postmenopausal women living in Palermo, Sicily, is presented to investigate the potential impact of a traditional Mediterranean diet on the risk of developing breast cancer. Of the 230 women who fulfilled specific eligibility criteria, 115 were enrolled in the study based on serum testosterone values equal to or greater than the median population value (0.14 µg/ml). Women were then individually randomized into a diet intervention ($n = 58$) and a control ($n = 55$) group. Women in the intervention group attended a weekly "cooking course" for 1 year, being trained by professional chefs in the correct use of the natural ingredients of the traditional Mediterranean diet, including whole cereals, legumes, seeds, fish, cruciferous vegetables, and many others. The intervention group was subsequently instructed to follow the learned diet at home, while the control group was only advised to increase the consumption of fruits and vegetables, as recommended by WHO. The following measures were taken at the beginning, middle, and end of the study: (a) fasting blood and 12-hour urine samples to assay defined hormonal endpoints; (b) height, weight, and circumference of the waist and hip; and (c) a food frequency and computerized 24-hour dietary recall questionnaire. After 1 year, both the control and the intervention groups showed satisfactory compliance rates (81 and 85%, respectively). In addition, preliminary results so far obtained reveal an unequivocal trend towards weight loss, a strong reduction in cholesterol levels, and a psychophysical feeling of well-being by women adopting the Mediterranean diet. The study is currently ongoing to verify the association of changes in serum and urine hormone levels and breast cancer risk in the intervention group.

KEYWORDS: Mediet Project; breast cancer; diet

Address for correspondence: Prof. Luigi Castagnetta, Unit of Experimental Oncology, Department of Clinical Oncology, "M. Ascoli" Cancer Hospital Centre, Via Parlavecchio 139, 90127 Palermo, Italy. Voice: +39-091-666-4346; fax: +39-091-666-4352.
 lucashbl@unipa.it

INTRODUCTION

Since the discovery of infertility or reproductive disorders in some wild or captivity-maintained animals living on a diet of specific herbs,[1] the socalled phytohormones have been a matter of investigation. Many studies have examined some of the biological actions exerted, their action mechanisms, and generally their potential role as endocrine disrupters. A major topic, however, has been the chemopreventive role of phytoestrogens,[2] especially soy derivatives, such as daidzein, genistein, and enterodiol. Interesting studies have been carried out either in Eastern countries, where soy is a popular nutrient, or in Western countries, where it is an unusual component of foodstuffs.[3]

The interest of nutritionists and epidemiologists in Mediterranean dietary profiles is derived from much evidence relating them to a substantially reduced risk of cancer.[4] The Mediterranean diet resembles the diet eaten in Southern Italy in the early 1960s, as described by the Euratom Study.[5] On this basis, it can be defined as a diet high in cereal (more than 60% of total energy), low in total fats (less than 30%), with moderate amounts of added fat, predominantly olive oil (representing more than 70% of the total lipids), with a high monosaturated/saturated ratio (greater than 2) and a moderate polyunsaturated/saturated ratio (about 0.4–0.5).[6]

The presence, amount, and interaction of various nutrients contained in plant foods as well as the mechanisms of action and regulation of supposed protective agents are currently under investigation in many countries. They could eventually better explain the benefical effects of specific diet in different areas, affected by a strongly different incidence and mortality rate of neoplasia.

BASIS OF THE MEDIET STUDY

For many years, evidence has indicated that Southern European populations experience a lower incidence of some types of cancer, including that of the breast.[7] Recent evidence from Palermo Provincial Cancer Registry shows that: (1) the incidence of breast cancer in Palermo has been increasing greatly, comparing 1993 with 1999; (2) the increase mainly regards specific cohorts of younger women;[8,9] and (3) the incidence of breast cancer in Palermo is more similar to that observed in Varese than in Ragusa.[10]

The incidence within the metropolitan area of Palermo was higher than that observed in rural areas of the same Province of Palermo (100.8 and 79.2 standardized rate, respectively), eventually suggesting significant differences between metropolitan and rural areas even in the southern part of the country.[9] Breast cancer mortality observed in the same areas and period confirms this evidence.[11]

This difference apparently is associated with a trend towards changing life style habits by metropolitan area residents. There is a net progressive "northernization" of the Mediterranean diet with a considerably decreased consumption of pasta and bread, a particular component of traditional Mediterranean nutrition, as opposed to a net increase in the consumption of milk and dairy products, meat, animal fat, and other oils.[12] This trend, reported in the early 1960s,[13] has repeatedly been confirmed (TABLE 1).[14,15]

TABLE 1. Comparison of food consumption between North and South in Italy from 1980–1984

Foods	North Median	South Median	Wilcoxon[a]	South vs. North fold difference
Animal fats	12	4	$p<0.001$	−3.00
Soft drinks	39	15	$p<0.001$	−2.60
Other vegetable oils	17	10	$p<0.001$	−1.70
Sugar and confectionery	76	56	$p<0.001$	−1.35
Milk and dairies	270	234	$p<0.001$	−1.15
Alcoholic beverages	167	151	$p<0.001$	−1.11
Meat	156	143	$p<0.001$	−1.09
Fruit	218	220	NSD	+1.01
Cereals	249	294	$p<0.001$	+1.18
Vegetables	21	30	$p<0.001$	+1.40
Pulses	714	321	$p<0.001$	+1.50
Fish	12	22	$p<0.001$	+1.83
Olive oil	10	29	$p<0.001$	+2.90

NOTE: Median values are expressed as gr/day/caput.
[a]Wilcoxon nonparametric test for differences. Data reported from A. Ferro-Luzzi *et al.* 1994.

Recent prospective studies provide consistent evidence that the risk of breast cancer is increased in postmenopausal women with high concentrations of testosterone and estradiol and low concentrations of estradiol bound to SHBG.[16–18] Much evidence is accumulating that Western dietary habits may contribute to the increased risk of breast cancer.[4]

The efficacy of dietary changes to reduce the availability of sex hormones has been observed in diet and androgens by the DIANA study, a controlled randomized trial mainly based on macrobiotic and Mediterranean vegetarian recipes.[19]

In our study, the ability to compel even a small portion of a Sicilian population to permanently introduce soy or soy derivatives in daily food was considered hopeless. However, many currently known active constituents in the primary prevention of cancer, that is, resveratrol, oleuropein, indole-3-carbinol, Ω-3, and Ω-9 unsaturated fatty acid, lignans, and the like, are present in true Mediterranean foods (TABLE 2).

Altogether, this evidence prompted us to plan a study of women in Palermo at normal risk of developing breast cancer, focusing on well-defined endocrine endpoints after a period of reeducation to a safe nutritional regimen, adopting exclusively a traditional Mediterranean diet (MEDIET) (FIG.1).

STUDY DESIGN: RANDOMIZED CONTROLLED TRIAL

Study Population and Methods

Subjects. Through a press campaign (newspaper and broadcasting advertisement), 300 healthy female volunteers aged 44–71 years from the Palermo area of

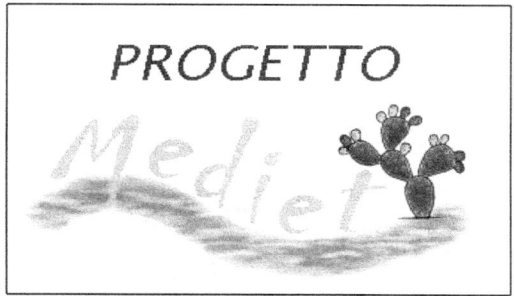

FIGURE 1. The Mediet Project logo.

TABLE 2. Chemopreventive agents as dietary constituents in recommended Mediterranean foods

Agent	Dietary constituent	Mediterranean foods
Lycopene	Carotenoid	Tomato
Tocopherols	Vitamin E	Almond, nut , pistachio, olive oil
Ascorbic acid	Vitamin C	Orange juice, red pepper chili
Ergosterol	Vitamin D	Tuna fish, swordfish, anchovy
Indol-3-carbinol	Indole	Cauliflower, broccoli
Resveratrol	Polyphenol	Red vine
Ellagic acid	Polyphenol	Redgrapes, figs, pomegranate, berries
Oleuropein	Glycosid	Olive oil
Oleic acid	Monounsaturated fatty acid (Ω-9)	Olive oil
Eicosanoids	Polyunsaturated fatty acid (Ω-3)	Blue fishes: tuna, sardines, mackerel etc.
Isoflavonoids	Phytoestrogens	Beens, chick peas, lupins, broad beans, peas, lentis etc.
Lignans	Phytoestrogens	Whole grain cereals : wheat, barley. Seads of: pumpkin, sesame, sunflower. Garlic, onion, fennel, carrot

Southern Italy contacted us to participate in our study in the summer of 1999. Eligibility criteria were: (1) postmenopausal for at least 2 years; (2) no history of bilateral ovariectomy; (3) no hormone replacement therapy for the previous 1 year; (4) no history of cancer; (5) no adherence to a vegetarian or macrobiotic diet or to any other medically prescribed diet; and (6) no treatment for diabetes, thyroid disease, and chronic bowel disease. Informed consent was obtained from all women. Among 300 women, 230 met eligibility criteria and were enrolled.

Experimental Design. The experimental design is shown in FIGURE 2. In July 1999 prebaseline serum levels of testosterone were determined in the 230 enrolled women, and 115 women were selected for the study, their serum testosterone value being equal to or greater than the median value (0.14 µg/ml). The selected 115 women were individually randomized into a diet intervention group ($n = 58$) and a control group ($n = 55$).

Women randomized to the intervention group were invited weekly to a "cooking course" and to a social dinner in collaboration with the Palermo Tourism School, with chefs addressing the principles of the traditional Mediterranean diet. The proposed recipes were based on a traditional Sicilian diet, including whole cereals, legumes, seeds, fish, cruciferous vegetables, and many other Mediterranean foods containing several active principles (TABLE 2). Furthermore, the women were asked to avoid refined carbohydrates, salt, and additional animal fat. This diet intervention trial was carried out for 1 year, the first period of 6 months, from January to June 2000, and then a second period of 3 months, from October to December 2000. Moreover, women were instructed to consume the same foods on a daily basis at home. The control women were advised to increase their consumption of fruits and vegetables but were not informed of the MEDIET diet principles.

Before the start, at the end of the first period of intervention, and at the end of the study, fasting blood samples and 12-hour urine samples were taken for hormone assay and stored at –80°C and –20°C, respectively. Height, weight, and circumference of the waist and hip were measured at the beginning and at the end of intervention.

Before randomization and at the end of the study, all of the women compiled a food frequency questionnaire developed for the EPIC[20] study, while a computerized 24-hour dietary recall system[21,22] was collected at the start, at the end of the first period, and at the end of the study.

PRELIMINARY RESULTS AND COMMENTS

Interestingly, mean plasma testosterone levels of both the dietary intervention and control groups in Palermo appeared significantly lower than those reported by the DIANA study in Milan. This agrees well with the lower incidence of breast cancer in postmenopausal women in the Palermo area.

As shown in FIGURE 3, compliance evaluated at 1 year after the start of the study, was good in both the dietary intervention group (81%) and the control group (85%). n the former, significant weight loss was observed at the end of the 6-month period; in fact, all subjects under study revealed this trend along with reduced cholesterol plasma levels in most of them.

Last but not least, all subjects under dietary intervention experienced a psychophysical feeling of well-being that motivated most of their relatives to adopt the samecourse of nutrition.

Whether these subjects have substantial modification of the endocrine end-point (TABLE 3) is currently under investigation in our laboratories. Certainly, most enjoyed the rediscovery of a true traditional Mediterranean diet, not only for its psychophysical beneficial effects but also for the adventure of any archeological discovery.I

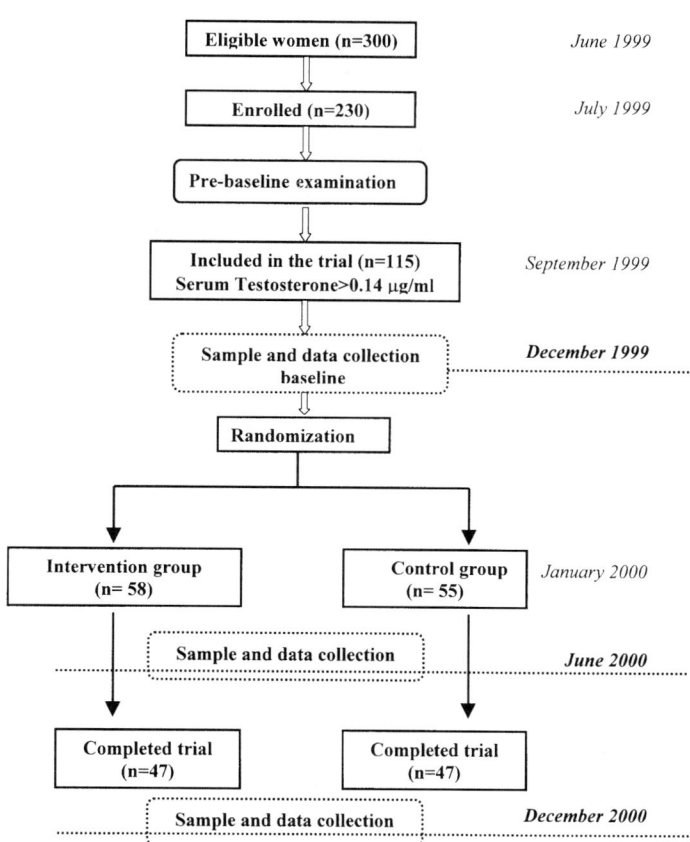

FIGURE 2. Experimental design.

TABLE 3. Endocrine end-points

Plasma levels	Urinary levels	Leukocyte DNA
Estradiol	Estrogens	DNA adducts
Testosterone	Phytoestrogens	GST M1 *gene*
DHEA	2/16 OH-estrone ratio	GST T1 *gene*
Insulin	...	...
Hormone binding proteins	...	...

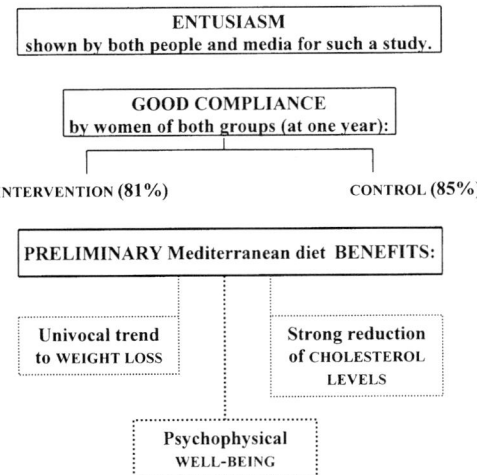

FIGURE 3. Main preliminary results.

ACKNOWLEDGMENTS

Our thanks are given to Dr. F. Berrino, Epidemiology Unit of Istituto Nazionale Tumori, Milan, Italy, for their essential collaboration. We also thank the teachers of the Palermo Tourism School 'P. Borsellino' and all of the participating women. This research was supported by a Special Project of City town and Province of Palermo and the Regional Agriculture Council of Sicily.

REFERENCES

1. SHUTT, D.A. & A.W.H. BRADEN. 1968. The significance of equol in relation to the oestrogenic responses in sheep ingesting clover with a high formononetin content. Austarlian Journal of agricultural research **19:** 545-553.
2. ADLERCREUTZ, H. 1995. Phytoestrogens: epidemiology and a possible role in cancer protection. Environ Health Perspect. **103:** 103-112.
3. ADLERCREUTZ, H. & W. MAZUR. 1997. Phytooestrogens and Western diseases. Ann. Med. **29:** 95-120.
4. FOOD, NUTRITION AND THE PREVENTION OF CANCER: a global perspective. 1997. World Cancer Research Fund / American Institute for Cancer Research.
5. CRESTA, M. *et al.* 1969. Etude des consommations alimentaires des populations de onze regions de la communaute europenne en vue de la determination des niveaux de contamination radioactive: rapport établì au Centre d'Etude Nucléaire de Fontenay-aux-Roses-France. EURATOM.
6. FERRO-LUZZI, A. & S. SETTE. 1989. The Mediterranean diet: an attempt to define its present and past composition. Eur. J. Clin. Nutr. **43:** 13-29.
7. PARKIN, D.M. *et al.* 1997. Cancer Incidence in Five Continents, Vol. VII. IARC Scientific Publications, N°143. Lyon, France.

8. CUSIMANO, R. et al. 1996. Breast cancer incidence in Palermo City (Italy). Ann. N.Y. Acad. Sci. **784:** 467-471.
9. TRAINA, A. et al. 2001. Collected abstract of 'V^a riunione scientifica annuale dell'Associazione Italiana Registri Tumori' (Alghero, Italy): 52. A.I.R.T. Italy.
10. ZANETTI, R. et al. 1997. Il Cancro in Italia. Il pensiero Scientifico Editore. Italy.
11. CUSIMANO, R. et al. 2001. Collected abstract of 'Dalla salute dell'individuo alla prevenzione nella collettività' Conference. Castelvetrano, Italy.
12. FERRO-LUZZI, A. & S. SETTE. 1989. The Mediterranean diet: an attempt to define its present and past composition. Eur. J. Clin. Nutr. **43:** 13-29.
13. FERRO-LUZZI, A. 1967. Problems in evaluating the nutritional level of ageing people. *In* Proceedings of the Seventh International Congress of Nutrition, Hamburg, 1966. Vol. 4. J. Kuhnau, ed. :193-203. Pergamon Press Ltd. Braunschweig.
14. FERRO-LUZZI, A. et al. 1994. The Mediterranean diet revisited. Focus on fruit and vegetables. Int. J. Food Sci. Nutr. **45:** 291-300.
15. DE LORENZO, A. et al. 2001. Food habits in a southern Italian town (Nicotera) in 1960 and 1996: still a reference Italian Mediterranean diet? Diabetes Nutr. Metab. **14:** 121-125.
16. TONIOLO, P.G. et al. 1995. A prospective study of endogenous estrogens and breast cancer in postmenopausal women. J. Natl. Cancer Inst. **87:** 190-197.
17. BERRINO, F. et al. 1996. Serum sex hormone levels after menopause and subsequent breast cancer. J. Natl. Cancer Inst. **88:** 291-296.
18. ZELENIUCH-JACQUOTTE, A. et al. 1997. Relation of serum levels of testosterone and dehydroepiandrosterone sulfate to risk of breast cancer in postmenopausal women. Am. J. Epidemiol. **145:** 1030-1038.
19. BERRINO, F. et al. 2001. Reducing bioavailable sex hormones through a comprehensive change in diet: the diet and androgens (DIANA) Randomized Trial. Cancer Epidemiol. Biomarkers Prev. **10:** 25-33.
20. PISANI, P. et al. 1997. Relative validity and reproducibility of a food frequency dietary questionnaire for use in the Italian EPIC centres. Int. J. Epidemiol. **26:** S152-S160.
21. SLIMANI, N. et al. 1999. Structure of the standardized computerized 24-h diet recall interview used as reference method in the 22 centres participating in the EPIC project. Comput. Methods Programs Biomed. **58:** 251-266.
22. SALVINI, S. et al. 1998. Banca dati di composizione degli alimenti per studi epidemiologici in Italia. Istituto Europeo di Oncologia. Milan, Italy.

Murine Models of Paroxysmal Nocturnal Hemoglobinuria

VITTORIO ROSTI

Laboratory of Organ Transplantation, IRCCS Policlinico San Matteo, Pavia, Italy

ABSTRACT: Paroxysmal nocturnal hemoglobinuria (PNH) is an acquired clonal disorder characterized by chronic intravascular hemolysis, cytopenia, and an increased tendency to thrombosis. All patients with PNH studied so far have a somatic mutation of phosphatidyl inositol glycan complementation group A (PIG-A), an X-linked gene involved initially in the biosynthesis of the glycosyl phosphatidylinositol (GPI) molecule, which serves as an anchor for many cell surface proteins. The mutation occurs in a hematopoietic stem cell, and consequently, all cells derived from the mutated stem cell are devoid of GPI-linked proteins. The absence of GPI-linked proteins explains some clinical symptoms of the disease but not the mechanism that allows the expansion of the mutated clone. By using targeted disruption of the PIG-A gene in mouse embryonic stem cells, some mice models of PNH have been generated. These animals have a discrete proportion of blood cells devoid of GPI-linked proteins, and although not anemic, they have evidence of hemolysis. The clinical course of these animals is benign, and there are no signs of a substantial expansion of the PNH clone, as observed in human patients. The fact that these animals do not develop the disease strongly supports the notion that a mutation of PIG-A is not sufficient per se to cause PNH and that another factor, namely, bone marrow failure, is necessary to allow proliferation and expansion of the PNH clone.

KEYWORDS: phosphatidyl inositol glycan complementation group A; PIG-A; knockout mice; Cre/loxP; paroxysmal nocturnal hemoglobinuria

INTRODUCTION

Over the last 20 years few diseases have been investigated at the cellular and molecular level as deeply and extensively as paroxysmal nocturnal hemoglobinuria (PNH). However, despite this effort a definitive model of its pathogenesis has not yet been proposed. This is in some way surprising, considering that the molecular defect underlying the disease has been well known since 1993. In this review we summarize our current knowledge of the biology of PNH. Some animal models that were generated in the last 5 years with the aim of reproducing a pathogenetic model of the disease are discussed.

Address for correspondence: Vittorio Rosti, M.D., Medicina Interna ed Oncologia Medica, IRCCS Policlinico San Matteo, Piazzale Golgi, 2, 27100 Pavia, Italy. Voice: 39 0382 502162; fax: 39 0382 525222.

virosti@tin.it

PAROXYSMAL NOCTURNAL HEMOGLOBINURIA: GENERAL ASPECTS

Paroxysmal nocturnal hemoglobinuria is defined as a clonal disorder of a hematopoietic stem cell. From a clinical point of view the disease presents with hemolytic anemia, cytopenia of variable degree (the most common feature), and venous thrombosis.[1] These are the symptoms that characterize the course of the disease, whereas cytopenia with underlying bone marrow failure and/or thrombotic events is the main cause of morbidity and mortality. Although spontaneous remissions have been reported, PNH is a chronic disease with a median survival of 14 years from diagnosis.[2,3] The main therapeutic approaches are immunosuppressive therapy and allogeneic bone marrow transplantation. The latter currently represents a unique therapy that can cure PNH. However, the procedure has an intrinsic mortality, which suggests that we should keep this approach for young patients with an available identical donor.[4]

SOMATIC MUTATION

It is now known that all patients with PNH have a somatic mutation, occurring in a hematopoietic stem cell, of an X-linked gene called PIG-A, which stands for phosphatidyl inositol glycan complementation class A.[5,6] The product of PIG-A is involved in the first step of the biosynthesis of the glycosylphosphatidylinositol (GPI) molecule, which serves as an anchor for many proteins tethered to the cell membrane.[7] The mutation of PIG-A impairs the function of the gene, and as a result the stem cell in which the mutation occurs and all its progeny are devoid of the GPI anchor and, in turn, of all GPI-linked proteins. Thus, in the peripheral blood of patients with PNH, two populations of cells exist, one normal and one deficient in all GPI-linked proteins. To date, more than 170 mutations of PIG-A have been described; they are spread all over the gene. Most mutations are insertions or deletions, but point mutations (nonsense and missense) have also been reported.[8] Often the mutation completely abrogates PIG-A activity, resulting in the total absence of GPI molecules, which in turn causes the total absence of GPI-linked proteins from the surface of the cells (socalled type III PNH cells). In some cases, however, the PIG-A mutation does not completely impair the function of the gene, resulting in residual PIG-A gene activity. This allows a small amount of GPI molecules to be synthesized, so that in this case red cells are only partially deficient in GPI-linked proteins (type II PNH cells). Type II and type III red cells sometimes coexist in the same patient, indicating that two different clones also exist. In addition, patients who have only type III red blood cells may also have two (or more) clones.[9,10]

CLINICAL FEATURES

The molecular defect explains some of the clinical features of PNH, namely, hemolytic anemia, which is due to the action of the complement on circulating red cells.[11] In normal individuals, red cells are protected from the action of the complement by the CD59 and CD55 molecules; in fact, both proteins are GPI linked and therefore they are lacking on PNH red cells. The presence of the PIG-A mutation, however, does not explain the presence of a certain degree of bone marrow failure and the frequent association of PNH with aplastic anemia. The occurrence of thrombotic events in patients with PNH does not have a definitive explanation; however, the defect of one or more GPI-linked proteins from the surface of platelets apparently accounts, at least in part, for the recurrence of thrombotic episodes in patients with PNH.[12]

PATHOGENESIS

Although the molecular defect has been clarified, the pathogenesis of PNH is not yet completely understood. Basically, the key to unraveling the pathogenetic mechanism seems to lie in the answer to the puzzling question: how it is possible that a hematopoietic stem cell and its progeny lacking all the GPI-linked proteins expand in the bone marrow and overwhelm their normal counterpart? In fact, in many patients with PNH, the PNH clone accounts for more than 50% of peripheral blood cells, and it is not uncommon to have patients in which 90% of circulating granulocytes lack GPI-linked proteins.

The simplest answer to this question is to assume that the mutated stem cell has an intrisic growth advantage, derived from the absence of one or more of these proteins. The advantage would result in expansion of the defective clone that takes over on normal hematopoiesis. This theory, which is based on some experimental evidence,[13] experiences some difficulties, however, in its validation on both a clinical and an experimental basis. First, spontaneous remissions of the disease have been reported.[2] Second, and different from leukemia (in which the pathologic clone has a real proliferative advantage), in many patients with PNH after initial expansion the PNH clone remains stable and in a sort of a balance with the remaining normal hematopoiesis.[2] Third, the *in vitro* growth of hematopoietic progenitor cells derived from patients with PNH is poor, and often low numbers of PNH CFC and/or LTC-IC are detected.[14,15] The main evidence in support of this theory is the finding that PIG-A-negative cells are more resistant to apoptosis than are their normal counterparts,[13] but the results have not been confirmed by others[16,17] and a relation between GPI-linked proteins and apoptosis has not been described. An alternative answer is based on the assumption that the molecular defect of PIG-A must be associated with another (extrinsic) factor that allows expansion of the PNH clone. This theory, called the dual pathogenesis of PNH,[18,19] stems from the observation that a variable degree of bone marrow failure is almost invariably associated with PNH and not infrequently one or more PNH clones are found in patients with aplastic anemia.[2,20,21] Based on this observation, it was speculated that failure of normal bone marrow due to injury that spares GPI-negative progenitor cells allows expansion of the PNH clone.[18,19,22] The real mechanism driving the entire process is actually unknown, but it is very likely that aplastic anemia is due to an (auto)immune attack towards normal stem cells.[23] Surmising that the immune attack is mediated through a GPI-dependent mechanism, the GPI-negative stem cell would easily escape injury and subsequently expand. Not surprisingly, treatment of PNH patients with immunosuppressive therapy often results in the recovery of normal hematopoiesis and the disappearance of the PNH clone. Moreover, in some patients treated with the monoclonal antibody

CAMPATH-1H, which is directed towards the GPI-linked protein CD52, GPI-negative T lymphocytes were detected during therapy and gradually disappeared when therapy was withdrawn.[24–26] Importantly, in some of these patients different mutations of PIG-A were documented, and in one case it was possible to show that the mutation was present before treatment was started.[26] In these cases as well as in patients with aplastic anemia who develop PNH, it is the positive selective pressure driven by either injury to normal bone marrow or antibody against CD52, respectively, that favors expansion of the PNH clone. The finding of PIG-A mutations in CD59-negative granulocytes of normal individuals further supports the notion that PIG-A mutation *per se* is not sufficient (although necessary) to cause PNH.[27] Finally, a defect in residual normal hematopoietic stem cells was also suggested in a recent report by Chen *et al.*[28] who found that *ex vivo* cultured PIG-A$^+$ CD34$^+$ cells display greater susceptibility to apoptosis than does their PIG-A-negative counterpart.

Besides all the findings that favor either hypothesis (intrinsic or conditional growth advantage), the need for an animal model to help understand the pathogenesis of the disease has compelled different groups to generate transgenic mice carrying the PIG-A mutation in their hematopoietic stem cells. Targeted disruption of the PIG-A gene in mouse embryonic stem (ES) cells, followed by their injection into blastocysts subsequently transplanted in pseudopregnant females, represents the simplest way to obtain animals chimeric for a nonfunctional gene.[29,30] In fact, in mice as in humans, PIG-A maps on the X chromosome, and only one recombination event is needed to inactivate the gene in male ES cells. In the first attempts, viable animals were obtained only when the contribution of PIG-A–negative ES cells to developing embryos was low.[31–33] In these animals the number of GPI-negative blood cells was low at birth and further decreased during the first weeks of life. Subsequently, with the Cre/*loxP* system, conditional inactivation of PIG-A in ES cells was obtained, so that animals with a higher contribution of PIG-A–negative stem cells to the hematopoietic system were generated.[34,35] These mice had a greater number of blood cells lacking GPI-linked proteins than did mice obtained with the previous approach, and the proportion of these cells was also more stable. Moreover, although they were not anemic and had a normal life span, their red cells had increased sensitivity to complement-mediated lysis and, as in PNH patients, they had two discrete populations of blood cells, one normal and one devoid of all GPI-linked proteins. In both models, however, GPI-negative blood cells did not show any intrinsic growth advantage compared to their normal counterpart but, rather, they either decreased with time or maintained their number unchanged. The absence of selective pressure in favor of the PNH clone (namely, a variable degree of normal bone marrow failure) would be the reason for the lack of expansion of PIG-A–negative hematopoietic stem cells in these animals. Thus, murine models of PNH seem to agree with the theory of the dual pathogenesis of PNH.

OTHER MURINE MODELS

Other murine models of PNH have also been generated in order to obtain animals in which most, if not all, blood cells are GPI negative. In addition, to shed further light on PNH pathogenesis, these animals were generated to allow functional studies on single different lineages of GPI-negative blood cells. In 1997 Nakamura and coworkers,[36] taking advantage of the Cre/*loxP* strategy with the Cre recombinase under the control of a T-cell–specific promoter, were able to specifically disrupt PIG-A function exclusively in T lymphocytes. In these animals, all T cells were GPI negative, whereas the other hematopoietic lineages were normal. Interestingly, these mice were healthy and their T cells, although devoid of all GPI-linked proteins, were functionally competent in exerting TCR-mediated immune responses both *in vitro* and *in vivo*. Based on these results it seems that GPI-linked molecules on T cells are not essential for their functional competence. It should be remembered that although a role for GPI-linked proteins in lymphoid cell function has been suggested,[37] patients with PNH do not have any evident deficit in immune function. However, in human patients the proportion of GPI-negative T lymphocytes usually does not exceed 50% of total T cells,[38] and therefore it is possible that the remaining GPI-positive T cells account for the integrity of the immune function. Recently, two other animal models of PNH have been generated. In both cases, PIG-A was inactivated selectively in the hematopoietic system by means of the Cre/*loxP* approach, but using different regulatory sequences for the control of the activity of the Cre recombinase.[39,40] When Cre was driven by regulatory sequences of the human gene c-FES, PIG-A inactivation was obtained exclusively in early hematopoietic progenitors. Newborn mice had low levels of GPI-negative cells in all hematopoietic lineages. However, their number increased with age, and in adult mice, blood cells were almost exclusively GPI negative.[39] These mice, in addition to mimicking the hematologic pattern observed in many PNH patients, represent a powerful tool for performing functional studies on PIG-A–negative blood cells. In a similar study, PIG-A was inactivated in the erythroid and megakaryocityc lineages selectively, by using the Cre/*loxP* system with the Cre recombinase under the control of the transcriptional regulatory sequences of GATA-1. In these mice, almost 100% of the peripheral red blood cells were deficient in GPI-linked proteins. Interestingly, a proportion of red cells expressed low levels of GPI-linked proteins, probably because the Cre-mediated recombination of PIG-A occurred late in erythroid differentiation, after the BFU-E stage.[40] These red cells with residual expression of GPI-linked proteins clearly resemble PNH type II cells, which are not uncommonly observed in many patients with PNH. As expected, PIG-A recombination was also observed in megakaryocytes but not in neutrophils and lymphocytes, according to the tissue specificity of expression of GATA-1 regulatory sequences. These mice neither were anemic nor showed signs of thrombosis or hemoglobinuria, although their red blood cell values were in the lower range of normal control values. Despite their apparent normality, the peripheral red blood cells of these animals were very similar to red cells of patients with PNH (both type II and type III cells), thus promising to be very helpful in future functional studies on GPI-linked proteins of red blood cells.

FUTURE RESEARCH

Many biological and molecular aspects of PNH have been clarified in recent years because of a great number of studies devoted to comprehending this disease. However, we are still far from a complete understanding of not only the pathogenesis of the disease (including the intrinsic biological behavior of the PIG-A–negative stem cell) but also the functions of many GPI-linked proteins and the GPI anchor itself. Thus, further *in vitro* and *in vivo* experiments, including new animal models, are necessary to answer the still open questions on PNH biology. The answer to these questions will, in turn, help to discover better treatments for patients with PNH.

REFERENCES

1. DACIE, J.V. & S.M. LEWIS. 1972. Paroxysmal nocturnal haemoglobinuria: clinical manifestations, haematology and nature of the disease. Ser Haematol **5:** 3–23.
2. HILLMEN, P., S.M. LEWIS, M. BESSLER, *et al.* 1995. Natural history of paroxysmal nocturnal haemoglobinuria. N Engl J Med **333:** 1253–1258.
3. SOCIE, G., J.Y. MARY, A. DE GRAMONT, *et al.* 1996. Paroxysmal nocturnal haemoglobinuria: long term follow up and prognostic factors. Lancet **348:** 573–577.
4. ARATEN, D. J., L. LUZZATTO. 2000. Allogeneic bone marrow transplantation for paroxysmal nocturnal hemoglobinuria. Haematologica **85:** 1–2.
5. MIYATA, T., J. TAKEDA, J. JIDA, *et al.* 1993. The cloning of PIG-A, a component in the early step of GPI-anchor biosynthesis. Science **259:** 1318–1320.
6. BESSLER, M., P.J. MASON, P. HILLMEN, *et al.* 1994. Paroxysmal nocturnal haemoglobinuria (PNH) is caused by somatic mutations in the PIG-A gene. EMBO J **13:** 110–117.
7. HILLMEN, P., M. BESSLER, P.J. MASON, *et al.* 1993. Specific defect in N-acetylglucosamine incorporation in the biosynthesis of the glyosylphosphatidylinositol anchor in cloned cell lines in patients with paroxysmal nocturnal haemoglobinuria. Proc Natl Acad Sci USA **90:** 5272–5276.
8. LUZZATTO, L. & K. NAFA. 2000. Genetics of PNH. *In* Paroxysmal nocturnal hemoglobinuria and GPI-linked proteins. N.S. Young et al, Eds.: 21–47. Academic Press. New York, NY.
9. BESSLER, M., P. MASON, P. HILLMEN AND L. LUZZATTO. 1994. Somatic mutations and cellular selection in paroxysmal nocturnal haemoglobinuria. Lancet **343:** 951–953.
10. NISHIMURA, J., N. INOUE, H. WADA, *et al.* 1997. A patient with paroxysmal nocturnal hemoglobinuria bearing four independent PIG-A mutant clones. Blood **89:** 3470–3476.
11. PARKER, C.J. 2000. Hemolysis in PNH. *In* Paroxysmal nocturnal hemoglobinuria and GPI-linked proteins. N.S. Young et al, Eds.: 49–100. Academic Press. New York, NY.
12. Luzzatto, L. 2000. Pathophysiology of paroxysmal nocturnal haemoglobinuria. *In* Educational book of the European Haematology Association: 203–209. 5th Congress of the European Haematology Association, Birmingham, UK.
13. BRODSKY, R.A., M.S. VALA, J.P. BARBER, *et al.* 1997. Resistance to apoptosis caused by PIG-A gene mutations in paroxysmal nocturnal hemoglobinuria. Proc Natl Acad Sci USA **94:** 8756–8760.
14. ROTOLI, B. & L. LUZZATTO. 1982. Decreased number of circulating BFU-E in paroxysmal nocturnal haemoglobinuria. Blood **60:** 157–159.
15. MACIEJEWSKI, J.P., E.M. SLOAND, T. SATO, *et al.* 1997. Impaired hematopoiesis in parosxysmal nocturnal haemoglobinuria/aplastic anemia is not associated with a selective proliferative defect in the glycosylphosphatidylinositol-anchored protein-deficient clone. Blood **89:** 1173–1181.
16. HORIKAWA, K., H. NAKAKUMA, T. KAWAGUCHI, *et al.* 1997. Apoptosis resistance of blood cells from patients with paroxysmal nocturnal hemoglobinuria, aplastic anemia and myelodisplastic syndrome. Blood **90:** 2716–2722.
17. WARE, R.E., J. NISHIMURA, M.A. MOODY, *et al.* 1997. The PIG-A mutation and absence of glycosylphosphatidylinositol-linked proteins do not confer resistance to apoptosis in paroxysmal nocturnal hemoglobinuria. Blood **92:** 2541–2550.
18. ROTOLI, B. & L. LUZZATTO. 1989. Paroxysmal nocturnal hemoglobinuria. Sem Haematol **26:** 201–207.
19. LUZZATTO, L. & M. BESSLER. 1996. The dual pathogenesis of paroxysmal nocturnal hemoglobinuria. Curr Op Hematol **3:** 101–110.
20. TICHELLI, A., A. GRATWOHL, A. WURSCH, *et al.* 1988. Late haematological complications in severe aplastic anaemia. Br J Haematol **69:** 413–418.

21. SCHREZENMEIER, H., B. HERTENSTEIN, B. WAGNER, et al. 1997. A pathogenetic link between aplastic and paroxysmal nocturnal hemoglobinuria is suggested by a high frequency of plastic anemia patients with a deficiency of phosphatidylinositol glycan anchored proteins. Exp Hematol **23:** 81–87.
22. BESSLER, M. & L. LUZZATTO. 1998. Somatic mutations and clonal selection in the pathogenesis and in the control of paroxysmal nocturnal hemoglobinuria. Sem Hematol **35:** 149–167.
23. YOUNG, N.S. & J.P. MACIEJEWSKI. 1997. The pathophysiology of acquired aplastic anemia. N Engl J Med **336:** 1365–1372.
24. HERTENSTEIN, B., B. WAGNER, D. BUNJES, et al. 1995. Emergence of CD52-, phosphatidylinositol-glycan-anchor-deficient T lymphocytes after in vivo application of Campath-1H for refeactory B-cell non-Hodgkin's lymphoma. Blood **86:** 1492–1497.
25. TAYLOR, V.C., M. SIMS, S. BRETT, et al. 1997. Antibody selection against CD52 produces a paroxysmal nocturnal haemoglobinuria phenotype in human lymphocytes by a novel mechanism. Biochem J **322:** 919–925.
26. RAWSTROM, A.C., S.J. ROLLINSON, S. RICHARDS, et al. 1999. The PNH phenotype cells that emerge in most patients after Campath-1H therapy are present prior to treatment. Br J Haematol **107:** 148–153.
27. ARATEN, D.J., K. NAFA, K. PAKDEESUWAN, et al. 1999. Clonal population of hemopoietic cells with paroxysmal nocturnal hemoglobinuria genotype and phenotype are present in normal individuals. Proc Natl Acad Sci USA **96:** 5209–5214.
28. CHEN, R., S. NAGARAJAN, G.M. PRINCE, et al. 2000. Impaired growth and elevated Fas receptor expression in *PIG-A+* stem cells in primary paroxysmal nocturnal hemoglobinuria. J Clin Invest **106:** 689–696.
29. CAPECCHI, M. 1989. The new mouse genetics: altering the genome by gene targeting. Trends Genet **5:** 70–76.
30. GALLI-TALIADORIS, L.A., J.D. SEDGURICK, S.A. WOOD, et al. 1995. Geno ko technology: a methodological overview for the interested novice. J Immunol Methods **181:** 1–5.
31. DUNN, D. E., J. YU, S. NAGARAJAN, et al. 1996. A knock-out model of paroxysmal nocturnal hemoglobinuria: Pig-a- hematopoiesis is reconstituted following intercellular transfer of GPI-anchored proteins. Proc Natl Acad Sci USA **93:** 7938–7943.
32. KAWAGOE, K., D. KITAMURA, M. OKABE, et al. 1996. Glycosylphosphatidyl inositol-anchor-deficient mice: implications for clonal dominance of mutant cells in paroxysmal nocturnal hemoglobinuria. Blood **87:** 3600–3606.
33. ROSTI, V., G. TREMML, V. SOARES, et al. 1997. Murine embryonic stem cells without *pig-a* gene activity are competent for hematopoiesis with the PNH phenotype but not for clonal expansion. J Clin Invest **100:** 1028–1036.
34. MURAKAMI, Y., T KINOSHITA, Y. MAEDA, et al. 1999. Different roles of glycosylphosphatidyl inositol in various hematopoietic cells as revealed by a mouse model of paroxysmal nocturnal hemoglobinuria. Blood **94:** 2963–2970.
35. TREMML, G., C. DOMINGUEZ, V. ROSTI, et al. 1999. Increased sensitivity to complement and a decrease red blood cells life span in mice mosaic fora non functional *Pig-a* gene. Blood **94:** 2945–2954.
36. TAKAHAMA, Y., K. OHISHI, Y TOKORO, et al. 1998. Functional competence of T cells in the absence of glycosylphosphatidylinositol-anchored proteins caused by T cell-specific disruption of the *Pig-a* gene. Eur J Immunol **28:** 2159–2166.
37. MARMOR, M.D. & M. JULIUS. 2000. The function of GPI-anchored proteins in T cell development, activation and regulation of homeostasis. **14:** 99–115.
38. TSENG, J.E., S. HALL, T.A. HOWARD, et al. 1995. Phenotypic and functional analysis of lymphocytes in paroxysmal nocturnal hemoglobinuria. Am J Hematol **50:** 244–253.
39. KELLER, P., J.L. PAYNE, G. TREMML, et al. 2001. FES-Cre targets phosphatidylinositol Glycan class A (PIGA) inactivation to hematopoitic stem cell in the bone marrow. J Exp Med **194:** 581–589.
40. JASINSKI, M., P. KELLER, Y. FUJIWARA, et al. 2001. GATA1-Cre mediates *Piga* gene inactivation in the erythroid/megakaryocitic lineage and leads to circulating red cells with a partial deficiency in glycosylphosphatidylinositol-linked proteins (paroxysmal nocturnal hemoglobinuria type II cells). Blood **98:** 2248–2255.

Molecular Genetics of Acute Myeloid Leukemia

PAOLO BERNASCONI, MARINA BONI, PAOLA MARIA CAVIGLIANO, SILVIA CALATRONI, ILARIA GIARDINI, BARBARA ROCCA, AND MARILENA CARESANA

Department of Blood, Heart and Lung Medical Sciences of the University of Pavia and Division of Hematology, Policlinico San Matteo IRCCS, Pavia, Italy

ABSTRACT: Recurring chromosomal abnormalities are detected in most patients with acute myeloid leukemia (AML). They may be associated with a distinct AML FAB subtype or may identify distinct clinicobiological entities within the same FAB subtype. Therefore, cytogenetic investigation has a pivotal role in AML diagnosis. In addition, it is one of the most valuable prognostic determinants of the disease, as recently demonstrated. The development of new molecular techniques, such as reverse transcriptase polymerase chain reaction and fluorescence in situ hybridization, has allowed perfect definition of the chromosome regions containing genes with a crucial role in normal hemopoiesis and leukemia. Understanding the action of such genes provides new insights into AML pathogenesis and has led us to envisage new therapeutic options.

KEYWORDS: acute myeloid leukemia; FAB subtype; genetics; chromosomal abnormalities

INTRODUCTION

Acute myeloid leukemia (AML), a clonal disorder due to an acquired somatic mutation in a hematopoietic progenitor cell, is a heterogeneous disease, showing variability in the degree of commitment and differentiation of the cell lineage involved. Two main classification schemes are currently available, the French-American-British (FAB) system, based on morphological, cytochemical, and immunological features of the blast cell population, and the cytogenetic system, based on the clonal chromosomal abnormality observed. The accuracy of chromosome analysis has progressively increased over the last 20 years since the introduction and refinement of high resolution banding techniques. Nowadays, conventional chromosome studies performed by skilled personnel can identify nonrandom clonal aberrations in at least 60–80% of AMLs.[1] Some of these clonal cytogenetic defects correlate with specific FAB subtypes, whereas others identify distinct morphological and clinical entities within the same FAB subtype. Therefore, cytogenetic investigation has a pivotal role in the diagnostic work-up of AML patients. In addition, it pro-

---

Address for correspondence: Prof. Paolo Bernasconi, Divisione di Ematologia, Policlinico San Matteo, IRCCS, 27100 Pavia, Italy. Voice: 0039 0382 526276; fax: 0039 0382 502250.
p.bernasconi@smatteo.pv.it

vides information on the possible clinical behavior and therapeutic response of a particular AML subtype.[2]

Despite the aforementioned technical improvements, however, an apparently normal chromosome pattern or no cytogenetic data are obtained from at least 20% and 10% of AML patients, respectively. These unsatisfactory cytogenetic results are due to the fact that the technique requires good quality metaphases. In some cases, however, conventional cytogenetics is unable to identify the rearrangement, as it involves chromosome regions (telomeric ends) weakly stained on G-banding. Since the late 1980s, the introduction of FISH has overcome some of these limitations, greatly enhancing the power of cytogenetics and creating a bridge between it and molecular biology.[3] The FISH technical principle is based on the ability of single-stranded DNA to anneal to complementary DNA. A variety of nucleic acid sequences can be employed as probes to cellular DNA targets, such as nuclear DNA of interphase cells or the DNA of metaphase chromosomes. The use of differently labeled probes has allowed the simultaneous detection of multiple target regions. In this way, FISH has discovered new cryptic chromosome aberrations and has pinpointed genomic regions containing genes that play a crucial role in normal hematopoiesis and which function is altered by the leukemogenic process. The advent of new resources and technical innovations, such as color karyotyping and comparative genomic hybridization, will shed light on AML pathogenesis and will uncover new clinical entities with distinct morphologic and prognostic features.

Clonal chromosome abnormalities can be subdivided into balanced defects, without loss or gain of chromosome material (translocations and inversions), and unbalanced defects, with loss or gain of chromosome material (deletions, nonreciprocal translocations, monosomies, and trisomies). All these aberrations are specific clonal markers that can identify the neoplastic cell population in any phase of the disease. They may be present on diagnosis, disappear on complete remission, and be associated with additional abnormalities on relapse. In the present report we review the most important cytogenetics and molecular genetic findings in AML, underlying their relevance in the diagnosis and prognosis of the disease.

BALANCED CHROMOSOMAL ABNORMALITIES

These balanced chromosomal abnormalities consisting of reciprocal translocation and para- or pericentric inversions are found in about 40% of patients with AML. These defects cause rearrangement of genomic regions containing either genes encoding for a variety of transcription factors or promoter/enhancer sequences governing the expression of such genes. The abnormality leads to the creation of a chimeric gene that interferes with growth, differentiation, and survival of hematopoietic progenitor cells. Translocations and inversions may be demonstrated not only with conventional cytogenetics but also with FISH and reverse transcriptase polymerase chain reaction (RT-PCR), a technique that amplifies the chimeric sequence formed by the rearrangement. Recently, the specific oncoprotein caused by the chromosomal abnormality may also be identified by a specific monoclonal antibody.

Genes involved in such translocations and inversions are the following: core binding factor (CBF), retinoic acid receptor alpha (RARA), mixed lineage leukemia (MLL), transcriptional coactivators (CBP/p3000), and other genes.

Core Binding Factor

These rearrangements involve a heterodimeric transcription factor essential for the formation of the definitive hematopoietic system. It is formed by two subunits, α (also called AML1) and β. AML1 is the DNA-binding subunit of CBF. Its affinity for DNA binding is increased by the creation of a heterodimer with the β subunit. The α subunit is involved in the t(8;21)(q22;q22), whereas the β subunit in the inv(16)(p13q22).

t(8;21)(q22;q22) AML1/ETO

This translocation has an incidence of 5–10% and is observed in AML of the child and young adult. It is strictly correlated with an AML-M2: almost all t(8;21) are associated with such a cytotype, and 30–40% of AML-M2 carry the translocation. Blast cells typically show prominent Auer rods, a cytoplasm containing large vacuoles and salmon-colored granules, and strong myeloperoxidase activity on cytochemistry. These cells are positive for CD19, CD13, CD34, and CD56 on immunophenotyping, and this finding is so characteristic that it alone suggests the presence of the translocation. Bone marrow examination demonstrates important dysgranulopoiesis and increased eosinophils. Some patients may show a blast cell percentage of less than 30%, but this finding may be misleading, masking quick evolution into frank leukemia.

The t(8;21) determines the rearrangement between the AML-1 gene, mapped at band 21q22, and the ETO gene, mapped at band 8q22. Both AML-1 and ETO breakpoints cluster within a single intron, and in every case a similar AML-1/ETO chimeric gene is created. This last, formed on the derivative of chromosome 8, der(8), is thought to be the critical genetic event. The AML-1/ETO protein is formed by the N-terminal 177 amino acids of AML-1 fused to the almost complete ETO protein. Normally, AML-1 activates transcription of numerous hematopoietic specific genes through p300/CBP binding. These last have intrinsic histone acetyltransferase activity. In this way, the normal AML-1 induces acetylation of lysine residues determining a change in chromatin structure and enhanced transcription. The leukemogenic activity of the AML-1/ETO protein is due in part to its dominant negative activity on the remaining normal AML1 allele and in part to an altered regulation of target gene transcription (homeobox genes). This last function is probably due to the fact that ETO may interact with the nuclear corepressors N-CoR and Sin3A, generating a histone deacetylase activity.[4]

The t(8;21), which may derive from variant translocations in about 5% of cases, is frequently observed in combination with additional cytogenetic abnormalities such as loss of the sex chromosomes, trisomy 8, and deletion of chromosome 9 long arm (9q–). It is associated with a good response to chemotherapy. The probability of obtaining complete remission is about 80–90%, and the overall 5-year survival rate is about 60–70%. However, outcome is unfavorable in t(8;21) patients with advanced age, hyperleukocytosis, and 9q– as additional chromosomal defects.

inv(16)(p13q22) CBFb/SMMHC

This is the second most frequent cytogenetic defect involving the β subunit of the CBF. It is discovered in at least 10–12% of all AMLs, even if its incidence seems to be higher with FISH or RT-PCR. This difference is due to the fact that inv(16) involves regions not easily visualized in poor quality metaphases. This type of AML is most frequently classified as M4, more rarely as M2 or M5. Bone marrow cytology is typical: myeloid and monocytoid blast cells are seen in combination with atypical eosinophils showing a mixture of eosinophilic and basophilic granules in the cytoplasm and monocytoid nuclei (AML-M4eo). The chromosome abnormality most frequently consists in a pericentric inversion of chromosome 16 and more rarely in a t(16;16)(p13;q22). Additional abnormalities (trisomy 8 or 22) are seen in 50% of patients.

The molecular defect of inv(16)/t(16;16) consists in the juxtaposition of CBF β subunit sequences, mapped at 16q22, with those of the smooth muscle heavy chain gene (SMMHC), mapped at 16p13. The breakpoints within CBFβ occur at either the end of exon 5 or, more rarely, the end of exon 4; the breakpoints within the SMMHC gene are variable. The chimeric protein has probably a dominant inhibitory action on the wild-type AML1 gene. Rearrangement of either subunit of the CBF determines an altered homeobox gene transcription, resulting in distinct acute leukemia phenotypes: in AML-M2 with maturation if the patient develops a t(8;21), in AML-M4 if the patient develops an inv(16), and in acute lymphoblastic leukemia (ALL) if the patient, almost always a child, develops a t(12;21). The unifying clinical feature is that all patients with these rearrangements have a chemosensitive disease with a favorable clinical outcome.

Retinoic Acid Receptor Alpha (RARA)

Virtually all patients with acute promyelocytic leukemia show a t(15;17)(q22;q12), which probably does not occur at the level of the most primitive hematopoietic stem cell, even if some progenitor cells containing the translocation may give rise, *in vitro,* to myeloid and erythroid colonies.

The t(15;17) causes a rearrangement between the PML gene, mapped at band 15q22, and the RARA gene, mapped at band 17q12. Three distinct breakpoints may occur within the PML gene, whereas the breakpoint within the RARA gene is always constant, being localized within the second intron of the gene. Normally, PML has pro-apoptotic and growth inhibitory activity and is localized to specialized nuclear pods. These last are changed into nuclear "speckles" by the t(15;17). Normally, RARA is a transcriptional factor that mediates the effect of retinoic acid at specific retinoid elements. It has differentiation-promoting and growth-suppressing activity and plays a crucial role in normal hematopoiesis. The PML-RARA chimeric gene, formed on 15q, may counteract PML functions and act as a dominant negative inhibitor on the wild-type RARA gene. The myeloid differentiation block determined is obtained through recruitment of co-repressor molecules and histone deacetylase activity that repress transcription of retinoic acid target genes. The demonstration that PML-RARA fusion gene plays a crucial role in leukemogenesis has been confirmed on transgenic mice that developed AML-M3 after a 6-month latency period.

Acute promyelocytic leukemia is a unique form of AML, being extremely sensitive to the cytotoxic effect of antracyclines and to the differentiative action of all-trans-retinoic acid. This latter can relieve the repression of retinoic acid target genes by releasing the corepressor/histone deacetylase activity complex from PML-RARA. Various clinical studies have demonstrated that such an association can cure most patients with acute promyelocytic leukemia, and hence assessment of the PML-RARA status in patients with morphologic acute promyelocytic leukemia is absolutely mandatory for their diagnosis and optimal management.

The role of conventional cytogenetics in confirming a morphologic diagnosis of acute promyelocytic leukemia is further underlined by involvement of the RARA gene in other balanced translocations having a different response to ATRA. These translocations are t(11;17)(q23;q21), t(5;17)(q35;q12-21), and t(11;17)(q13;q21) and cause rearrangement of the RARA gene with PLZF, mapped at band 11q23, with NPM, mapped at band 5q35, and with NuMA, mapped at band 11q13. AML patients carrying these translocations may be morphologically classified as either M2 or M3 and have a different clinical behavior from that of classic M3. AMLs harboring the t(11;17) have a blast cell population with a hypergranular cytoplasm, rare Auer rods, and a regular nuclear outline. This last characteristic, when present in at least 30% of the cells, is the key feature for distinguishing patients with the t(11;17) from those with the standard t(15;17), but it is also present in other variant RARA rearrangements. Moreover, the latter, like t(11;17) patients, show an increased number of hypogranular Pelger-like cells. Therefore, variant RARA translocations, cannot be morphologically distinguished and the immunophenotype, demonstrating CD56 positivity, is the only factor that can identify t(11;17) patients. It has therefore been proposed that a regular nuclear outline and CD56 positivity should alert on the possibility of an underlying PLZF/RARA rearrangement. This datum is of utmost importance because t(11;17) patients are unresponsive to ATRA. This phenomenon, due to the PLZF gene's ability to bind in a retinoid-insensitive fashion the co-repressor complex, can be overcome by administration of ATRA combined with arsenic trioxide.

Mixed Lineage Leukemia

These karyotype abnormalities are in most cases translocations involving band 11q23, where the mixed lineage leukemia (MLL) gene is mapped. As band 11q23 is rearranged with at least 40 different chromosomal loci, MLL is considered a "promiscuous" gene. MLL translocations are particularly frequent in infant leukemia (50–60% of cases). The incidence of these rearrangements is about 4–5% in de novo AMLs, but it increases to 80% in AMLs occurring after treatment with topoisomerase II inhibitors (such as etoposide), antracyclines, and cisplatinum. The t(9;11)(p21;q23) was initially reported in patients with monoblastic leukemia without differentiation (AML-M5a). However, it was later evident that 11q23 rearrangement may be discovered in acute leukemia of either myeloid or lymphoid lineage (mixed lineage leukemias). The t(9;11) is still associated with AML-M5a, whereas the t(4;11)(q21;q23) and t(11;19)(q23;p13.3) with a lymphoid phenotype in infant patients. The t(6;11)(q27;q23) may be associated with a myelodysplastic syndrome. Some other 11q23 translocations have frequently been reported in AML, showing lymphoid markers. Recently, it was observed that patients with a normal karyotype or with trisomy 11 may harbor a "tandem duplication" of the MLL gene.

The highly conserved 100-kb long MLL gene is expressed as a 15-kb transcript containing 23 exons and coding for a protein of 3,972 amino acids. MLL has homology with the trithorax gene, which directs the development along the anteroposterior axis during *Drosophila* embryogenesis. In humans the MLL gene is crucial for normal hematopoiesis, regulating the early differentiation of the most primitive hematopoietic stem cells. Normally the MLL gene controls expression of homeobox genes. MLL alters local chromatin structure or facilitates the recruitment of transcription factors by binding to enhancer sites of the minor groove of DNA through its AT hook and methyltransferase domains.

Translocation and tandem duplication breakpoints fall within an 8.3-kb region, containing exons 5-11 (now numbered as 8-14), rich in ALU repeats and harboring a topoisomerase II cleavage site. In de novo AML the breakpoints are localized within the 5′ part of the 8.3-kb region, whereas in infants and therapy-related AML within its 3′ part. The critical chimeric gene created onto the der(11) is formed by the amino terminus of MLL with its AT hook and methyltransferase domains fused to the carboxy terminus of the partner gene. The role of this last gene in the transformation process is still unknown, but it has been proposed that the partner gene might alter the expression patterns of homeobox genes, leading to distinct leukemia phenotypes. The latter are responsible for the heterogeneous clinical behavior of AML patients with band 11q23 rearrangements. Recent data suggest that t(9;11) is correlated with an intermediate prognosis, whereas other 11q23 translocations, such as the t(11;19), with an unfavorable outcome.

Transcriptional Coactivators (CBP/p3000)

These karyotype abnormalities consist of translocations and inversions, including the t(8;16)(p11;p13), inv(8)(p11;q13), t(11;16)(q23;p13), and t(11;22)(q23;q13). The t(8;16) occurs in 0.4% of AMLs and identifies a peculiar clinicobiologic entity within the M5 cytotypes. The blast cell population has a monocytoid appearance and displays erythrophagocytic activity. Clinically, these patients frequently show central nervous system (CNS) involvement and a high tendency to hemorrhage, even if they do not develop intravascular disseminated coagulation (DIC).

Recently, the t(8;16) has been cloned and the genes involved in such a karyotype defect have been identified. The rearrangement determines the fusion between the cyclic-adenosine monophosphate-responsive element binding protein (CBP), mapped at 16p13, and the MOZ gene, mapped at 8p11. CBP is a transcriptional coactivator, interacting with a broad spectrum of transcriptional factors and having histone acetyltransferase activity. MOZ encodes for a zinc finger protein, also having histone acetyltransferase activity. The mechanism of action of the chimeric gene MOZ-CBP is unknown, but it probably depends on a gene dosage effect. This hypothesis is suggested by patients affected with the Rubistein-Taybi syndrome with loss of one CBP allele, who have an increased risk of cancer, and by those patients who harbor a biallelic p300 mutation and develop gastric and colon cancer.

Until now the t(11;16) has been identified only in patients with therapy-related AML or MDS, who display a blast cell population with M5 morphology and without erythrophagocytosis activity. The chimeric gene 5′MLL-3′ CBP is critical for the leukemogenic process. All transcription coactivator abnormalities are correlated with an unfavourable clinical outcome.

Other Genes

DEK-CAN: t(6;9)(p23;q34)

This chromosome rearrangement, which is not easily recognized in metaphases of suboptimal quality, is found in about 1–2% of AMLs. Firstly, the 6;9 translocation was associated with a M2 FAB cytotype with basophilia. Later it was evident that such a karyotype defect might also be present in M1 and M4 cytotypes and was not constantly correlated with basophilia. In addition, as the t(6;9) was also found in MDS and in acute agnogenic myeloid metaplasia, it was proposed that the translocation may mark a group of myeloid malignancies originating from the myeloid stem cell. The t(6;9) more frequently occurs in patients exposed to environmental carcinogens or treated for a previous malignancy. Dysplastic features are frequently found in these patients, suggesting that the chromosome defect develops in an actively proliferating stem cell compartment, particularly sensitive to carcinogeneic agents.

The t(6;9) causes a rearrangement between the DEK gene, mapped at band 6p23, and the CAN gene, mapped at band 9q34. The chimeric gene, critical for the leukemogenic process, resides on der(6) and is the DEK-CAN gene. Normally DEK functions as a negative transcription regulator, whereas CAN encodes for a protein that carries mRNA and proteins from the nucleus to the cytoplasm. CAN overexpression might lead to a block in cellular cycle at the G0 phase.

EVI1-Ribophorin: t(3;3)(q21;q26)/inv(3)(q21q26)

These chromosome defects are observed in about 2–5% of AML, usually classified as M1 with a high number of platelets. On bone marrow examination an elevated number of megakaryocytes with dysplastic features is detected. The 3;3 translocation is frequently accompanied by a chromosome 7 monosomy or an interstitial long arm deletion of number 5. Prognosis is always unfavorable because of chemoresistance. Molecular studies have demonstrated overexpression of the EVI1 gene, mapped at band 3q26. This event is due to the juxtaposition of the gene with the enhancer of the ribophorin gene, mapped at 3q21. EVI1 is a protein interacting with DNA and regulating the expression of genes crucial for cell differentiation. EVI1 overexpression causes an in vitro maturation block of hematopoietic progenitor cells.

Translocations of the TEL Gene

Rearrangements of the TEL gene, a transcription factor, are difficult to determine on conventional cytogenetics, as the gene resides within band 12p13 which is very weakly stained by G-banding. TEL translocations are therefore discovered by either FISH or molecular biology techniques. TEL has been found rearranged with at least 41 different chromosomal bands and, therefore, it is considered a "promiscuous" gene. Initially, TEL was involved in the t(5;12)(q33;p13) observed in patients with chronic myelomonocytic leukemia. Later it was noted that 16–30% of pediatric ALLs may show a t(12;21)(p13;q22) in which TEL creates a chimeric protein with AML-1. Since then, other rearrangements with several tyrosine kinases have been reported. All these translocations are frequently part of a complex karyotype.

The TEL gene is 240 kb long and is constituted of eight exons. It encodes for a protein with a "helix-loop-helix" (HLH) domain at its amino terminal end and an ETS domain (DNA binding) at its carboxy terminal end. The first domain is encoded by exons 3 and 4, whereas the second by exons 6, 7, and 8. TEL breakpoints may fall within the 5' end of the gene above the exons encoding for the HLH domain, as it occurs in the t(3;12)(q26;p13), or within the 3' end of the gene above the exons encoding for the TEL "DNA-binding" domain, as it happens in the t(5;12), t(9;12), and t(12;21).

Translocations of the NUP98 Gene

These balanced 11p15 rearrangements are rarely but recurrently seen in patients with AML. The NUP98 gene may rearrange with numerous chromosomal regions containing homeobox genes. All these translocations, except for t(4;11), occur in AML or MDS either de novo or secondary. Among them the most frequent is the t(7;11). NUP98 encodes a nucleoporin (a nuclear pore complex protein) of 98 kd, which transports RNA and proteins between the cytoplasm and the nucleus.

Unbalanced Chromosome Abnormalities

Trisomies

These defects are due to nondisjunction events that may be caused by submicroscopic alterations of genes involved in the mitotic process. AML carrying these numerical abnormalities show a great heterogeneity in hematologic features (TABLE 1) .Except for trisomy 11, there is no demonstration about which type of gene lesion is correlated with trisomies.

Deletions and Monosomies

Deletions of part or the whole chromosome (monosomies), especially in elderly patients, are primary AML cytogenetic lesions and are specifically correlated with peculiar hematologic features (TABLE 2).

It has been proposed that the loss of a tumor suppressor gene(s) associated with subsequent mutation of the other apparently normal allele(s) is a crucial mechanism

TABLE 1. Clinicohematologic characteristics of chromosomal abnormalities

Chromosome defects	Incidence	Clinicohematologic characteristics
+8	3–5%	Secondary abnormality Different incidence in relation to the FAB cytotype: M5>M2 Frequent extramedullary localizations in patients with a trisomy/tetrasomy mosaicism Intermediate prognosis if present alone; otherwise, prognosis depends on primary change
+11	1%	AML-M4 or M2 with MLL tandem duplication. AML involving the multipotent stem cell
+4	1%	AML-M4
+13	1%	Biphenotypic AML with unfavorable prognosis

TABLE 2. Molecular analysis of clinicohematologic characteristics of chromosomal defects

Chromosomal defect	Incidence	Molecular analysis	Clinicohematologic characteristics
-5/5q-, -7/7q-	10–15%	Minimally deleted regions: 5q31, 7q21, and 7q31	AML with unfavorable prognosis, especially in patients with a complex karyotype; proximal 7q deletions have a better prognosis than distal ones
Cryptic del(12p)	1–2%	Minimally deleted region: 12p12.2–p13.2	Secondary AML with a complex karyotype
Del(17p)	1–5%	Loss of TP53	Part of a complex karyotype, frequent in advanced phase of the disease; very poor prognosis

in the leukemogenesis process. Many deletions involve chromosomal regions containing genes with a crucial role in normal hematopoiesis. These regions may undergo genetic damage, as they are actively transcribed in the myeloid stem cell or, alternatively, the loss of many of these alleles may cause neoplastic transformation through a gene dosage effect.

REFERENCES

1. ROWLEY, JD. 1999 The role of chromosome translocations in leukemogenesis. Semin. Hematol. **36:** 59–72.
2. SLOVAK, M.L. et al. 2000. Karyotypic analysis predicts outcome of preremission and postremision therapy in adult acute myeloid leukemia: a Southwest Oncology Group/Eastern Cooperative Oncology Group study. Blood **96:** 4075–4083.
3. KEARNEY, L. 1999. The impact of the new FISH technologies on the cytogenetics of haematological malignancies. Br. J. Haematol. **104:** 648–658.
4. REDNER, RL. et al. 1999. Chromatin remodeling and leukemia: new therapeutic paradigms. Blood **94:** 417–428.

From Genes to Therapy: The Case of Philadelphia Chromosome-Positive Leukemias

DANIELA CILLONI, ANGELO GUERRASIO, EMILIA GIUGLIANO, PATRIZIA SCARAVAGLIO, GISELLA VOLPE, GIOVANNA REGE-CAMBRIN, AND GIUSEPPE SAGLIO

Department of Clinical and Biological Sciences, University of Turin, Hospital S. Luigi Gonzaga, 10043, Orbassano-Torino, Italy

ABSTRACT: The Philadelphia chromosome (Ph-chromosome) has long represented the only cytogenetic abnormality known to be associated with a specific malignant disease in humans, being present in more than 95% of patients with chronic myelogenous leukemia. This abnormality is the result of a reciprocal translocation between the long arms of chromosome 9 and 22, t(9;22)(q34;q11), and its presence is not restricted to chronic myelogenous leukemia, but can also be found in 30% of cases of acute lymphoblastic leukemia in adults. In the 1980s, the molecular counterpart of the chromosomal rearrangement was identified to consist of the juxtaposition of parts of the BCR and ABL genes to form a BCR-ABL hybrid gene. The resulting chimeric proteins (P210 and P190), which retain constitutively activated tyrosine kinase activity, have demonstrated a causative role in the genesis of the leukemic process. Although many aspects of the BCR-ABL driven transformation remain unsolved, great advances in understanding the molecular pathology of Ph-positive leukemias resulted in meaningful improvement in the clinical setting. Molecular tools to diagnose disease (PCR, FISH, and southern blot) and to monitor minimal residual disease after potential curative treatment are now in current practice, and new powerful therapeutic tools have emerged that target the molecular oncogenic pathways activated in Ph-positive cells. Among them, specific ABL tyrosine kinase inhibitors recently obtained extraordinary results in many clinical protocols. This review summarizes the most recent advances in this field with special focus on the putative mechanisms of the transformation and progression of chronic myelogenous leukemia and on the major impact that understanding the molecular biology of these diseases is having in clinical practice.

MOLECULAR BIOLOGY OF PH-POSITIVE LEUKEMIAS

Besides sporadic cases showing peculiar types of rearrangements, it is well known that two main types of BCR/ABL rearrangements occur in Ph-positive leukemias, depending on the breakpoint position within the BCR gene on chromosome 22.[1,2] When the breakpoint takes place in the socalled "major breakpoint cluster" or "Mbcr" region of the BCR gene, the BCR/ABL hybrid gene contains approximately

---

Address for correspondence: Giuseppe Saglio, M.D., Department of Clinical and Biological Sciences, University of Turin, San Luigi Hospital, Gonzole 10, 10043 Orbassano-Torino, Italy. Voice: +39-011-9026610; fax: +39-11-9038636.
saglio@csi.it

half the BCR coding sequences and is transcribed in mRNA in which the mBCR region exon 2 or 3 is joined to ABL exon 2 (b2a2 or b3a2 types of junction, respectively).[3] When the breakpoint takes place within the first intron of the BCR gene, only the BCR exon 1 coding sequences still remain on derivative chromosome 22; therefore, transcripts derived from this type of hybrid gene contain an e1a2 type of junction, in which the BCR exon 1 is joined directly to ABL exon 2.[3] The first type of rearrangement leads to the production of BCR/ABL proteins of approximately 210 kd in molecular weight, called P210, whereas the latter leads to a hybrid protein of a lower molecular weight, P190. The two main types of BCR/ABL rearrangements are not equally distributed among Ph-positive hematologic malignancies. Whereas in chronic myelogenous leukemia (CML) only the first type of BCR/ABL rearrangement is generally found, both types of genic rearrangements can be present in Ph-positive acute lymphoblastic leukemias (Ph+ALLs).

A third rare variant of the BCR-ABL rearrangement was found in CML cases frequently showing a milder phenotype overlapping the clinical picture of chronic neutrophilic leukemia (CNL) and denominated Ph-positive CNL.[4,5] In these cases, the breakpoint takes place at the very 3' end of the BCR gene joining BCR exon e19 to ABL exon2 a2, and the resulting fusion transcript, which is translated in the P230 protein, contains the same ABL sequences as the other BCR-ABL transcripts, but includes almost all the BCR coding sequence. The relation between the type of molecular rearrangement and the consequent hybrid transcripts and proteins is still waiting to be fully elucidated.[6]

MECHANISM OF PHILADELPHIA CHROMOSOME TRANSLOCATION

Although the molecular mechanisms leading to BCR and ABL gene rearrangement are entirely obscure, this event seems to occur frequently in humans. Biernaux et al.,[7] using a very sensitive polymerase chain reaction (PCR) technique, found BCR-ABL transcripts in about 20% of the "normal" subjects with a positive correlation with increasing age, overlapping roughly the age distribution of CML. This important finding, later confirmed by Bose et al.,[8] has a profound implication in the postulated mechanisms of Ph-induced leukemogenesis, suggesting that the occurrence of BCR-ABL rearrangement is not by itself able to induce leukemia.

Recent data suggest that the rearrangement process is not a simple balanced translocation but is associated, at least in one third the cases, with large and variable deletions of chromosome 9 and 22;[9] more importantly, deletions are associated with a poor prognosis, suggesting the possible presence of tumor suppressor genes in the deleted sequences. In the remaining two thirds of patients, no significant deletions are observed, thus matching very well the reported incidence of the presence of "reciprocal" ABL/BCR transcripts in patients with CML. The role, if any, of this "reciprocal" transcript is not known.[10]

MOLECULAR MECHANISMS OF NEOPLASTIC TRANSFORMATION

BCR-ABL fusion proteins not only represent a specific "marker" of Ph-positive leukemias but also play a key role in the mechanism of neoplastic transformation.

Definitive evidence of this assumption is derived from transfection studies of BCR-ABL P210-type transcript in mice bone marrow cells: Daley et al.[11] reproduced in this way a CML-like disease that frequently changed into an acute lymphoid phenotype, thus overlapping the characteristic biphasic course of the human disease. However, the molecular mechanisms underlying the BCR-ABL induced transformation remain elusive despite the large body of data accumulated in recent years; this is a direct consequence of the uncertainty concerning the normal role of ABL and BCR products in the physiology of the cell. Although the absence of ABL protein is lethal in knockout mice for ABL genes,[12] its precise function currently remains enigmatic. ABL protein, a nonreceptor tyrosine kinase located at both cytoplasmic and nuclear levels, interacts with many substrates and proteins in both subcellular compartments; however, its precise role is largely unknown.[13] The N-terminal segment of ABL includes two SRC homology domains, SH3 and SH2, which regulate the function of the SH1 domain, that is, the tyrosine kinase domain. SH3 has a suppressive effect on tyrosine kinase function; experimental evidence suggests that SH3 deletion enhances the enzymatic and transforming activity of ABL. On the contrary, mutations that decrease SH2 binding to phosphotyrosine residues reduce Abl-transforming activity. In rare cases of CML, a junction between BCR exons b2 or b3 and Abl exon a3, thus deleting from fusion protein SH3 sequences included in ABL exon 2, have been described;[14] however, a more aggressive clinical phenotype, as would expected, was not reported in these cases. The C-terminal portion of ABL contains several domains with poorly defined functions that include binding sites to F-actin, DNA, and nuclear proteins.

In recent years accumulating data indicate that ABL protein is an important element of the cellular machinery involved in DNA protection from genotoxic agents.[15,16] In particular, c-ABL protein kinase activation occurs in response to a variety of DNA-damaging treatments (except ultraviolet light), and its overexpression causes cell cycle arrest at the G1 phase through a mechanism that depends on tumor suppressor protein p53. On the contrary, the BCR-ABL hybrid proteins are consistently found only in the cytoplasm, suggesting that the mechanisms of neoplastic transformation and progression may derive in part from the loss of ABL nuclear functions.

At cytoplasmic level P210, protein interacts with "adapter" molecules such as GRB-2 and SHC, endowed with SH2 and SH3 domains and, through them, to SOS, which activates the RAS signaling pathway and the MAP kinases.[17] A second putative proliferation pathway is activated by binding another adapter protein, CRKL, which links P210 to the PI-3 kinase pathway;[18] also, however, the JAK-STAT kinase system is activated in BCR/ABL transformed cells. In particular, the importance of RAS signaling pathway activation in CML has been pointed out by *in vitro* studies showing that a block of RAS function suppresses the transforming properties of BCR-ABL fusion proteins.[19] This agrees with the low incidence of RAS mutations in CML, whereas a high incidence of RAS mutation is usually detected in BCR-ABL negative acute and chronic myeloproliferative disorders.[20] An increasing set of data suggest that p210 fusion protein is also implicated in the well-known defective adhesive capacity of CML cells; BCR-ABL fusion proteins form multimeric complex with adhesion proteins such as Paxillin[21] and can bind to F-actin, thus suggesting a direct action on cytoskeletal function.

Another postulated "target" of the transforming activity of P210 protein is represented by the protooncogene MYC, which is expressed at high levels in CML cells and whose action seems independent from RAS activation; an *in vitro* complementation study revealed that the ABL SH2 region is probably involved in the mechanism of MYC upregulation.[22]

In conclusion, the foregoing studies indicate that a multiplicity of molecular interactions implicated in the transforming activity of BCR-ABL hybrid protein can profoundly modify cellular behavior, leading to neoplastic transformation.

MECHANISMS OF CELL EXPANSION AND CLONAL PROGRESSION

The chronic phase of CML is the result of massive expansion of a clone derived from a Ph-positive pluripotent stem cell, which retains the ability to differentiate into various hematopoietic lineages (myeloid, erythroid, megakaryocytic, and T and B lymphoid); however, the BCR-ABL gene produces initially and for unclear reasons a preferential expansion of the myeloid and megakaryocytic compartments, leading to the well-known clinical phenotype of the disease. Mechanisms inducing the advantageous growth of Ph-positive progenitors over normal ones are not completely clear, but a large body of data in past years has elucidated some important features of the biological behavior of the leukemia clone. Several lines of evidence suggest that Ph-positive precursors are resistant to apoptosis induced by deprivation of growth factors;[23] inhibition of apoptosis was observed in both cell lines transfected with the BCR-ABL gene and in CFU-GM (granulocytes-macrophages colony-forming units) from CML patients.[24,25] Furthermore, Ph-positive progenitors seem more resistant to irradiation or cytotoxic drugs than are normal ones, suggesting that the mechanisms of programmed cell death after exposure to DNA's damaging agents, perhaps induced by normal ABL protein, as just reported, are not fully operative in BCR-ABL rearranged cells.

Understanding the mechanisms that trigger the transition from chronic to acute phase is of utmost importance, because the timing of this event is the major determinant of patient survival in CML. Several factors have been implicated as causative agents for acute transformation; however, no consistent molecular pathways leading to the acute leukemia phenotype have been recognized so far. When the disease progresses to acute phase, about 80% of patients show additional chromosomal abnormalities.[26] These include trisomy 8, isochromosome 17q, trisomy 19, and the additional Ph chromosome. Likewise, a growing number of molecular changes has been found during the transition to the blastic phase, including p53 mutations, retinoblastoma gene deletion, and RAS activation.[27,28] However, no specific alteration has been observed even if the deletion of another tumor suppressor gene, p16 or cyclin-dependent kinase 4 inhibitor, seems associated with lymphoid transformation.[29] The more frequent molecular abnormality is represented by a p53 deletion or mutation detected in about 30% of cases of myeloid blast crisis.[30] However, it seems that an important role in the transition to acute phase might be played by the duplication of the Ph chromosome or by an increase in expression of the BCR-ABL transcript, which has been reported to precede in some cases the progression of the disease.[31] Overall, the genetic alterations observed suggest that a large spectrum of molecular mechanisms are involved in the clonal progression of CML; thus, BCR-ABL transformed cells seem endowed with intrinsic genetic instability, leading to progressive accumulation of genetic lesions that ultimately induce an acute leukemic phenotype.

IMPACT OF MOLECULAR BIOLOGY IN THE CLINICAL SETTING OF PH-POSITIVE LEUKEMIAS

Great advances in understanding the molecular pathology of CML in the last 10 years have not only had a major impact on the comprehension of the biological and cellular processes underlying the phenotypic manifestations of the disease but also resulted in meaningful improvement in the clinical setting. Molecular tools to diagnose the disease (PCR, FISH, and southern blot) and to monitor the minimal residual disease after potential curative treatment (allogeneic bone marrow transplantation or interferon) are now in current practice in hematology laboratories. Considerable debate persists on the clinical use of basing the therapeutic decision-making on the PCR-derived results of minimal residual disease.[32] The new concept of "functional cure," as opposed to "molecular cure," has emerged with the possibility that molecular eradication of the disease may not be mandatory in every case and every disease.

Finally, new powerful therapeutic tools have emerged that target the oncogenic pathways of the Ph-positive cell; of particular interest among them are the ABL tyrosine kinase selective inhibitors,[33] whose activity could be of great use in potentiating the more conventional therapies available. The recent introduction of these drugs in clinical trial represents the best-awaited outcome of basic research in a clinical setting. In the early 1990s, knowing that the constitutively activated kinase had a major role in CML, a new drug, a phenylamin pyrimidine molecule, called STI571, which occupies the kinase pocket of the BCR-ABL protein and blocks access to ATP, thereby preventing phosphorylation of any substrate, was developed.[33] Preclinical studies showed that the molecule was highly effective in blocking the tyrosine kinase activity of ABL as well as a number of other tyrosine kinases. These encouraging results led to clinical studies in patients with CML in chronic phase, in blast crisis, or with Ph-positive ALL.[34,35] The reports of these trials document the impressive capacity of STI571 (for signal-transduction inhibitor) to rapidly reverse the clinical and hematologic abnormalities of CML in the chronic phase and, in many cases, to reduce to zero or to low levels the proportion of Ph-positive cells in the bone marrow. The toxicity profile seems very mild. STI571 apparently has considerable advantages versus interferon alfa. It can be given by mouth, and hematologic responses as well as the rate of cytogenetic response seem more rapid and probably more frequent with fewer adverse effects. However, follow-up of patients given the drug is still very short, and no direct evidence exists that STI571 prolongs life or at least produces complete molecular eradication of the disease. Important clinical problems could still emerge. These points provide the rationale for ongoing prospective clinical trials with different combination therapies. More recently, the idea that targeting other pathways in BCR/ABL-transformed cells could also provide enhanced activity of chemotherapy in this disease has also emerged.[36] Genetic and biochemical data argue that Ras activation plays a central role in leukemogenic transformation by BCR/ABL (see above), and new inhibitors of the RAS activity have been developed. Ras function depends on proper subcellular localization to the plasma membrane, which is facilitated in part by the addition of a 15-carbon isoprenoid moiety to the carboxy terminus, a reaction catalyzed by the farnesyl protein transferase enzyme. Farnesyl protein transferase inhibitors (FTIs) are a class of drugs designed to specifically block oncogenic Ras signaling and Ras-dependent cellular transformation. Recent studies have already established that FTIs might be active agents in the treatment of BCR/ABL-induced leukemia and identify FTIs as promising clinical candidates for the treatment of BCR/ABL-induced leukemia.[36] This further suggests the key role that socalled molecular therapy will have in the near future in possibly curing human leukemias. As always, Ph-positive leukemias have been a model disease for hematologic advances.

ACKNOWLEDGMENTS

This work was supported by grants from CNR (Progetto Finalizzato Biotecnologie), MURST-COFIN 2000, Associazione Italiana contro le Leucemie (AIL), and Associazione Italiana per la Ricerca sul Cancro (AIRC). D.C. is supported by a fellowship of the Associazione Italiana Amici di Josè Carreras.

REFERENCES

1. FADERL, S. *et al.* 1999. The biology of chronic myeloid leukemia. N. Engl. J. Med. **341:** 164–172.
2. SAWYERS, C.L. 1999. Chronic myeloid leukemia. N. Engl. J. Med. **340:** 1330–1340.
3. MELO, J. 1996. The diversity of BCR-ABL fusion proteins and their relationship to leukemia phenotype. Blood **88:** 2375–2384.
4. SAGLIO, G. *et al.* 1990. New type of BCR/ABL junction in Philadelphia chromosome-positive chronic myelogenous leukemia. Blood **76:** 1819–1824.
5. PANE, F. *et al.* 1996. Neutrophilic chronic myeloid leukemia: a distinct disease with a specific molecular marker (BCR/ABL with C3/A2 junction). Blood **88:** 2410–2414.
6. SAGLIO, G. *et al.* 1997. BCR/ABL transcripts and leukemia phenotype: an unsolved puzzle. Leukemia Lymphoma **26:** 281–286.
7. BIERNAUX, C. *et al.* 1995. Detection of major BCR-ABL gene expression at very low levels in blood cells of some healthy individuals. Blood **86:** 3118–3122.
8. BOSE, S. *et al.* 1998. The presence of typical and atypical BCR/ABL fusion genes in leucocytes of normal individual: biologic significance and implications for the assessment of minimal residual disease. Blood **92:** 3362–3367.
9. SINCLAIR, P.B. *et al.* 2000. Large deletions at the (9;22) breakpoint are common and may identify a poor prognosis subgroup of patients with chronic myeloid leukemia. Blood **95:** 738–744.
10. MELO, J.V. *et al.* 1993. The ABL/BCR fusion gene is expressed in chronic myeloid leukemia. Blood **81:** 158–165.
11. DALEY, G.Q. *et al.* 1990. Induction of chronic myeloid leukemia in mice by the p210 BCR/ABL gene of the Philadelphia chromosome. Science **247:** 824–830.
12. SCHWARTZMBERG, P.L. *et al.* 1991. Mice homozygous for ABL m1 mutation shows poor viability and depletion of selected B and T population. Cell **65:**1165–1176.
13. LANEUVILLE, P. Abl tyrosine protein kinase. Semin. Immunol. **7:** 255–266.
14. IWATA, S. *et al.* 1994. Heterogeneity of the breakpoint in ABL gene in cases with BCR/ABL transcript lacking ABL exon a2. Leukemia **8:** 1696–1702.
15. YUAN, Z.M. *et al.* 1996. Role for cABL tyrosine kinase in growth arrest response to DNA damage. Nature **382:** 272–274.

16. LIU, Z.G. et al. 1996. Three distinct signalling responses by murine fibroblasts to genotoxic stresses. Nature **384:** 273–276.
17. PUIL, L. et al. 1994. BCR-ABL oncoproteins bind directly to activators of Ras signalling pathway. Embo J. **13:** 764–773.
18. SATTLER, M. et al. 1996. The protoncogene product p120 CBL and the adaptor protein-sCRKL and CRK link c-ABL, p190BCR-ABL and p210 BCR-ABL to phosphatidyl-inositol-3' kinase pathway. Oncogene **12:** 839–845.
19. SAWYERS, C.L. et al. 1995. Genetic requirement for RAS in the transformation of fibroblasts and hematopoietic cells by the BCR-ABL oncogene. J. Exp. Med. **181:** 307–313.
20. GAIDANO, G.L. et al. 1993. Mutations in the p53 and RAS family genes are associated with tumor progression of BCR-ABL negative chronic myeloproliferative disorders. Leukemia **7:** 946–953.
21. SALGIA, R. et al. 1996. p210 BCR-ABL induces formation of complexes containing focal adhesion proteins and the protooncogene product p120cCBL. Exp. Hematol. **24:** 310–313.
22. AFAR, D.E.H. et al. 1994. Differential complementation of BCR-ABL point mutation with c-MYC. Science **264:** 424–426.
23. BEDI, A. et al. 1994. Inhibition of apoptosis by BCR-ABL in chronic myeloid leukemia. Blood **83:** 2038–2044.
24. DALEY, G.Q. & D. BALTIMORE. 1988. Transformation of an interleukin-3 dependent hematopoietic cell line by the chronic myelogenous leukemia-specific BCR-ABL protein. Proc. Natl. Acad. Sci. **85:** 9312–9315.
25. BEDI, A. et al 1995. BCR-ABL mediated inhibition of apoptosis with delay of G2/M transition after DNA damage: a mechanism to resistence to multiple cancer agents. Blood **86:** 1148–1158.
26. BERNSTEIN, R. 1988. Cytogenetics of chronic myeloid leukemia. Semin. Hematol. **25:** 20–34.
27. AHUJA, H. et al. 1991. The spectrum of molecular alterations in the evolution of chronic myelocytic leukemia. J. Clin. Invest. **87:** 2042–2047.
28. GAIDANO, G. et al. 1994. Genetic analysis of p53 and RB1 tumor suppression genes in blast crisis of chronic myeloid leukemia. Ann. Hematol. **68:** 3–7.
29. SERRA, A. et al. 1995. Involvement of cyclin-dependent kinase-4 inhibitor (CDKN2) gene in the pathogenesis of lymphoid blast crisis of chronic myelogenous leukemia. Br. J. Haematol. **91:** 625–629.
30. STUPPIA, L. et al. 1997. p53 loss and point mutation are associated with suppression of apoptosis and progression of CML into myeloid blast crisis. Cancer Genet. Cytogenet. **98:** 28–35.
31. GAIGER, A. et al. 1995. Increase of BCR-ABL chimeric mRNA expression in tumor cells of patients with chronic myeloid leukemia precedes disease progression. Blood **86:** 2371–2378.
32. FADERL, S. et al. 1999. Should polymerase chain reaction analysis to detect minimal residual disease in patients with chronic myelogenous leukemia be used in clinical decision making? Blood **93:** 2755–2759.
33. DRUKER, B.J. et al. 1996. Effects of a selective inhibitor of the ABL tyrosine kinase on the growth of BCR-ABL positive cells. Nature Med. **2:** 561–566.
34. DRUKER, B.J. et al. 2001. Efficacy and safety of a specific inhibitor of the BCR-ABL tyrosine kinase in chronic myeloid leukemia. N. Engl. J. Med. **344:** 1031–1037.
35. DRUKER, B.J. et al. 2001. Activity of a specific inhibitor of the BCR-ABL tyrosine kinase in the blast crisis of chronic myeloid leukemia and acute lymphoblastic leukemia with the Philadelphia chromosome. N. Engl. J. Med. **344:** 1038–1042.
36. PETERS, D.G. et al. 2001. Activity of the farnesyl protein transferase inhibitor SCH66336 against BCR/ABL-induced murine leukemia and primary cells from patients with chronic myeloid leukemia. Blood **97:** 1404–1412.

Multidimensional Flow Cytometry Immunophenotyping of Hematologic Malignancy

GUIDO PAGNUCCO,[a,b] LAURA VANELLI,[b] AND FRANCESCO GERVASI[a]

[a]*Division of Hematology, Department of Oncology, A.R.N.A.S. Civico-Benfratelli, G. Di Cristina e M. Ascoli, 90100 Palermo, Italy*

[b]*Division of Hematology, Department of Hematology, Policlinico San Matteo I.R.C.C.S., 27100 Pavia, Italy*

> ABSTRACT: Immunophenotyping of hematologic malignancies represents one of the most relevant clinical applications of flow cytometry. Classically, leukemic/lymphomatous cells have been considered to reflect the immunophenotypic characteristics of different precursors and mature healthy cells blocked at certain differentiation stages. Recently, accumulating evidence has shown that neoplastic cells display several aberrant phenotypic patterns. These aberrant phenotypes are believed to reflect genetic abnormalities present in pathologic cells, and recent data have shown that at least in acute leukemias, myelodysplastic syndromes, chronic lymphoproliferative disorders, and plasma cell dyscrasias, they may be present in almost all patients. The aim of this work is to review recent advances in flow cytometry and the role of gating strategies more useful in the identification and characterization of neoplastic cells of different hematologic malignancies.
>
> KEYWORDS: flow cytometry; immunophenotyping; hematologic malignancy

INTRODUCTION

Although morphologic studies are still the mainstay of the practicing hematologist and may be sufficient to establish a diagnosis of hematologic malignancies, discrepancies still exist in many cases because of the subjectivity of this type of analysis even among experts. Therefore, other methodologic approaches to the study of neoplastic hematopoietic cells have been developed, with the emergence of immunophenotyping together with conventional and molecular cytogenetics as an increasingly relevant approach to the diagnosis and classification of hematologic malignancies. Consequently, immunophenotyping of hematologic malignancies has been of great help in providing answers to the major specific problems posed in current clinical practice: (1) recognition of lymphocytosis as a chronic lymphoproliferative disorder, both T- and B-cell lineages; (2) distinction between lymphoid and myeloid hemato-

---

Address for correspondence: Dr. Guido Pagnucco, Unit of Hematology, Department of Clinical Oncology, A.R.N.A.S. Civico, Via Parlavecchio 139, 90127 Palermo, Italy. Voice: +39 333 2057967; fax: +39 091 666-422.

poietic cell lineages of blast cells present in a certain sample; (3) subclassification of acute lymphoblastic leukemias; (4) diagnosis of M0, M6, and M7 acute myeloblastic leukemias FAB morphologic subtypes; (5) association of a monoclonal component with a malignant disease condition; and (6) presence of residual leukemic cells in a sample that is in morphologically complete remission.[1]

Over the last decade, multiparametric flow cytometry has evolved from a promising new technology to an indispensable tool in the diagnosis of hematologic malignancies and has replaced fluorescence microscopy and microscopic immunocytochemistry techniques in the immunologic characterization of surface antigen expression in neoplastic cells from patients with hematologic malignancies.[1-3] Furthermore, the recent availability of reliable flow cytometric techniques for analysis of intracellular markers, both nuclear and cytoplasmic, has meant that even in this area morphologic studies will play a secondary role.[4-8]

The clinical use of immunophenotyping for the classification, prognostic stratification, and monitoring of residual disease of hematologic malignancies is well established.[1-3] Major progress in the technology of flow cytometry and in the availability of a large series of monoclonal antibodies against surface membrane and intracellular antigens have made possible the specific and sensitive identification, enumeration, and phenotypic characterization of leukemic/lymphomatous cells.[4-8]

CHARACTERIZATION OF LEUKEMIC/LYMPHOMATOUS CELLS AND ABERRANT PHENOTYPES

Classically, leukemic/lymphomatous cells are thought to reflect the immunophenotypic characteristics of different precursors and mature healthy cells blocked at certain differentiation stages and, therefore, represent clonal expansion of either lymphoid or myeloid cells blocked at various stages of differentiation.[9]

Accumulating evidence, however, suggests that although these neoplastic cells reflect to a certain extent the normal maturation features of hematopoietic cells, they frequently display aberrant phenotypes as defined by cross-lineage antigen expression, asynchronous antigen expression, antigen overexpression, ectopic phenotypes, and abnormal differentiation pathways. These aberrant phenotypes are believed to reflect, to a certain extent, the underlying genetic abnormalities in pathologic cells. Since the report on the existence of an association between the common phenotype (CD10$^+$, cytoplasmic Ig$^-$, and surface Ig$^-$) and the presence of DNA hyperploidy in acute lymphoblastic leukemia, an increasing list of associations has been reported, including, among others: t(8;21) and expression of CD19 and less often CD56 in the context of acute myeloid leukemia (AML) with maturation (M2 FAB subtype);[11] t(15;17) and CD2 expression in HLADR$^-$ AML;[12] and abnormalities of chromosome 16 and CD2 expression in M4Eo FAB subtype.[13]

Careful analysis of these associations, however, indicates that although some phenotypes are present at higher frequency in certain groups of hematologic malignancies, they are not specific. The possible explanations for these findings are the wide range of different reagents and methods used and the technical aspects such as instrument set-up and calibration, the potential component of subjectivity introduced during data analysis or on interpretation of results, and the fact that morphology continues to be the standard of reference for the immunophenotypic characterization of hematologic malignancies.[4–6,14–16]

A major advance in this field was achieved by the definition of the normal patterns of myeloid, B-, and T-cell differentiation in bone marrow using multiparameter flow cytometry, in which triple antibody combinations were used together with sensitive data acquisition methods ("live gate").[5,17–20] With this approach, detailed information was obtained on the different cell subsets present in normal bone marrow that may remain undetected by conventional methods of analysis. Furthermore, when immunophenotypically defined precursor subpopulations from normal bone marrow samples are projected in fluorescence dot-plots, templates for the normal myeloid, B-, and T-cell differentiation pathways can be defined and so-called "empty spaces" where no cell populations are located become evident, allowing discrimination between normal and malignant precursor cells, because cells appearing in the empty spaces can easily be identified as neoplastic cells at diagnosis and in follow-up samples during and after treatment.

These considerations have in recent years led to an effort by several groups to obtain new specific protocols for the immunophenotyping of hematologic malignancies and common criteria for data interpretation and reporting, taking into account three main rules: (1) phenotypic characteristics should be analyzed on the basis of genetic abnormalities in all cases and not just those selected on the basis of morphology; (2) multivariate phenotypic patterns should be taken into account, rather than individual markers considered positive or negative, dim or strong; and (3) phenotypic patterns of healthy cells present in all types of samples used for diagnosis of hematologic malignancies should be well established, considering their phenotypic characteristics, which define a precise place for these cells in a multidimensional space created by the different light scatter and fluorescence-associated markers analyzed.

These rules have been used as the basis for a new way of understanding the immunophenotype of hematologic malignancies. More work is needed, however, before an international consensus can be reached between the international groups involved in immunophenotyping and the laboratory concerned. As a consequence of this approach using appropriate multiple-staining techniques, the incidence of aberrant phenotypes has been reported to be extremely frequent: 90% of acute lymphoblastic leukemia cases, 75% of acute myeloblastic leukemia, 80% of chronic lymphoproliferative disorders, 90% of multiple myeloma, and monoclonal gammopathies of undetermined significance, among others.[17–21]

GATING STRATEGIES

From a practical point of view, flow cytometric identification of pathologic cells now cannot be achieved by selecting them exclusively on the basis of the morphologically related parameters, i.e. forward and side light scatter, as was initially proposed for the analysis of peripheral lymphoid subsets. This approach, though very useful, is not sufficient to specifically identify and distinguish pathologic cells from their normal counterparts. Thus at least one additional parameter, a monoclonal antibody reagent, has to be used in combination with the two light scatter parameters for the specific identification of hematopoietic neoplastic cells by flow cytometry.

TABLE 1. Gating strategies more useful for the identification and characterization of neoplastic cells of different hematologic malignancies

Gated cells	Additional staining within gated cells	Diagnosis
CD45 blast/SSC	CD34, CD33, CD13, CD19, CD7, CD10, CD14, DR	AML vs ALL
	DR/CD33, CD15/CD34, CD45/CD117, CD7/CD13	PML/RARα
	CD34/CD19, CD13/CD56 or CD33/CD56	AML1-ETO
CD19+/SSC	CD10/CD20, CD34, CD20, CD34/CD38, CD34/CD22, TdT/CD10	B-ALL
	CD10/CD13, CD34/CD38, CD34/CD45	B-ALL Ph+
	CD34/CD45, CD45/CD135, CD10/CD20, CD2/DR	TEL-AML1
	CD5/CD79b, CD22/CD79b, CD79b/CD45	B-CLL
CD7+/SSC	TdT/cyCD3, CD5/CD3, CD4/CD8, CD2/CD3, CD38/CD34	T-ALL
CD38^{bright}/SSC	CD138/CD45, CD19/CD56	MM, MGUS

Once the main cell population has been selected, additional staining performed simultaneously within that particular cell subset will contribute to a precise discrimination between the healthy and pathologic counterparts.

TABLE 1 summarizes the gating strategies more useful in the identification and characterization of neoplastic cells of different hematologic malignancies. Examples of useful markers include: CD45/orthogonal light scatter (SSC) gating in acute myeloblastic leukemia, CD19+/SSC gating in both B lineage acute lymphoblastic leukemias and B-cell chronic lymphoproliferative disorders, CD7+/SSC gating in T lineage acute lymphoblastic leukemias, and CD38+ ^{bright}/intermediate SSC gating in multiple myelomas and monoclonal gammopathies of undetermined significance. Once the main cell population has been selected, additional stainings performed simultaneously within that particular cell subset will contribute to a precise discrimination between the healthy and neoplastic counterparts. Therefore, the use of multiple staining is essential because the same information cannot be obtained using corresponding single staining, and indirect immunofluorescence methods, in principle, avoided because of inherent technical problems.

CD45/SSC Gating

CD45/SSC gating has been proposed as a helpful tool for obtaining more specific and sensitive identification of blasts cells of acute leukemia from normal differentiating cells, because leukemic blast cells usually appear in a position where few healthy cells are located.[22,23] This kind of approach makes it easier to distinguish lymphoid and erythroid subpopulations and monocytic and myeloid cells in the different steps of their differentiation pathways. The CD45 characteristic intensity of expression in normal populations (more intense in lymphocytes and monocytes, less intense in granulocytes and maturing myeloid cells, and absent in erythroid precursors and platelets) made it possible to discriminate leukemic cells of any origin from normal mature cells and facilitate analysis of leukemic blast cells present at low frequencies. Lymphoblasts are typically CD45 low or negative with a low SSC level; myeloid blasts have intermediate CD45 expression and a higher SSC value. Using the CD45/SSC blast cell, gating strategy was superior to the conventional FSC/SSC procedure in quantifying leukemic cells with aberrant antigen expression as well as increasing the sensitivity for detection of minimal residual disease. In most patients with acute leukemia in complete remission after induction chemotherapy or during maintenance, relapse was predicted by evaluation of minimal residual disease using this method.[24] These results indicate that this is a powerful tool for evaluating the quality of complete remission and predicting disease progression and that more aggressive treatment may be necessary in patients with high minimal residual disease. This procedure was also useful in detecting minimal residual disease during complete remission after allogeneic bone marrow transplantation. When the minimal residual disease was detected after bone marrow transplantation, discontinuation of immunosuppressive agent induced graft-versus-leukemia effect in association with graft-versus-host disease, resulting in a lower minimal residual disease.[24]

Recent reports have also indicated the existence of an important association between specific genetic alterations and the immunophenotypic characteristics of leukemic cells in both AML and ALL, particularly using multivariate phenotypic patterns and considering the extent of antigen expression and its pattern of reactivity (homogeneous vs heterogeneous, unimodal vs multimodal).[23–27] As a matter of fact, in a recent study of 111 patients with AML in whom multivariate information provided by the use of multiple staining analyzed at flow cytometry was obtained, it was shown that the combination of three phenotypic variables (number of major blast cell populations, pattern of CD34/CD15 expression, and reactivity for CD13) was highly sensitive (100%) and specific (99%) for the selection of AML cases carrying PML/RAR-α gene rearrangements, as demonstrated by the combined use of the reverse transcription-polymerase chain reaction and fluorescent in situ hybridization (FISH) analysis.[25]

Furthermore, some nonspecific myeloid markers such as CD2 expression in AML-M4-Eo with inv(16)[13] and CD19 and CD56 expression in AML-M2 with t(8:21)[24,26,27] are useful in recognizing new immunophenotypic subgroups associated with these genetically defined subtypes.

A recent study addressed the potential contribution of the CD45/SSC gating strategy to the diagnosis of myelodysplastic syndromes in 45 patients with straightforward myelodysplastic syndrome.[28] The results were compared with those obtained in a series of patients with aplastic anemia, healthy donors, and patients with a history of nonmyeloid neoplasia in complete remission. A series of different double-staining combinations were used to detect immunophenotypic abnormalities associated with myeloid (CD11b/CD16, CD13/CD16), erythroid (CD71/glycophorin A), and megakaryocytic (CD41a/CD61) dysplasia of the different bone marrow cell populations within the gates drawn on the dot-plot CD45/SSC. Such an approach could detect immunophenotypic abnormalities in cases in which combined morphology and cytogenetics were nondiagnostic. In addition, flow cytometric analysis was informative even when aspirates collected for morphology were inadequate and was very helpful in differentiating hypocellular myelodysplastic syndromes from aplastic anemia.

CD19+/SSC Gating

Analysis of the sequence of antigen expression among normal human $CD19^+$ B cells from adult bone marrow using the $CD19^+$/SSC gating strategy has shown that the various B-cell precursor subpopulations display constant patterns of maturation as regards both their phenotypic characteristics and their relative distribution.[18] Investigation of abnormalities in these patterns may provide a potentially useful tool for monitoring minimal residual disease in precursor-B-ALL patients who achieve cytomorphologic complete remission, because the persistence of residual leukemic cells may induce abnormalities in the precursor B-cell compartment in bone marrow.[29] This hypothesis was confirmed by a study of a total of 180 bone marrow samples from 45 consecutive precursor-B-ALL patients in morphologic complete remission, showing that a significant increase of two subpopulations of immature B cells ($CD34^+/CD19^+$ and $CD20^-/CD19^+$ cells) or an altered overall B-cell differentiation using CD19/CD10/CD20 triple-staining predicted a high relapse rate and shorter disease-free survival.[19] Analyzing normal B-cell differentiation to predict relapse has additional benefits compared to traditional flow cytometric phenotyping to detect minimal residual disease such as its relative simplicity, relatively low cost, and applicability in all precursor-B-ALL patients, independent of the existence of leukemia-associated phenotypes.

The immunophenotyping of precursor-B-ALL with the multiparametric quantitative approach seems able to identify homogeneous groups of ALL also corresponding to genotypically determined types such as $t(12;21)(p13;q22)^+$ childhood ALL[30] and BCR/ABL^+ adult ALL.[31] The $t(12;21)^+$ ALL showed a peculiar pattern in CD19 gated cells characterized by bimodal distribution of CD34, high intensity of HLA-DR expression, high expression of CD10 and low intensity of CD20, and low/absent CD135 and CD45 expression. A multivariate analysis disclosed that $t(12;21)^+$ cases can be identified with a sensitivity of 86% and a specificity of 100%. BCR/ABL^+ adult ALL constantly displayed homogeneous expression of CD10 and CD34 but low and relatively heterogeneous CD38 expression together with an aberrant reactivity for CD13. These data further support the notion that the phenotypic features of leukemic B cells blocked in their maturation at a relatively early differentiation stage to a large extent reflect the underlying genetic aberration carried by neoplastic cells and that multidimensional immunophenotyping could provide rapid, sensitive, and specific screening for identifying cases carrying specific genetic lesions.

The possible value of flow cytometric minimal residual disease detection of surface expression of CD79b in B-cell chronic lymphocytic leukemia was explored using a "live gate" drawn on $CD19^+/SSC$ cells, because this marker is absent or underexpressed in chronic lymphocytic leukemia cells and thus could be considered as a "tumor phenotype" associated with chronic lymphocytic leukemia.[32] Lymphocytes from peripheral blood were analyzed using simultaneous triple labeling with either CD5/CD79b/CD19 or CD22/CD79b/CD19. Because normal immature bone marrow B cells are $CD79b^{-/dim+}$ as chronic lymphocytic leukemia cells, the combination CD19/CD79b/CD45 was used in all bone marrow samples, selecting mature B lymphocytes according to their bright CD45 intensity. Dilution experiments indicated that the detection limit with this marker almost reached the levels obtained by molecular biology methods as the polymerase chain reaction technique. In addition, quantitative studies may be useful in samples with a low percentage of $CD19^+$ lymphocytes, and the different intensity of expression of CD79b in normal B lymphocytes and chronic lymphocytic leukemia cells can be exploited to identify both populations separately.

CD7⁺/SSC Gating

Flow cytometric characterization of T-cell subsets in normal bone marrow using five triple stains based on CD7⁺/SSC gating strategy allowed definition of "empty spaces" in multidimensional dot-plots of each studied antigen combination, as has been reported for precursor B cells.[20] All 65 consecutive T-ALL cases analyzed using the same triple antibody combinations and flow cytometry protocols were located in empty spaces and could be discriminated from normal T cells. The most informative triple staining was TdT/CD7/cyCD3, which was aberrant in 91% of the cases. Application of the five proposed combinations in T-ALL contributes to standardized detection of minimal residual disease, because leukemic cells persistent or reappearing in the empty spaces can easily be identified in bone marrow samples during and after treatment.

CD38⁺bright/Intermediate SSC Gating

Plasma cell multiparametric immunophenotyping can differentiate between neoplastic cells and their normal counterpart. The strong reactivity for CD38 and the positivity for Syndecan-1 expression (CD138) are the two best markers for identifying plasma cells. For consistent sensitive detection of low levels of plasma cells a combination of high CD38 and CD138 with low CD45 expression should be used for identification.[33] Of interest, it is also possible to distinguish myeloma from normal plasma cells by differential expression of CD19 and CD56: normal plasma cells are consistently CD19⁺/CD56⁻, whereas myeloma plasma cells are predominantly CD19⁻/CD56⁺.[17,33] A clear example of this is the value that has been associated with assessment of the percentage of bone marrow plasma cells corresponding to healthy residual polyclonal plasma cells in the differential diagnosis between monoclonal gammopathy of undetermined significance and multiple myeloma.[17] Using a flow cytometric technique based on simultaneous triple labeling with CD38/CD56/CD19 and a two-step acquisition procedure it is possible to acquire and study for the relative expression of CD19 and CD56 only those events included in a "live gate" drawn on the CD38/SSC bright fraction. In patients with monoclonal gammopathy of undetermined significance, two clearly defined and distinct plasma cell subpopulations were identified. One of these plasma cell subpopulations showed phenotypic characteristics identical to those of normal plasma cells, including a very strong reactivity for the CD38 antigen and intermediate/low scatter characteristics and positivity for CD19, in the absence of CD56, and corresponds to the residual normal bone marrow plasma cell. The second plasma cell subpopulation showed an immunophenotype similar to that of myelomatous plasma cells, characterized by slightly lower reactivity for CD38 and strong CD56 expression, in the absence of positivity for CD19, these plasma cells corresponding to the clonal plasma cell. Moreover, as shown by multivariate analysis, the number of residual polyclonal plasma cells was the single parameter for the discrimination between cases of monoclonal gammopathy of undetermined significance and multiple myeloma at diagnosis, even when only stage I multiple myeloma cases were considered.

REFERENCES

1. JENNINGS, C.D. & K.A. FOON. 1997. Recent advances in flow cytometry: application to the diagnosis of hematologic malignancy. Blood **90:** 2863–2892.
2. DAVIS, B.H., K. FOUCAR, W. SZCZARKOWSKI, et al. 1997. U.S.-Canadian consensus recommendations on the immunophenotypic analysis of hematologic neoplasia by flow cytometry: medical indications. Cytometry **30:** 249–263.
3. BENÉ, M.C., M. BERNIER, G. CASTOLDI, et al. on behalf of EGIL, European Group on Immunological Classification of Leukemias. 1999. Impact of immunophenotyping on management of acute leukemias. Haematologica **84:** 1024–1034.
4. ROTHE, G. & G. SCHMITZ. 1996. Consensus protocol for the flow cytometric immunophenotyping of hematopoietic malignancies. Working Group on Flow Cytometry and Image Analysis. Leukemia **10:** 877–895.
5. BOROWITZ, M.J., R. BRAY, R. GASCOYNE, et al. 1997. U.S.-Canadian consensus recommendations on the immunophenotypic analysis of hematologic neoplasia by flow cytometry: data analysis and interpretation. Cytometry **30:** 236–244.
6. RUIZ ARGUELLES, A., R.E. DUQUE & A. ORFAO. 1998. Report on the first Latin American consensus conference for flow cytometric immunophenotyping of leukemia. Cytometry **34:** 39–42.
7. BRAYLAN, R.C., A. ORFAO, M.J. BOROWITZ, et al. 2001. Optimal number of reagents required to evaluate hematolymphoid neoplasias: results of an international consensus meeting. Cytometry **46:** 23–27.
8. BASSO, G., P. BERNASCONI, R. CHIANESE, et al. 2001. Monoclonal antibody panels for acute leukemia and myelodysplastic sindrome diagnosis. Results of a co-operative quality control group. J. Biol. Regul. Homeostatic Agents **15:** 145–155.
9. VAN DONGEN, J.J.M. & H.J. ADRIAANSEN. 1996. Immunobiology of leukemia. In Leukemia. E.S. Henderson, T.A. Lister & M.F. Greaves, eds. :83–130. Saunders. Philadelphia, PA.
10. PUI, C.H., D.L. WILLIAMS, P.K. ROBERSON, et al. 1988. Correlation of karyotype and immunophenotype in childhood acute lymphoblastic leukemia. J. Clin. Oncol. **6:** 56–61.
11. READING, C.L., E.H. ESTEY, Y.O. HUH, et al. 1993. Expression of unusual immunophenotype combinations in acute myelogenous leukemia. Blood **81:** 3083–3090.
12. CLAXTON, D.F., C.L. READING, L. NAGARAJAN, et al. 1992. Correlation of CD2 expression with PML gene breakpoints in patients with acute promyelocytic leukemia. Blood **80:** 582–586.
13. ADRIAANSEN, H.J., P.A.W. TE BOEKHORST, A.M. HAGEMEIJER, et al. 1993. Acute myeloid leukemia M4 with bone marrow eosinophilia (M4Eo) and inv(16) (p13q22) exhibits a specific immunophenotype with CD2 expression. Blood **81:** 3043–3051.
14. BENE, M.C., G. CASTOLDI, W. KNAPP, et al. 1995. Proposals for the immunological classification of acute leukemias. European Group for the Immunological Characterisation of Leukaemias. Leukemia **9:** 373–385.
15. STELZER, G.T., G. MARTI, A. HURLEY, et al. 1997. U.S.-Canadian consensus recommendations on the immunophenotypic analysis of hematologic neoplasia by flow cytometry: standardization of laboratory procedures. Cytometry **30:** 214–230.
16. STEWART, C.C., F.G. BEHM, J.L. CAREY, et al. 1997. U.S.-Canadian consensus recommendations on the immunophenotypic analysis of hematologic neoplasia by flow cytometry: selection of antibody combinations. Cytometry **30:** 231–235.
17. OCQUETEAU, M., A. ORFAO, J. ALMEIDA, et al. 1998. Immunophenotypic characterization of plasma cells from monoclonal gammopathy of undetermined significance patients. Implications for the differential diagnosis between MGUS and multiple myeloma. Am. J. Pathol. **152:** 1655–1665.
18. LUCIO, P., A. PARREIRA, M.V. VAN DEN BEEMD, et al. 1999. Flow cytometric analysis of normal B cell differentiation: a frame of reference for the detection of minimal residual disease in precursor-B-ALL. Leukemia **13:** 419–427.
19. CIUDAD, J., J.F. SAN MIGUEL, M.C. LOPEZ-BERGES, et al. 1999. Detection of abnormalities in B-cell differentiation pattern is a useful tool to predict relapse in precursor-B-ALL. Br. J. Haematol. **104:** 695–705.

20. PORWIT-MACDONALD, A., E. BJORKLUND, P. LUCIO, et al. 2000. BIOMED-1 concerted action report: flow cytometric characterization of CD7+ cell subsets in normal bone marrow as a basis for the diagnosis and follow-up of T cell acute lymphoblastic leukemia (T-ALL). Leukemia **14**: 816–825.
21. SAN MIGUEL, J.F., M. GONZALES & A. ORFAO. 1998. Minimal residual disease in acute myeloid malignancies. *In* Textbook of Malignant Hematology. L. Degos, F. Herman, D. Linch & B. Lowenberg, eds. :871–891. Martin Dunitz. London.
22. STELZER, G.T., K.E. SHULTS & M.R. LOKEN. 1993. CD45 gating for routine flow cytometric analysis of human bone marrow specimens. Ann. N.Y. Acad. Sci. **677**: 265–280.
23. BOROWITZ, M.J., K.L. GUENTER, K.E. SHULTS, et al. 1993. Immunophenotyping of acute leukemia by flow cytometric analysis: use of CD45 and right-angle light scatter to gate on leukemic blasts in three-color analysis. Am. J. Clin. Pathol. **100**: 534–540.
24. ITO, S., Y. ISHIDA, K. MURAI, et al. 2001. Flow cytometric analysis of aberrant antigen expression of blasts using CD45 blast gating for minimal residual disease in acute leukemia and high-risk myelodysplastic syndrome. Leuk. Res. **25**: 205–211.
25. ORFAO, A., M.C. CHILLON, A.M. BORTOLUCCI, et al. 1999. The flow cytometric pattern of CD34, CD15, and CD13 expression in acute myeloblastic leukemia is highly characteristic of the presence of PML-RARalpha gene rearrangements. Haematologica **84**: 405–412.
26. GARCIA VELA, J.A., M. MARTIN, I. DELGADO, et al. 1999. Acute myeloid leukemia M2 and t(8;21)(q22;q22) with an unusual phenotype: myeloperoxidase (+), CD13 (–), CD14 (–), and CD33 (–). Ann. Hematol. **78**: 237–240.
27. FERRARA, F., R. DI NOTO, A. VIOLA, et al. 1999. Complete remission in acute myeloid leukaemia with t(8;21) following treatment with G-CSF: flow cytometric analysis of *in vivo* and *in vitro* effects on cell maturation. Br. J. Haematol. **106**: 520–523.
28. STETLER-STEVENSON, M., D.C. ARTHUR, N. JABBOUR, et al. 2001. Diagnostic utility of flow cytometric immunophenotyping in myelodysplastic syndrome. Blood **98**: 979–987.
29. CIUDAD, J., A. ORFAO, B. VIDRIALES, et al. 1998. Immunophenotypic analysis of CD19+ precursors in normal human adult bone marrow: implications for minimal residual disease detection. Haematologica **83**: 1069–1075.
30. DE ZEN, L., A. ORFAO, G. CAZZANIGA, et al. 2000. Quantitative multiparametric immunophenotyping in acute lymphoblastic leukemia: correlation with specific genotype. I. ETV6/AML1 ALLs identification. Leukemia **14**: 1225–1231.
31. TABERNERO, M.D., A.M. BORTOLUCI, I. ALAEJOS, et al. 2001. Adult precursor B-ALL with BCR/ABL gene rearrangements displays a unique immunophenotype based on the pattern of CD10, CD34, CD13 and CD38 expression. Leukemia **15**: 406–414.
32. GARCIA VELA, J.A., I. DELGADO, L. BENITO, et al. 1999. CD79b expression in B cell chronic lymphocytic leukemia: its implication for minimal residual disease detection. Leukemia **13**: 1501–1505.
33. RAWSTRON, A.C., R.G. OWEN, F.E. DAVIES, et al. 1997. Circulating plasma cell in multiple myeloma: characterization and correlation with disease stage. Br. J. Haematol. **97**: 46–55.

Androgen Receptor Status in Nontumoral and Malignant Human Colorectal Tissues

L. CASTAGNETTA,[a,b] A. TRAINA,[c] I. CAMPISI,[a] M. CALABRÒ,[a] A. MARATTA,[a] A. SAETTA,[b] B. AGOSTARA,[c] AND N. MEZZATESTA[c]

[a]*Unit of Experimental Oncology & Palermo Branch of IST-GE,*
[c]*Cancer Registry,* [d]*Unit of Medical Oncology, and* [e]*Unit of Surgery, Department of Clinical Oncology, "M. Ascoli" Cancer Hospital Centre, A.R.N.A.S., Civico, Palermo, Italy*

[b]*Department of Experimental Oncology and Clinical Application, University Medical School, Palermo, Italy*

ABSTRACT: Data on androgen receptor (AR) status of nontumoral and malignant human colorectal tissues are compared using ligand binding assay in 22 patients who underwent surgery for colorectal cancer at the "M. Ascoli" Cancer Hospital Centre in Palermo, Sicily. In nontumoral tissues, ARs were predominantly (67%) positive, with 25% of cases having a 0/+ status. Conversely, malignant tissues showed only 32% of cases with a positive (+/+) AR status, with a proportional increase of 0/+ cases (from 25% to 55%); the extent of AR-negative (0/0) cases remained fairly constant (8–9%). Overall, our evidence indicates that nontumoral colorectal tissues have a predominantly positive (+/+) AR status and that this condition shifts towards a significant decrease of AR-positive cases in cancer tissues. Studies on the relation between status of sex steroid receptors and specific biomolecular markers in human colorectal tumors are currently being carried out in our laboratories.

KEYWORDS: androgen; receptors; colorectal tissues

INTRODUCTION

Human colorectal cancer should be considered a major human tumor. Epidemiologic data indicate that both incidence and mortality rates have continuously been increasing in recent years; colorectal carcinoma accounts for 8.5% of all new cancer cases per year and represents the fourth most common type of cancer and cause of death from cancer throughout the world.[1,2] Human colorectal cancer was regarded as a hormone-independent tumor until recent experimental and clinical data indicated that steroid hormones, retinoids, vitamin D3, epidermal growth factor, and transforming growth factor α and β may profoundly affect the biological features of epi-

---

Address for correspondence: Prof. Luigi Castagnetta, Experimental Oncology, Department of Clinical Oncology, "M. Ascoli" Cancer Hospital Centre, Via Parlavecchio 139, 90127, Palermo, Italy. Voice: +39 091 666-4346; fax: +39 091 666-4352.
lucashbl@unipa.it

TABLE 1. Tumor size, nodal status, and grading of colorectal cancer tissues

		Frequency	Valid percent
Primary tumor	T2	9	40.9
	T3	8	36.4
	T4	2	9.1
	TX	3	13.6
Regional lymph nodes	N0	17	77.3
	N1	2	9.1
	N2	1	4.5
	N3	1	4.5
	NX	1	4.5
Grading	G2	18	81.8
	G3	1	4.5
	GX	3	13.6

thelial cells in the large intestine.[3,4] The presence of steroid receptors, including altered isoform expression,[5] has been reported by different groups.[6,7] In the present work, we compare preliminary data on androgen receptor status of nontumoral and malignant human colorectal tissues, using ligand binding assay.

MATERIAL AND METHODS

Patients. Both nontumoral and malignant tissue specimens were collected in 22 patients who underwent surgery for colorectal cancer at the "M. Ascoli" Cancer Hospital Centre in Palermo. All patients had histologically confirmed adenocarcinoma of the colorectum. Patients with prior or concomitant cancer at another site or organ as well as those with prior chemotherapy or radiotherapy were not included. At entry in the study, patients had a median age of 69.6 years (range 50–85).

Ligand Binding Assay of Androgen Receptors. The ligand binding assay procedures for assaying androgen receptors have been extensively described elsewhere.[8,9] Briefly, fragments of tissue (20–50 mg/ml) were homogenized in buffer (Hepes 10 mM, EDTA 1.5 mM, dithiothreitol 0.5 mM, sodium molybdate 10 mM, and glycerol 30% v/v) using a glass/glass homogenizer. The homogenate was spun at $3,600 \times g$ for 5 minutes to separate the particulate (nuclear) from the supernatant (soluble) fraction. Aliquots (150 ml) of each fraction were incubated overnight at 4°C with increasing concentrations (0.1–5 nM) of the relevant radioligand (mibolerone). A 100-fold excess of cold triamcinolone acetonide (AR) was also used for competition studies. Receptor data were processed using Scatchard analysis and a modification of a least-square fit routine,[9] yielding both dissociation constant and concentration values. A positive androgen receptor status is defined by the concurrent presence of receptor in both soluble and nuclear cell fractions, whereas the absence of androgen receptor in one or both fractions identifies a negative receptor status.

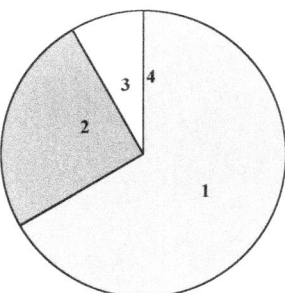

FIGURE 1. Distribution of androgen receptor status of nontumoral human colorectal tissues. (1) +/+; (2) 0/+; (3) 0/0; (4) +/0.

TABLE 2. Frequency of androgen receptor status in nontumoral human colorectal tissues

S/N	Frequency	Percent
+/+	8	66.7
0/+	3	25.0
0/0	1	8.3
+/0	0	0.0
Total	12	100.0

RESULTS AND CONCLUSIONS

Overall, 12 female and 10 male patients were included in the study. As reported in TABLE 1, most tumors were T2–T3 (89.5%), with no regional lymph node involvement (81%) and G2 grading (94.7%). For each patient, androgen receptor status was analyzed by ligand binding assay in fragments of either nontumoral or cancer tissue. In the former, androgen receptor status was predominantly (67%) positive, with 25% of cases having a 0/+ status (TABLE 2; FIG. 1). On the other hand, in malignant tissues the positive (+/+) androgen receptor status significantly decreased 32%, with a proportional increase of 0/+ cases (from 25–55%); the extent of androgen receptor-negative (0/0) cases remained fairly constant (8–9%) (TABLE 3; FIG. 2).

This evidence, although preliminary, suggests that the role exerted by male sex steroids in carcinogenesis and/or progression of colorectal cancer could be argued. Further studies are needed to confirm our experimental evidence and to ascertain whether a relative reduction in androgen receptor content is accompanied by a loss of response to androgens and whether other hormonal factors (estrogens?) may be involved.

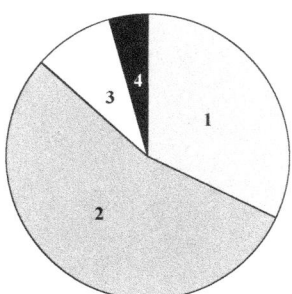

FIGURE 2. Distribution of androgen receptor status of human colorectal tumor tissues. (1) +/+; (2) 0/+; (3) 0/0; (4) +/0.

TABLE 3. Frequency of androgen receptor status in human colorectal tumor tissues

S/N	Frequency	Percent
+/+	7	31.8
0/+	12	454.5
0/0	2	9.1
+/0	1	4.5
Total	22	100.0

REFERENCES

1. WHO. 1997. World Health Report 1997. WHO. Geneva.
2. WORLD CANCER RESEARCH FUND/AMERICAN INSTITUTE FOR CANCER RESEARCH. 1997. Food, Nutrition and the Prevention of Cancer: A Global Perspective. American Institute for Cancer Research. Washington.
3. TUTTON, P.J.M. & D.H. BARKLA. 1988. Steroid hormones as regulators of the proliferative activity of normal and neoplastic intestinal epithelial cells. Anticancer Res. **8:** 451–456.
4. HUANG, S.A. et al. 1991. Growth modulation by epidermal growth factor (EGF) in human colonic carcinoma cells: constitutive expression of the human EGF gene. J. Cell Physiol. **148:** 220–227.
5. CATALANO, M.G. et al. 2000. Altered expression of androgen-receptor isoforms in human colon-cancer tissues. Int. J. Cancer **86:** 325–330.
6. CASTAGNETTA, L. et al. 1992. Soluble and nuclear type I and II androgen-binding sites in benign hyperplasia and cancer of the human prostate. Urol. Res. **20:** 127–132.
7. WALISZEWSKI, P. et al. 1997. Molecular study of sex steroid receptor gene expression in human colon and in colorectal carcinomas. J. Surg. Oncol. **64:** 3–11.
8. CUTOLO, M. et al. 1992. Evidence for the presence of androgen receptors in the synovial tissue of rheumatoid arthritis patients and healthy controls. Arthritis Rheum. **35:** 1007–1015.
9. CASTAGNETTA, L. et al. 1991. Androgen receptor assay in specimens of prostatic tissue obtained by transurethral resection and transvesical adenomectomy. Urol. Res. **19:** 337–341.
10. LEAKE, R.E. et al. 1987. In Steroid Hormones: A Practical Approach. B. Green & R.E. Leake, eds. :93-97. IRL Press. Oxford.

Correlation between *Helicobacter pylori* Infection and IL-18 mRNA Expression in Human Gastric Biopsy Specimens

M.T. FERA,[a] M. CARBONE,[a] C. BUDA,[b] M. ARAGONA,[b] S. PANETTA,[b]
M. GIANNONE,[a] F. LA TORRE,[b] A. GIUDICE,[c] AND E. LOSI[c]

[a]*Dipartimento di Patologia e Microbiologia Sperimentale and*

[b]*Dipartimento di Patologia Umana, U.O. di Oncologia Medica, Facoltà di Medicina e Chirurgia, Università di Messina, Messina, Italy*

[c]*Istituto Nazionale per la Ricerca sul Cancro – Genova, Unità Satellite di Messina, Messina, Italy*

> ABSTRACT: Our data indicate that *H. pylori* infection is associated with active interleukin-18 production in patients with chronic gastritis. Different cell types appear to be involved in this activity and may play a role in the development of immunopathologic damage.
>
> KEYWORDS: *Helicobacter pylori*; interleukin-18; infection; mRNA; gastritis

INTRODUCTION

The microaerophilic bacterium *Helicobacter pylori* is a causative agent of chronic gastritis and is strongly associated with peptic ulcer disease.[1,2] Furthermore, *H. pylori* is a significant risk factor in the development of gastric adenocarcinoma.[3] Gastric inflammation is an invariable finding in patients infected with *H. pylori* and represents the host immune response to the bacterium.[4]

The mucosal inflammatory reaction induced by *H. pylori* consists of infiltration of many polymorphonuclear and mononuclear cells, including monocytes, T cells, and plasma cells, and at mucosal sites also involves an array of mediators, such as prostaglandins, mast cells, proteases, leukotrienes, and cytokines.[5,6] As extracellular signaling molecules that coordinate the inflammatory and immune responses, cytokines have many roles in the normal process of host defense against infection and injury. However, cytokines exert these responses either directly or indirectly by stimulating production of other effector molecules.[7] Interleukin-18 (IL-18) is a cytokine recently described as a member of the IL-1 cytokine family and initially defined as a gamma interferon (IFN-γ)-inducing factor in mice after endotoxin shock.[8] Il-18 and IL-1 do not appear to share significant biologic actions.[9] Because of its property

---

Address for correspondence: Dr. M.T. Fera, Dipartimento di Patologia e Microbiologia Sperimentale, Policlinico Universitario, Torre Biologica, 2d piano, 98125 Messina, Italy. Voice: 39-090-2213313; fax: 39-090-2213312.

mtfera@unime.it

to induce IFN-γ, IL-18 is by default a member of the TH1-inducing family of cytokines (IFN-γ, IL-2, IL-12, and IL-15). Il-18 is a pleiotropic cytokine with a broad array of effector functions beyond lymphocyte activation that implicates IL-18 as an important regulator of both innate and acquired immune responses. Little is known about the gastric cells associated with expression of this cytokine.

MATERIAL AND METHODS

This study evaluates IL-18 gene expression by reverse transcriptase-polymerase chain reaction (RT-PCR) and localizes immunohistologically the cellular origin of IL-18 protein in antral biopsy specimens from 25 *H. pylori*-infected and *H. pylori*-uninfected patients. Of the 25 symptomatic patients, 5 had no evidence of *H. pylori* on culture and were urease negative. All of these patients were also negative for anti-*H. pylori* immunoglobulin G by ELISA and had histologically normal results on antral biopsy. Therefore, these five patients were used as controls. The remaining 20 patients were affected by chronic gastritis. Twelve (60%) of these were culture positive and 8 (40%) were culture negative.

Of the 20 patients affected by chronic gastritis, 15 had active gastritis and 5 had quiescent gastritis as determined by histologic criteria. Among the 12 patients positive for *H. pylori*, 10 (83.3%) had histologic evidence of active gastritis.

RESULTS

Interleukin-18 mRNA expression showed no differences in biopsies of patients with active gastritis relative to those with quiescent gastritis and to controls. IL-18 mRNA expression is present in the mucosa of *H. pylori*-infected and *H. pylori*-uninfected subjects and controls. IL-18 positivity by immunohistochemistry mainly correlated with the presence of *H. pylori*, but it was not necessarily associated with disease activity. However, there was a tendency for a higher frequency of IL-18–positive elements in active gastritis than in quiescent gastritis. IL-18–positive cells were mostly epithelial cells, located in clusters around the neck and at the surface in the antral glands, and occasionally mononuclear inflammatory elements. In biopsies from patients without evidence of *H. pylori* infection, only slight IL-18 staining was occasionally found in epithelial cells. Neutrophils were unreactive in all samples examined.

DISCUSSION

These data show that IL-18 mRNA expression is present in the mucosa of *H. pylori*-infected and *H. pylori*-uninfected subjects and controls. Our findings are in contrast to those of Tomita et al.[10] who detected greater IL-18 mRNA expression in *H. pylori*-positive than in *H. pylori*-negative patients with normal mucosa.

It is known that IL-18 mRNA is constitutively expressed in various organs and macrophage lineage cells and cell lines in contrast to other cytokines that have to be stimulated to produce mRNA. In particular, IL-18 gene expression seems to be controlled by two distinct promoters, TATA-less and G+C poor type, both characteristically observed in a wide spectrum of cell types. Accordingly, IL-18 is expressed as the biologically inactive precursor in a wide range of cell types, including not only macrophages but also non-immune cells.[11–13] IL-18, like IL-1β, exists in precursor form and needs cleavage to an active form by the IL-1β–converting enzyme (ICE), which is also known as caspase-1. Furthermore, Tone et al.[12] observed concordant expression of IL-18 and ICE mRNAs in many cell types. Biologically active, mature IL-18 secretion might also be regulated by intracellular processing mechanisms. IL-18 is a potent proinflammatory cytokine that has pathophysiologic roles in several inflammatory conditions. Therefore, IL-18 can stimulate innate immunity and both TH1- and TH2-mediated responses.[13]

In our study, the immune reaction for IL-18 in epithelial cells is evidence that IL-18 may be produced not only by inflammatory cells, but also by other specialized cells. Therefore, the gastric epithelium contributes substantially to the antral cytokine response of the proinflammatory cytokine IL-18. The presence of IL-18 protein in the uninfected gastric epithelium indicates that this cytokine might also affect normal epithelial cell functions.

REFERENCES

1. MARSHALL, B.J. & J.R. WARREN. 1984. Unidentified curved bacilli in the stomach of patients with gastritis and peptic ulceration. Lancet i: 1311–1314.
2. DUNN, B.E., H. COHEN & M.J. BLASER. 1997. Helicobacter pylori. Clin. Microbiol. Rev. 10: 720–741.
3. MAGNUSSON, P.K.E. et al. 2001. Gastric cancer and human leukocyte antigen: distinct DQ and DR alleles are associated with development of gastric cancer and infection by Helicobacter pylori. Cancer Res. 61: 2684–2689.
4. CRABTREE, J.E. 1996. Gastric mucosal inflammatory responses to Helicobacter pylori. Aliment. Pharmacol. Ther. 10: 29–37.
5. GIONCHETTI, P. et al. 1994. Enhanced mucosal interleukin-6 and -8 in Helicobacter pylori positive dyspeptic patients. Am. J. Gastroenterol. 89: 883–887.
6. BODGER, K, J.I. WYATT & R.V. HEATLEY. 1997. Gastric mucosal secretion of interleukin-10: relations to histopathology, Helicobacter pylori status, and tumor necrosis factor-alpha secretion. Gut 40: 739–744.
7. AGGARWAL, B.B. & R.K. PURI. 1995. Human Cytokines: Their Role in Disease and Therapy. Blackwell Sci. Cambridge, MA.
8. OKAMURA, H. et al. 1995. Cloning of a new cytokine that induces IFN-gamma production by T cells. Nature 378: 88–91.
9. DINARELLO, C.A. 1998. Interleukin-1β, interleukin-18, and the interleukin-1β converting enzyme. Ann. N.Y. Acad. Sci. 856: 1–11.
10. TOMITA, T. et al. 2001. Expression of interleukin-18, a Th1 cytokine, in human gastric mucosa is increased in Helicobacter pylori infection. J. Infect. Dis. 183: 620–627.
11. MCINNES, I.B. et al. 2000. Interleukin-18: a pleiotropic participant in chronic inflammation. Immunol. Today 21: 312–315.
12. TONE, M. et al. 1997. Regulation of IL-18 (IFN-γ-inducing factor) gene expression. J. Immunol. 159: 6156–6163.
13. NAKANISHI, K. et al. 2001. Interleukin-18 regulates both TH1 and TH2 responses. Annu. Rev. Immunol. 19: 423–474.

p53 and Anti-p53 Antibodies as Possible Markers of a Switch Towards a Neoplastic Phenotype in Patients Infected by *Helicobacter pylori*

E. LOSI,[a] A.M. MOLINARI,[b] P. GAZZERRO,[b] L. ORTEGA DE LUNA,[c] M.T. FERA,[d] M. CARBONE,[d] M.R. CATANIA,[c] D.L. HASTY,[e] AND F. ROSSANO[c]

[a]*Istituto Nazionale per la Ricerca sul Cancro - Genova, Unità Satellite di Messina, Messina, Italy*

[b]*Istituto di Patologia Generale,* [c]*Istituto di Microbiologia, Facoltà di Medicina e Chirurgia, Seconda Università degli Studi di Napoli, Naples, Italy*

[d]*Dipartimento di Patologia e Microbiologia Sperimentale, Facoltà di Medicina e Chirurgia, Università di Messina, Messina, Italy*

[e]*Departments of Anatomy and Neurobiology of Medicine, University of Tennessee, Memphis, Tennessee 38063, USA*

> ABSTRACT: *Helicobacter pylori* is a definite carcinogen whose mechanism of action is still unknown. The aim of this work was (1) to determine the presence of p53 protein and related antibodies in patients affected by various gastric pathologies and chronically infected with *H. pylori*, and (2) to try to discover a test to be used as a marker of a possible switch towards a neoplastic phenotype.
>
> KEYWORDS: p53; anti-p53; antibodies; *Helicobacter pylori*

INTRODUCTION

Helicobacter pylori has been indicated by the World Health Organization International Agency for Research on Cancer as a definite carcinogen,[1] but its mechanism of action is still unknown. Chronic inflammation by *H. pylori* can lead to mucosal disorders due probably to the production of ammonia,[2] cytokines,[3] and toxic radicals.[4] The transformation could be enhanced through cycles of degeneration and regeneration. Epithelial cell proliferation in association with genetic alterations or other additional factors, such as oncoprotein expression, can promote carcinogenesis. p53 is a key element in the control of genome stability and the regulation of cell cycle. Functional p53 arrests cycle progression in the late G1 phase, allowing the DNA to be repaired, or it induces apoptosis and cell death. Point mutations in the

---

Address for correspondence: Dr. F. Rossano, Istituto di Microbiologia, Facoltà di Medicina e Chirurgia, Seconda Università degli Studi di Napoli, Larghetto S. Aniello a Caponapoli, 2 80138 Naples, Italy. Voice/fax: 39-081-5665661.
fabio.rossano@unina2.it

p53 tumor suppression gene have been the most common genetic modifications in many human cancers.[5,6] Mutant alleles usually have a single missense mutation within exons 5–8 and code for altered growth regulatory proteins. Protein stability is increased by gene mutations, which leads to overexpression of p53 protein. p53 missense mutations can change the conformation of protein, leading to an increase in its half-life and resulting in the accumulation of p53 protein, which can be more easily revealed. Good agreement between the frequency of positive samples and that of tumors was indicated.[7] Another approach to the problem is the evaluation of p53 antibodies. Many authors[8,9] have found these antibodies in cancer patients; their presence seems associated with p53 mutations[10] and is connected to its overexpression. In addition, the presence of p53 antibodies has been correlated with a poor prognosis, with high histologic grade and absence of hormonal receptors.[11]

The aim of our work was (1) to determine the presence of p53 protein and related antibodies in patients affected by various gastric pathologies and chronically infected with *H. pylori*, and (2) to try to point out a test to be used as a marker of a possible switch towards a neoplastic phenotype.

MATERIAL AND METHODS

Our study was carried out in 117 patients, among those undergoing diagnostic gastroscopy. Diagnosis included: anthral gastritis (31 cases), gastric ulcer (42 cases), and gastric carcinoma (20 cases). The remaining 24 patients, who exhibited no pathologies, were used as controls. In the diagnosis of *H. pylori* infection, positivity of any test results 6 months after treatment proved it had not been eradicated; instead, eradication was determined when all findings were negative. The relations between p53 and gastric cancer were studied as follows. The parameters considered were (1) the presence of *H. pylori* checked on gastroscopies, (2) the presence of mutant p53 protein in gastric biopsies, and (3) the detection of circulating p53 antibodies.

RESULTS

The contemporaneous presence of all three parameters was observed in only a few cases (14 of 17), independent of the pathology studies. With our sensitive technique, biopsies of healthy patients almost always showed small amounts of p53; however, *H. pylori* and especially p53 antibodies were regularly absent. A relevant number of cases of gastritis (32%), ulcer (28%), and carcinoma (60%) were negative for both *H. pylori* and p53 antibodies; however, most gastritis and ulcer cases showed positivity for *H. pylori*, but they were negative for p53 antibodies. Almost all of the aforedescribed cases were negative for mutant p53 protein, with the exception of gastric carcinoma cases. In our patients the presence of p53 antibodies was always associated with positive biopsy specimens of mutant p53 protein. Instead, detection of p53 protein was only occasionally associated with the presence of p53 antibodies in the tested serum samples.

It should also be underlined that the presence of p53 antibodies seems associated with higher values of p53 protein. In other words, the contemporaneous presence of the three parameters considered is indicative of chronic inflammation independent of the pathologies studied. Nevertheless, many questions about the role of *H. pylori* in gastric cancer are left unanswered, and experimental evidence is still unclear. The action of the p53 gene in tumor suppression is of great importance. Its mechanism of action is mainly to repair DNA damage or lead to cell death through apoptosis. Persistent *H. pylori*-associated gastritis enhances DNA damage, particularly through the mechanisms just described, and the presence of p53 protein has been described in degenerating cells. Specific mRNA was also detected in gastric glands with incomplete gastric metaplasia.[12]

Our experiments confirmed the presence of p53 protein and related antibodies in chronic *H. pylori*-dependent gastropathies. Furthermore, these findings were observed with notable frequency in cases of gastric carcinoma. p53 antibody detection alone for routine screening does not seem likely to identify subjects at potential risk; however, genetic instabilities, which are connected to increased DNA damage and are revealed through the appearance of mutant p53, are early events in the pathogenesis of gastric cancer. In this sense the presence of chronic *H. pylori* infection, which might favor additional alterations, can enhance the possible development of cancer.

REFERENCES

1. IARC WORKING GROUP on the Evaluation of Carcinogenic Risks to Humans, Schistosomes, Liver Flukes and *Helicobacter pylori*. 1994. *In* IARC Monogr. Eval. Carcinog. Risk Hum. 1–241.
2. TSUJII, M. *et al.* 1992. Mechanism of gastric mucosal damage induced by ammonia. Gastroenterology **102:** 1881–1888.
3. Moss, S.F. *et al.* 1994. Cytokine gene expression in *Helicobacter pylori*-associated antral gastritis. Gut **35:** 1567–1570.
4. DAVIES, G.R. *et al.* 1994. *Helicobacter pylori* stimulates antral mucosal reactive oxygen metabolite production *in vivo*. Gut **35:** 179–185.
5. HOLLSTEIN, M. 1991. p53 mutations in human cancers. Science **253**: 49–53.
6. LEVINE, A.J., J. Momand & C.A. Finlay. 1991. The p53 tumour suppressor gene. Nature **351:** 453–456.
7. HALL, P.A. *et al.* 1991. p53 immunostaining as a marker of malignant disease in diagnostic cytopathology. Lancet **338:** 513.
8. SCHLICHTHOLZ, B. *et al.* 1994. Analyses of p53 antibodies in sera of patients with lung carcinoma define immunodominant regions in the p53 protein. Br. J. Cancer **69:** 809–816.
9. LABRECQUE, S. *et al.* 1993. Analysis of the anti-p53 antibody response in cancer patients. Cancer Res. **53:** 3468–3471.
10. RYDER, S.D. *et al.* 1996. Use of specific ELISA for the detection of antibodies directed against p53 protein in patients with hepatocellular carcinoma. J. Clin. Pathol. **49:** 295–299.
11. SCHLICHTHOLZ, B. *et al.* 1992. The immune response to p53 in breast cancer patient is directed against immunodominant epitopes unrelated to the mutational hot spot. Cancer Res. **52:** 6380–6384.
12. IMATANI, A. *et al.* 1996. *In situ* analysis of tissue dynamics and p53 expression in human gastric mucosa. J. Pathol. **179:** 39–42.

Cytokine Induction in Murine Bladder Tissue by Type 1 Fimbriated *Escherichia coli*

M. CARBONE,[a] D.L. HASTY,[b] K.C. YI,[b] J. RUE,[b] M.T. FERA,[a] F. LA TORRE,[c] M. GIANNONE,[a] AND E. LOSI[d]

[a]*Dipartimento di Patologia e Microbiologia Sperimentale, Facolta di Medicina e Chirurgia, Universita di Messina, Messina, Italy*

[b]*Departments of Anatomy and Neurobiology, University of Tennessee, Memphis, Tennessee 38063, USA*

[c]*Dipartimento di Patologia Umana, U.O. di Oncologia Medica, Facolta di Medicina e Chirurgia, Universita di Messina, Messina, Italy*

[d]*IST - Genova, Unita Satellite di Messina, c/o , U.O. di Oncologia Medica, Policlinico Universitario, Messina, Italy*

ABSTRACT: The local cytokine response to uropathogenic phenotype *Escherichia coli* KBC211 infection exhibits characteristics of both TH1 and TH2 profiles. Interleukin (IL)-6, MIP-2, IL-12, IL-18, and tumor necrosis factor-alpha (TNF-α) are expressed, but IL-4, IL-5, and IL-10 are also present at low levels. This is clearly a complex response that should be explored more fully. The relative contributions of the bladder epithelium and other cells of the bladder wall should also be determined. Epithelial cytokine responses may be considerable, and because these cells are the first to encounter the pathogen, they will be of great importance in the immune response to pathogenic *E. coli*.

KEYWORDS: cytokines; bladder; *Escherichia coli*

INTRODUCTION

Escherichia coli inhabit the large intestine of humans and other animals as a small but consistent part of normal microbiota. Sometimes *E. coli* also colonize the urinary bladder, elicit a host response, and thereby contribute to and determine the course of urinary tract infections (UTIs), such as cystitis and acute pyelonephritis. About 60% of the use of antibiotics is for treatment of UTIs; therefore, prevention of *E. coli* UTIs, especially recurrent infections, is clearly an important goal. The characterization of virulence factors of pathogenic strains will improve our understanding of the infectious process.

One important group of virulence factors involved in *E. coli* pathogenicity are the tissue-specific adhesive factors, namely, heteropolymeric surface organelles, called

---

Address for correspondence: Dr. M. Carbone, Dipartimento di Patologia e Microbiologia Sperimentale. Policlinico Universitario, Torre Biologica, 2¡ piano, 98125 Messina, Italy. Voice: 39-090-2213313; fax: 39-090-2213312.
elosi@unime.it

fimbriae. More than 95% of all isolates of *E. coli* express type 1 fimbriae,[1] also called D-mannose–sensitive (MS) or common fimbriae.[2] Type 1 fimbriae are composed primarily of the structural subunit FimA and minor amounts of at least three ancillary subunits, FimF, FimG, and FimH.[3] The 30-kD FimH subunit is the MS adhesin.[4] All type 1 fimbriae FimH phenotypes can also be functionally subdivided into either low M_1-binding (M_1L) or high M_1-binding (M_1H). These two basic phenotypes have been found predominantly in different habitats. *E. coli* FimH (M_1H) is present in more than 70% of cystitis and pyelonephritis isolates.[5] The transition from commensal to virulent phenotype has been attributed to the acquisition of distinct virulence genes, but allelic variation also clearly contributes. In addition to the possibility that some strains might be more pathogenic than others, the nature of the host immune response also contributes to the different outcomes of infection by this microrganism. Local inflammation in *E. coli* infection is characterized by infiltration of neutrophils and specific lymphocytes into the bladder mucosa and by increased production of several cytokines.[6]

The immunoregulatory and proinflammatory cytokines induced by *E. coli* may influence the nature of the local T-cell response. T (Th) cells can be divided into two subsets, Th1 and Th2. The Th1 subset promotes cell-mediated immunity by producing mainly interleukin-2 (IL-2), gamma interferon (IFN-γ), and IL-18, and the Th2 subset, which is important for antibody responses and also for downregulation of chronic inflammatory reactions, produces IL-4, IL-5, IL-6, IL-10, and IL-13.

MATERIAL AND METHODS

This study evaluates whether an association exists between increased levels of one or more cytokines in a C3H/HeN mouse bladder after inoculation of one of two different isogenic *E. coli* strains, one expressing a uropathogenic FimH phenotype (*E. coli* KBC211) and one expressing a normal fecal FimH phenotype (KBC213). The levels of cytokine transcript were assessed by reverse transcriptase polymerase chain reaction (RT-PCR). The cytokines measured were: tumor necrosis factor-alpha (TNF-α), IL-1, IL-2, IL-4, IL-5, IL-6, IL-8 or macrophage inflammatory protein-2 (MIP-2), IL-10, IL-12, IL-18, and IFN-γ, and the beta-actin transcript was used as the control.

RESULTS

Cytokine mRNA levels in C3H/HeN mice determined by RT-PCR using specific primers were as follows: 2 hours after inoculation, message for IL-1β and IL-4 was not detected, whereas message for IL-2, IL-5, IL-6, IL-10, IL-12, and IFN-γ was detected at low levels in two experimental groups after bladder stimulation. MIP-2, TNF-α, and IL-18 levels were clearly positive at this early time point. Six hours after inoculation, the message level for IL-4 began to be detected in the group of mice injected with uropathogenic phenotype *E. coli* KBC211 but not in mice inoculated with *E. coli* KBC213. No differences were found for message among mRNA levels of IL-2, IL-5, IL-10, IL-12, MIP-2, TNF-α, IL-18, and IFN-γ in both experimental groups of mice with respect to the 2-hour time point. At 6 hours, the message level of IL-6 was increased only in response to *E. coli* KBC211. Twenty-four hours after inoculation, the message for IL-2, IL-4, IL-6, IL-10, IL-12, IFN-γ, and TNF-α was strongly increased only in response to uropathogenic phenotype *E. coli* KBC211 compared to KBC213 or the phosphate-buffered saline control. No differences were found for IL-5, MIP-2, and IL-18. Interestingly, expression for IL-1β appeared only in the group of mice injected with uropathogenic phenotype *E. coli* KBC211 at the 24-hour time point.

DISCUSSION

Virulent microrganisms start the disease process by activating host responses that may affect mucosal integrity. In fact, bacterial adherence and invasion of epithelial cells are often the initial steps in the establishment of an infection. After adhesion has occurred, an inflammatory response with the production of cytokines is noted. Surface organelles produced by strains of *E. coli*, such as type 1 fimbriae, lead to adhesion and enhance bladder epithelial cytokine production in response to infection. Cytokines exert these responses either directly or indirectly by stimulating production of other effector molecules.

The present study demonstrates that levels of MIP-2, TNF-α, and IL-18 mRNA expression were positive in mice C3H/HeN after bladder inoculation with both isogenic strains. The local production of TNF-α from bladder may be responsible for epithelial MIP-2 expression. TNF-α is the first cytokine to be produced in many models of inflammatory responses,[7] and it triggers the release of other important mediators, including IL-1, IL-6, and MIP-2.[8]

It has been suggested that direct interactions between type 1 fimbriae and specific host receptors on bladder epithelial cells can activate IL-6 transcription, but lipopolysaccharide is also involved in stimulating a response. In agreement with several recent studies,[9] we found IL-18 mRNA to be present in all samples. IL-18 mRNA is constitutively expressed in various organs, cells of the macrophage lineage, and several cell lines, in contrast to the other cytokines that have to be stimulated before their mRNA is transcribed. Because of its property to induce IFN-γ, IL-18 is considered a member of the TH1-inducing family of cytokines (IFN-γ, IL-2, IL-12, and IL-15). The message level for IL-4 was detected only in response to *E. coli* strain KBC211 and not KBC213. IL-4 is generally expressed in TH2 cells, but also at minimal levels in TH1 cells.[10] The late IL-4 response during infection is probably promoted by IL-12 and TNF-α secretion by infected macrophages, which stimulates natural killer cells to produce IFN-γ.

Recent studies have documented that the immunoregulatory functions of IL-12 may either play a role in promoting endogenous protective responses during infections and/or contribute to pathology resulting from unregulated cytokine expression. Pathogen induction of IL-12 elicits interferon-γ production by natural killer cells, which contributes to early defense during certain bacterial, parasitic, and viral infections. IL-12 also facilitates the development of T helper type 1 (Th1) lymphocytes required for late protection against bacteria, parasites, and fungi. In this study, expression of IL-10 mRNA, detected at high levels after infection, may be explained as an attempt of the tissues to downregulate the proinflammatory cytokines, such as IL-1β, IL-6, MIP-2, IL-12, IL-18, and TNF-α.

REFERENCES

1. OFEK, I. & R.J. DOYLE. 1994. Bacterial Adhesion to Cells and Tissues. Chapman & Hall. New York.
2. OFEK, I. & E.H. BEACHEY. 1978. Mannose binding and epithelial cell adherence of *Escherichia coli*. Infect. Immunol. **22:** 247–254.
3. HULL, R.A. *et al.* 1981. Construction and expression of recombinant plasmids encoding type 1 or D-mannose resistant pili from a urinary tract infection *Escherichia coli* isolate. Infect. Immunol. **33:** 933–938.
4. SOKURENKO, E.V. *et al.* 1994. FimH family of type 1 fimbrial adhesins: functional heterogeneity due to minor sequence variations among *fimH* genes. J. Bacteriol. **176:** 748–755.
5. SOKURENKO, E.V. *et al.* 1995. Quantitative differences in adhesiveness of type1 fimbriated *Escherichia coli* due to structural differences in *fimH* genes. J. Bacteriol. **177:** 3680–3686.
6. SVANBORG, C., G. GODALY & M. HEDLUND. 1999. Cytokine responses during mucosal infections: role in disease pathogenesis and host defense. Curr. Opin. Microbiol. **2:** 99–105.
7. CUSUMANO, V. *et al.* 1997. Neonatal hypersusceptibility to endotoxin correlates with increased tumor necrosis factor production in mice. J. Infect. Dis. **176:** 168–176.
8. VASSALLI, P. 1992. The pathophysiology of tumor necrosis factors. Annu. Rev. Immunol. **10:** 411–452.
9. MCINNES, I.B. *et al.* 2000. Interleukin-18: a pleiotropic participant in chronic inflammation. Immunol. Today **21:** 312–315.
10. ZHENG, W. & R.A. FLAVELL. 1997. The transcription factor GATA-3 is necessary and sufficient for TH2 cytokine gene expression in CD4 T cells. Cell **89:** 587–596.

Closing Remarks

The series of Advanced Courses on *Biology and Biochemistry of Normal and Cancer Cell Growth* held every 2 years at the "Ettore Majorana Foundation and Centre for Scientific Culture" in Erice (Sicily) has become an established forum for international experts and young scientists to discuss and debate the most recent advances in either basic and translational or clinical research on major issues in oncology.

This 6th Course has focused on *Classical and Non-Classical Issues from Prevention to Treatment of Hormone-Related Tumors*. Topics covered ranged from cancer genetics to receptors and signals, from genes and phenotypes to therapy, and from epidemiology and prevention to the molecular basis for innovative strategies in the treatment of cancer patients. Among others, breast and prostate tumors were extensively discussed. In addition, hepatocellular carcinoma, colorectal cancer, neuroblastoma, and hematologic malignancies were also covered by lectures and posters in dedicated specific sections.

The introductory lectures on gene therapy and genomic instability provided the Course with a convenient opening. Thereafter, recent advances in materials and methodologies, from serial analysis of gene expression (SAGE) to knockout models and cDNA arrays, were introduced.

In addition, crucial aspects of genetic alterations (with special emphasis on oncogenes, tumor suppressor genes and their products), transcriptional and translational control mechanisms, as well as signaling pathways and triggering factors of either cell proliferation or apoptosis, were thoroughly dealt with by several presenters.

At the same time, clinical inference from either basic or translational research, eventually leading to the design of novel drugs and therapeutic strategies, accommodated highly stimulating findings and opened new grounds by back fertilization of basic research itself.

Most of the results presented in the various segments of this Course offer evidence for our expanding knowledge of tumorigenic processes and some dramatic new treatments, such as the use of Gleevec in hematologic disorders. Progress reported in studies on nutrition point again to the importance of micronutrients as protective agents against cancer. The studies on hepatocarcinogenesis point to a role for hormones in the initiation and promotion of these cancers. The segment on the prostate covered a broad span, from nutritional approaches to molecular changes in intercellular communication, cell proliferation, and apoptotic pathways during prostate carcinogenesis and tumor progression.

Because of the Majorana Centre's unique and extremely stimulating environment, this Course enjoyed a close association and a vigorous cross-fertilization between prestigious speakers and newcomer oncologists, basic researchers and clinicians, younger and less young scientists. Our hope is to fulfill everyone's enthusiastic expectation for the next Course by recreating this highly productive and enchanting milieu.

— The Editors

Index of Contributors

Agostara, B., 91–97, 98–103, 322–325
Alaimo, G., 122–139
Amoroso, M., 213–217
Andriani, F., 191–203
Aragona, M., 326–328
Auricchio, F., 185–190

Barbera, A., 1–5
Barrow, D., 104–115
Bernasconi, P., 297–305
Bilancio, A., 185–190
Blasi, L., 91–97
Boni, M., 297–305
Bradlow, H.L., 247–267
Bruzzi, P., 144–147
Buck, M., 140–143
Buda, C., 326–328
Buendia, M.A., 21–36
Buttafoco, P., 37–45

Calabrò, M., 98–103, 322–325
Calatroni, S., 297–305
Campisi, I., 98–103, 322–325
Cancemi, P., 122–139
Carbone, M., 326–328, 329–331, 332–335
Caresana, M., 297–305
Carlomagno, F., 116–121
Carruba, G., 98–103, 156–168, 213–217
Castagnetta, L., 13–20, 85–90, 98–103, 156–168, 213–217, 282–289, 322–325
Castoria, G., 185–190
Catania, M.R., 329–331
Cavigliano, P.M., 297–305
Cervello, M., 13–20, 46–52, 53–58
Chen, S., 229–238, 239–246
Cilloni, D., 306–312
Cocciadiferro, L., 156–168
Cohen, L.A., 148–155
Colantoni, A., 37–45
Conte, M., 74–84
Cusano, R., 74–84
Cusimano, R., 85–90, 282–289

D'Alessandro, N., 46–52, 53–58
Dantona, F., 13–20
de Falco, A., 185–190
De Maria, N., 37–45
Devoto, M., 74–84
Di Cristina, A., 156–168, 213–217, 282–289
Di Domenico, M., 185–190

Eng, E.T., 229–238, 239–246

Faucher, F., 221–228
Fera, M.T., 326–328, 329–331, 332–335
Ferretti, I., 37–45
Ferrigno, V., 85–90
Fontana, S., 122–139
Fusco, A., 116–121

Galosi, A.B., 204–212, 218–220
Gazzerro, P., 329–331
Gee, J.M.W., 104–115
Gervasi, F., 313–321
Giammanco, A.M., 85–90
Giannitrapani, L., 13–20, 46–52, 53–58
Giannone, M., 326–328, 332–335
Giardini, I., 297–305
Giudice, A., 326–328
Giugliano, E., 306–312
Granata, O.M., 282–289
Grottola, A., 37–45
Grube, B., 229–238
Guerrasio, A., 306–312
Guttadauro, A., 85–90

Hamel, P., 282–289
Harper, M.E., 104–115
Hasty, D.L., 329–331, 332–335
Hutcheson, I.R., 104–115

Iovanna, J.L., 53–58

Jones, H.E., 104–115

Kaaks, R., 268–281
Kao, Y.-C., 229–238
Kirma, N., 239–246
Knabbe, C., 140–143
Knowlden, J.M., 104–115
Kwon, A., 229–238

La Rosa, M., 46–52, 53–58
La Torre, F., 326–328, 332–335
Lacoste, L., 221–228
Laudani, A., 91–97
Leonardi, V., 91–97
Lévy, L., 21–36
Liquori, M., 85–90, 282–289
Longo, L., 74–84
Losi, E., 326–328, 329–331, 332–335
Lukanova, A., 268–281
Luu-The, V., 221–228

Mandava, U., 239–246
Manenti, F., 37–45
Marasà, L., 98–103
Maratta, A., 322–325
Marcelli, M., 191–203
Massimo, L., 59–62
Mazzucchelli, R., 169–184
McClelland, R.A., 104–115
McConville, C., 74–84
Melillo, R.M., 116–121
Mezzatesta, N., 322–325
Miele, M., 98–103, 282–289
Migliaccio, A., 185–190
Minafra, S., 122–139
Molinari, A.M., 329–331
Montalto, G., 13–20, 46–52, 53–58
Montironi, R., 169–184
Muzzonigro, G., 204–212, 218–220

Nan, B., 191–203
Nicholson, R.I., 104–115
Notarbartolo, M., 46–52, 53–58

Okubo, T., 229–238

Ortega De Luna, L., 329–331

Pagnucco, G., 313–321
Panetta, S., 326–328
Perri, P., 74–84
Polito, L., 282–289
Prieto, J., 6–12
Prosa, L., 1–5
Pucci-Minafra, I., 122–139

Qian, C., 6–12
Quader, S.T.A., 156–168, 213–217

Ravazzolo, B., 85–90, 282–289
Rees, S.A., 74–84
Rege-Cambrin, G., 306–312
Renard, C.A., 21–36
Rocca, B., 297–305
Romeo, G., 74–84
Rossano, F., 329–331
Rosti, V., 290–296
Rue, J., 332–335

Saetta, A., 322–325
Saglio, G., 306–312
Saladino, F., 156–168, 213–217
Sangro, B., 6–12
Santoro, M., 116–121
Savio, G., 91–97
Scaravaglio, P., 306–312
Scarpelli, M., 169–184
Schmitz, V., 6–12
Schwab, M., 63–73
Sepkovic, D.W., 247–267
Seri, M., 74–84
Snabboon, T., 191–203
Soresi, M., 46–52
Stefano, R., 156–168

Tekmal, R.R., 239–246
Terranova, A., 13–20
Tokar, E., 156–168
Tonini, G.P., 74–84
Traina, A., 85–90, 98–103, 282–289, 322–325

INDEX OF CONTRIBUTORS

Vanelli, L., 313–321
Vecchio, G., 116–121
Villa, E., 37–45
Virruso, L., 46–52, 53–58
Volpe, G., 306–312
von der Fecht, J., 140–143

Wakeling, A.E., 104–115
Webber, M.M., 213–217
Webber, M.T., 156–168
Wei, Y., 21–36

Williams, D., 239–246

Yang, C., 229–238
Yi, K.C., 332–335
Yu, B., 229–238
Yu, J., 191–203

Zhang, Y., 191–203
Zhou, D., 229–238

OHIO UNIVERSITY LIBRARY
Please return this book as soon as you have finished with it. In order to avoid a fine it must be returned by the latest date stamped below. All books are subject to recall after two weeks or immediately if needed for reserve.

CF